D0477881

Developmental Reading Disabilities: A Language Based Treatment Approach

Second Edition

Developmental Reading Disabilities:
A Language Based Treatment Approach

Second Edition

Candace L. Goldsworthy, Ph.D.

THOMSON

™

DELMAR LEARNING

Australia Canada Mexico Singapore Spain United Kingdom United States

THOMSON

DELMAR LEARNING ™

Developmental Reading Disabilities: A Language Based Treatment Approach, Second Edition
by Candace L. Goldsworthy

Health Care Publishing Director:
William Brottmiller

Executive Editor:
Cathy L. Esperti

Developmental Editor:
Darcy M. Scelsi

Editorial Assistant:
Chris Manion

Executive Marketing Manager:
Dawn F. Gerrain

Channel Manager:
Gretta Oliver

Production Editor:
Mary Colleen Liburdi

For permission to use material from this text or product, contact us by
Tel   (800) 730-2214
Fax   (800) 730-2215
www.thomsonrights.com

Library of Congress Cataloging-in-Publication Data

Goldsworthy, Candace L.
    Developmental reading disabilities: a language based treatment approach / Candace L. Goldsworthy -- 2nd ed.
        p. ; cm.
    Includes bibliographical references and index.
    ISBN 0-7693-0100-2
    1. Reading disability. 2. Language disorders in children. I. Title
    [DNLM: 1. Dyslexia--Child. 2. Dyslexia--Infant. 3. Dyslexia--therapy--Child. 4. Dyslexia--therapy--Infant. 5. Language Development Disorders--Child. 6. Language Development Disorders--Infant. 7. Language Therapy--Child. 8. Language Therapy--Infant. WL 340.6 G624d 2003]
    LB1050.5 .G65 2003
    372.43--dc21
                                                    2002035053

NOTICE TO THE READER

CONTENTS

ABOUT THE AUTHOR

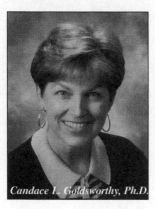

Candace L. Goldsworthy, Ph.D.

Candace L. Goldsworthy, Ph.D., Professor at California State University, Sacramento, and Vice-Chair of the Department of Speech–Language Pathology and Audiology, received her doctorate from Case Western Reserve University in Cleveland, Ohio. Dr. Goldsworthy is Co-Director of the Sacramento Scottish Rite Clinic for Childhood Language Disorders and is a partner in the private practice of Speech–Language–Learning Associates. Her publications through Thomson Delmar Learning include: *Developmental Reading Disabilities, Sourcebook of Phonological Awareness Activities: Children's Classic Literature, Sourcebook of Phonological Awareness Activities: Children's Core Literature*, and is co-authoring *Sourcebook of Phonological Awareness Activities: Children's Core Literature Grades 3–5*. Dr. Goldsworthy was named Fellow of the California Speech–Language–Hearing Association. She won the Outstanding Teaching Award for the College of Health and Human Services at California State University, Sacramento in the Spring of 2001.

FOREWORD

com•pe•tence (kom'p_t_ns) n. The state or quality of being properly or well qualified; capable.

Clinicians crave competence. They pursue it through education and experience, through emulation and innovation. Some are more successful than others in attaining what they seek. A major element in maintaining competence is being current. Dr. Candace Goldsworthy keeps us current with the second edition of her book **Developmental Reading Disabilities: A Language Based Treatment Approach**. She brings us up to date in our appraisal, diagnosis, and treatment of a variety of reading disabilities. As in the first edition, Dr. Goldsworthy extends our reach across the language modalities by adding reading and writing to the traditional focus on auditory comprehension and oral-expressive language. She provides additional appraisal techniques and expanded treatment programs to those that resided in the first edition. And, she justifies the "what" to do by a sound "why"—additional theoretical rationale to drive appraisal and therapeutic intervention. Certainly, Dr. Goldsworthy assists speech-language pathologists in fitting into the current national initiatives on literacy. Your attention to what she provides indicates your competence and your efforts to improve it, because competent clinicians seek competence as much for what it demands as for what it promises.

Robert T. Wertz, Ph.D.
Series Editor

PREFACE

I was honored when Delmar Learning asked me to author the second edition of this book. My first thoughts about revising the book were to update some of the topics and to add a few more. However, as I studied the books and articles I had compiled on developmental reading disabilities since 1996, I realized this revision was not merely a matter of "tweaking here and there." On the contrary, this edition of *Developmental Reading Disabilities* is much more than an expansion of the first edition. I will mention the primary changes here.

- In Chapter 1, results of follow-up studies of children with early speech and language problems are summarized to underscore the need for early identification and follow-up.

- Chapter 2 includes expanded discussion of the development of oral–written literacy. Locke's theory of neurolinguistic development, Frith's three-stage and Chall's 6-stage theories of reading acquisition are juxtaposed with the four-stage model of reading, writing and spelling development of Bear et al. Adams' model of reading acquisition is again presented to help organize the myriad aspects that will be considered under assessing and treating developmental reading disabilities.

- Chapter 3 includes a discussion of the many faces of phonology and a description of three types of developmental reading disabilities: specific reading disability (developmental dyslexia), generalized reading problem, and hyperlexia. In addition, the growing body of information on the contribution of verbal naming speed to reading is considered. Finally, the impact of phonological awareness and verbal naming speed on reading is examined through a description of single versus double deficit views of developmental reading disabilities.

- Information on assessment in Chapter 4 is considerably more extensive than in the first edition. Adams' model is used to help organize the many areas in need of examination in language based reading problems.

Domains to assess are presented under the phonologic, orthographic, meaning, and context processors with suggested tests and subtests for each area.

- Treatment methods for developmental reading disabilities are presented in Chapters 5 and 6. To extend the continuity of this edition, instructional goals, methods, and suggested materials are presented for the phonological processor in Chapter 5, and for the orthographic, meaning, and context processors in Chapter 6. While the emphasis of the first edition of this text was on the phonological processor core of developmental reading disabilities, the contribution of phonological processing and verbal naming speed are considered in this edition.

- Chapter 7 considers practical information as to what constitutes good instruction, curriculum IEP based goals to support literacy, collaboration, a personal story, and future directions.

This book is written for practitioners who work with students who display subtle or overt oral and written language problems. Assessment tools and suggested teaching goals, methods, and materials are suggested for preschool through adolescent-aged students. This book is designed for graduate students in speech–language pathology and those in regular and special education who plan to work with students experiencing oral and written language problems.

ACKNOWLEDGMENTS

I cannot imagine what it would be like to have my view of the world limited by a reading disability. For some reason, maybe a good one, my professional life as a speech–language pathologist gravitated toward students with reading problems over 20 years ago. During those years, I discovered how Speech–Language Pathology can contribute to children and adults whose oral language problems evolve into written language problems. Over the years, I jotted down ideas that worked and some that did not. This book started with a desire to share some of the ideas and experiences I have had with students with reading disabilities. That desire became more and more compelling as time went on. However, the "jotted" ideas would never have taken form without the assistance of too many people to mention in this limited space. I gratefully acknowledge the editorial staff of Delmar Learning for their insightful critiques and comments on the manuscript. Their recommendations added significantly to the quality of the book.

Special thanks are extended to my colleagues and friends for their continual ideas and support. I want to specially acknowledge Robert A. Pieretti, M.S., for his work on a modified RAVE-O program, his enthusiasm for developmental reading disabilities, and for his help with editing this manuscript. I wish to thank the students with developmental reading disabilities and their families with whom I have had the good fortune to work. You have taught me so much. And to my husband, Jim Everett, for being my constant source of encouragement. I am truly blessed.

Years ago I worked with a 10-year-old named Tim who had a specific reading disability. After I explained how the lesson we were working on would help, Tim asked for a pen and paper and drew the following sketch. When I asked what his drawing meant. Tim explained:

"Well, you see, this house is me and the open windows are questions I have about me and my reading and why I have so much trouble. Your answer just helped me to close one of the windows so I understand me better."

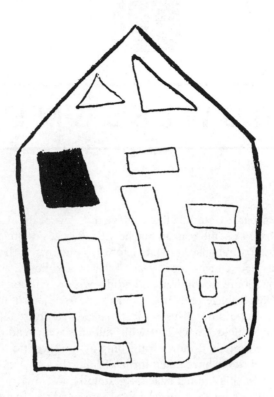

Thank you, Tim. This book is dedicated to those individuals who, like Tim, have been my students, my teachers, and my inspiration. May the information in this book close some of your "windows," and may a few doors be opened for you along the way.

CHAPTER

1

Language Based Reading Disabilities and Speech–Language Specialists

OUTLINE

I. SCOPE OF THE PROBLEM

Why do some children learn to read easily and others struggle so with the printed word? Parents of early readers are filled with pride when their child begins reading street signs, cereal boxes, and candy wrappers. Other parents, whose child stumbles over words attempting to read aloud, are bewildered as to what is going on. Their child stands bravely in front of the class slowly sounding out words: "/c/..../a/...." Beginning again, this student timidly says: "/k/.../ae/.../kae/." With other students glaring, heads turning, laughter erupting, this student, whose voice is now barely audible, continues: "/t/..../k/.../ae/.../kae/..../t/.../kae/..../t/.../kae/../t/............CAT!" And if this continues for the next few words or sentences, this student is clueless as to what was just "read."

Most children learn to read without problems. However, for at least 20–30% of American children, learning to read is an arduous task (Lyon, 1995a). Without help, the problem worsens over the course of the child's educational career. According to the National Institute of Child Health and Human Development (NICHD) (2000): "approximately 10 million students experience problems learning to read; 10–15% of these drop out of high school; approximately 2% complete four-year college programs; approximately 50% of adolescents and young adults with criminal records have a history of reading problems, and 50% of youths with substance abuse histories have reading problems" (p. 1). These figures are staggering, and add credence to the fact that these reading disabilities are not isolated problems. Indeed, language-based reading problems are a national epidemic.

II. WHO DEVELOPS LANGUAGE BASED READING PROBLEMS?

Many students referred to speech–language specialists during their preschool years are later identified as having reading, writing, and spelling problems. Follow-up studies of young children with overt oral language problems clearly and consistently indicate that many early oral language problems evolve into or resurface as written language problems. For every young child with identified oral language problems, there are many others with subtle language problems left undetected until they manifest as a language-based reading–writing–spelling problem.

A. The Kaleidoscopic Nature of Language Problems.

Language disabilities take on different forms over time as students face varying demands of school curriculum. Students whose overt oral language problems were identified during preschool may go on to experience problems following classroom directions, expressing thoughts orally, reading chapter books, and writing about increasingly difficult subject matter. For others, subtle language problems go undetected until they are unveiled by increased demands for oral and written language proficiency. When students with language problems attempt to map print onto their weak phonological processing systems, the underlying language-based problem becomes apparent. Bashir and Scavuzzo (1992) proposed that the "academic vulnerability" of children with language disorders stems from the "lifelong need to acquire language, to learn with language, and to apply accrued knowledge of language to learning tasks, such as reading and writing" (p. 53). Students with histories of oral language problems that evolved into written language problems "often fail to process and comprehend the information because of their poor mastery of semantic, syntactic, and pragmatic aspects of language" (Norris, 1991, p. 71). Torgesen (1998) noted that "one of the most compelling findings from recent reading research is that children who get off to a poor start in reading rarely catch up" (p.1). Citing an NICHD statistic, Viall (2000) noted: "If a child leaves 3rd grade not reading at grade level—that child has only a 'one-in-seven' chance of EVER reading at grade level" (p. 3).

Nelson (1994) suggested that if fifth through eighth grade students continue to experience difficulty understanding or using abstract meanings and complex syntax, they may become "overwhelmed by increased linguistic demands of school discourse. When complexity factors are compounded by social-interaction and self-esteem issues, the challenges are multiplied" (p. 126). In her discussion of language problems during adolescence, Ehern (1994) suggested that ignoring or deemphasizing language intervention for adolescents is "counterproductive" and "should be a core consideration when trying to understand academic failure" (p. 394). According to Butler (2000), strong evidence indicates that children with oral language problems are at risk for reading and writing problems, and if left untreated, "they become prone to academic failure throughout their school years, from preschool to postsecondary setting" (p. iv).

B. Follow-up of Children with Early Speech-Language Problems.

In their summary of follow-up studies, Lewis, Freebairn, and Taylor (2000) explained "40% to 100% of children with early speech and language disorders have persistent language problems, and 50% to 75%

have academic difficulties" (p. 434). To predict which groups of children with early speech and language problems develop later reading, writing, and spelling problems, research over the past decade has examined a number of relationships. Some relevant findings are summarized in the following section.

According to NICHD "the best predictor in K or 1st grade of a future reading disability in grade 3 is a combination of performance on measures of phonemic awareness, rapid naming of letters, numbers, and objects, and print awareness" (Grossen, 1997). Estimating children's risk for reading difficulties, Catts, Fey, Zhang, and Tomblin (2001) administered a battery of language, early literacy, and nonverbal cognitive measures to 604 kindergartners with follow-up reading achievement testing in second grade (see Table 1-1).

Of the children included in this study, 183 were identified with reading problems using the criterion of reading scores at least 1 SD below the mean. Five kindergarten variables predicted reading outcome in second grade: letter identification, sentence imitation, phonological awareness, rapid naming, and mother's education. Catts et al. (2001) concluded that children with histories of speech–language problems should be assessed in these areas: Letter Identification, Sentence Imitation, Deletion, and Rapid Automatized Naming (in this study using animal names). These children should be assessed as early as possible during kindergarten as "their history of speech–language problems places them at risk for reading difficulties that are four to five times greater than those of children from the general population" (p. 45). The researchers also concluded that children without histories of speech–language problems should be referred to speech–language specialists for potential reading problems if classroom teachers notice these students falling behind in the following kindergarten curriculum: familiarity with books, speech and oral language development, and the ability to rhyme and perform other phonological awareness tasks (p. 45).

Examining the "very early" language deficits in 52 children later diagnosed with dyslexia, Scarborough (1990) grouped 30-month-old subjects into three sets: 1) 20 children from families with an incidence of dyslexia who subsequently became disabled readers; 2) 12 children from families with incidence of dyslexia who became normal readers; and 3) 20 normally achieving children who had no history of dyslexia. Scarborough found that children who demonstrated dyslexia usually experienced difficulty with the following three emergent literacy skills during the preschool period.

Table 1-1. Areas Tested and Assessment Tools Presented by Catts et al. (2001).

Areas tested	Assessment tools
	In Kindergarten
Receptive and expressive vocabulary	Picture Vocabulary, Oral Vocabulary, Grammatical Understanding, Sentence Imitation, and Grammatical Completion (*Test of Language Development: Primary—2,* Newcomer & Hammill, 1988)
Narration	Comprehending and retelling major details of a story (Culatta, Page, & Ellis, 1983)
Phonological Awareness	Syllable/phoneme deletion task (Catts, 1993)
Automatized Naming	Rapid Automatized Naming of Animals task (Catts, 1993)
Letter Identification	Letter Identification subtest (*Woodcock Reading Mastery Tests—Revised,* Woodcock, 1987)
Nonverbal Cognitive Abilities	Block Design and Picture Completion subtests (*Wechsler Preschool and Primary Scale of Intelligence—Revised,* Wechsler, 1989) These measure visual attention, visual recognition, visual—motor coordination, and spatial reasoning.
	In Second Grade
Reading Comprehension	Passage Comprehension (*Woodcock Reading Mastery Test—Revised,* 1987) Comprehension component (*Gray Oral Reading Test—3,* Wiederholt & Bryant, 1992) Reading comprehension subtest (*Diagnostic Achievement Battery—2,* Newcomer, 1990)

At 2 1/2 years of age, they produced shorter, syntactically simpler sentences with less accurate word pronunciations than other typical 2-year-olds while demonstrating normal lexical or speech discrimination skills. At 3 years of age, they began to demonstrate deficits in receptive vocabulary and object-naming abilities. At 5 years of age, they exhibited problems in object-naming, poor rhyme recitation abilities, poor letter–sound knowledge, and phonemic awareness deficits.

C. Specific relationships between speech/language problems and later reading/writing problems.

1. Phonological processing deficits and reading problems.

Examining cognitive profiles of reading-disabled children, Shankweiler et al. (1992) found that reading problems consistently co-occur with phonological processing problems regardless of whether children had isolated reading problems or if they coexisted with other semantic, syntactic, and/or phonological language problems. According to Magnusson and Naucler (1990) and Menyuk (1991), phonological coding, converting what is heard through the auditory channel into phonemes, is a metalinguistic ability. Phonological coding ability predicts later reading achievement more accurately than semantic and syntactic abilities, although these are related to reading ability later. Vellutino et al. (1996) found that children who were most difficult to remediate differed from readily remediated and normal readers on phonological but not semantic skills. Lombardino et al. (1997) concluded "it appears that weak phonological representations affect both speech and language processing and production in children with reading disabilities" (p. 73).

Poor readers frequently score lower than good readers on verbal short-term memory, verbal working memory, and speech production tasks. Stone and Brady (1995) found less skilled third grade readers scored significantly lower than their peers and younger reading-age controls on two verbal memory measures: pseudoword imitation (repeating nonsense words), and word span (repeating monosyllabic words, e.g., "rose, plate" in the order presented). Furthermore, poor readers scored lower than the other two groups on two speech production accuracy measures: word-pair repetition (repeating pairs e.g., car/hat; banana/elephant), and tongue twister tasks (repeating two-syllable pseudowords, e.g., "seeshee"). The untimed pseudoword repetition task correlated most closely with word attack and word identification scores. When subjects were asked to repeat real words, the less skilled readers scored between the two comparison groups. Stone and Brady noted that one of the important research conclusions to date is that underlying phonological processes differentiate skilled and less skilled reading when the task includes novel phonological patterns. Stated differently, tasks that place demands on encoding phonological information, that is, when there is minimal top-down information or when the input is difficult to analyze because of noise, are more difficult for poor readers (p. 73).

2. **Isolated expressive phonology problems versus expressive phonology plus other language and reading problems.**

More than half of a group of 6 year olds with speech and language disorders later encountered language, reading, and spelling problems (Shriberg & Austin, 1998). Noting that later reading achievements were related to the nature of speech errors in young children, Magnusson and Naucler (1990) explained that earlier rule-based, nonsegmental speech errors (crossing phonemic boundaries) resulted in lower reading scores than did isolated segmental errors (articulatory-only problems). Lewis, Freebairn, and Taylor (2000) followed 52 children diagnosed at 4 to 6 years with moderate to severe expressive phonology disorders. In third and fourth grades, these subjects were assigned to one of two groups based on initial language status: isolated phonology problem (P) and phonology disorder and other language problems (PL). Lewis et al. concluded that children with isolated phonology disorders have better outcomes than children with phonological disorders in addition to other language problems. Furthermore, the PL group performed more poorly than the P group on two phonological processing tasks: Elision (Torgesen & Wagner, 1994) and Sound Analysis subtest of *Goldman–Fristoe–Woodcock Sound Symbol Test* (GFWSS: Goldman, Fristoe, & Woodcock, 1974). An Elision task measures a subject's ability to delete a sound in a word, and then to replace the sound with another sound. The Sound Analysis subtest measures a subject's ability to identify sounds in nonsense (made-up) words, while the Sound Blending subtest measures a subject's ability to blend sounds to form real words. The Sound Blending task of the GFWSS did not differentiate the two groups of children. Lewis et al. suggested that sound blending requires competence in phonological synthesis, while elision requires competence in phonological analysis *and* synthesis. The PL group's poorer performance suggested that "a deficit in phonological processing may in part be responsible for the reading problems" observed in this group (p. 10). Initial testing using the *Test of Language Development—Primary, Second Edition* (TOLD-P:2: Newcomer & Hammill, 1988) identified subjects with language impairment. Twenty-four of the subjects obtained total TOLD-P:2 scores less than 85, and all these subjects obtained higher Receptive than Expressive Language scores. Follow-up testing revealed the PL group performed more poorly than the P group on receptive and expressive language abilities as measured by the *Clinical Evaluation of Language Fundamentals—Revised* (CELF-R: Semel, Wiig, & Secord, 1987). Only 11 subjects (46%) of the PL group scored one or more standard deviations below the mean on reading measures suggesting that an early language disorder, using the CELF-R, does not necessarily predict a later reading disorder (Lewis et al., 2000, p. 10). Performance on the *Goldman–Fristoe Test of Articulation*, Sounds in Words subtest (GFTA: Goldman & Fristoe, 1986), revealed only 1 subject in the P group (4%) and 6 children in the PL group (22%) continued to demonstrate articulation disorders at follow-up. Lewis et al. "found no evidence for associations between comorbid language or reading problems and residual articulatory problems" (p. 100). The P group performed more poorly on age-adjusted scores on follow-up testing on the *Test of Written Spelling, Third Edition* (TWS-3; Larsen & Hammill, 1994) than on language and reading tests. (See later section on Phonological disorders and spelling). Lewis et al. explained "poor spelling skills may be a residual consequence of an early expressive phonology disorder" (p. 10).

3. **Rapid automatized naming and reading problems.**

Rapid automatized naming, the ability to rapidly name a small number of items (colors, numbers, letters, or objects) as quickly as possible, has proven to be one of the best predictors of a student's printed word recognition. According to Catts (1993), "phonological awareness and rapid-naming deficits lie near the core of reading disabilities in young children" (pp. 955–956). Wolf and Bowers (2000) explained that substantial cross-sectional, longitudinal and cross-linguistic research documents that children and adults diagnosed with dyslexia "are slower than most other readers to access and retrieve verbal labels for visually presented stimuli especially when the stimuli are serial letters and numbers" (p. 322). Wolf and Obregon (1989) found significant differences between dyslexic and average readers each year between kindergarten and 4th grade on picture naming tasks (confrontation naming task) and rapid automatized naming of letters, digits, and common objects. Color naming did not differentiate the two reading groups in 4th grade. Wolf (1991) concluded: "Thus it appears that there is a persistent naming-rate deficit among most dyslexic readers well into middle childhood" (p. 133). Meyer, Wood, Hart and Felton (1998) found that performance on rapid naming tasks had predictive power from 3rd through 8th grades for poor but not average readers, suggesting that "impaired readers are qualitatively different from the normal-reading population and are not simply the 'tail' of a normal distribution of reading ability" (p. 106).

4.   Oral motor factors and naming skills in poor readers.

Wolf (1991) proposed that reading and verbal naming speed may have similar underlying processes and a deficit in these sub-processes may explain the correlation between reading problems and slow verbal naming speed. More specifically, Wolf suggested that automatization of responses requiring precise timing may lie at the core of reading problems and slower-rapid naming ability. This automatization is "characteristic of both the language and motor domains and hence, the paired problems observed in the motor coordination required for rapid continuous naming and for rapid manual tasks such as tapping patterns" (Snyder & Downey, 1995, p. 33).

Snyder and Downey (1995) hypothesized that the serial rapid-naming problems in children with reading disabilities were caused both by word finding difficulty *and* oral–motor output problems. In their study, 30 students with reading disabilities (15 younger students with mean age of 9 years, 4 months, and 15 older with a mean age of 12 years, 7 months) were compared with similar aged groups of normally reading students on a number of measures (See Table 1-2).

Snyder and Downey found that students with reading disabilities (RD) scored significantly lower than students with normal reading achievement (NRA) in serial naming; however, the two groups did not score significantly different from each other on serial naming accuracy. The RD group named significantly fewer animals than NRA students; and older students in each group named more animals than younger students. Finally, the reading disabled group's slower reaction times may be related to access related processes while their extended production durations and corresponding articulatory speed problems suggest factors involved after accessing words may be implicated (p. 47).

Table 1-2. Assessment Measures Used by Snyder and Downey (1995).

General cognitive abilities	*Wechsler Intelligence Scale for Children—Revised* (Wechsler, 1974)
Reading comprehension	*Reading Test of the Metropolitan Achievement Test* (Harcourt, Brace, Jovanovich, 1976)
Word Recognition	*Reading Recognition subtest of Peabody Individual Achievement Test* (Dunn & Markwardt, 1970)
Serial Naming	*Producing Names on Confrontation of Clinical Evaluation of Language Fundamentals* (CELF, Wiig & Semel, 1980)
Verbal Fluency	*Producing Word Associations* (CELF)
Word Retrieval	*Controlled Word Association (Neuropsychological Battery,* Benton, 1973)
Articulatory Speed	*Oral Diadochokinetic Measure* (Fletcher, 1972)

5.   **Phonological disorders and spelling.**

Implicit and explicit phonological awareness are "fundamental to spelling acquisition" (Clarke-Klein, 1994, p. 44). Lewis, Freebairn, and Taylor (2000) followed 52 children diagnosed at 4 to 6 years with moderate to severe expressive phonology disorder. In third and fourth grades, these subjects were assigned to one of two groups based on initial language status: isolated phonology problem (P) and phonology disorder and other language problems (PL). The P group performed more poorly on age-adjusted scores on follow-up testing on the *Test of Written Spelling, Third Edition* (TWS-3; Larsen & Hammill, 1994) than on language and reading tests. Because the PL group performed more poorly than the P group on TWS-3 Lewis et al. concluded that "weaknesses in phonological processing and/or other language deficiencies are additional barriers to the development of spelling skills" (p. 100).

Clarke-Klein (1994) presented the case study of Matthew, who, as a preschooler, demonstrated a severe expressive phonological disorder. At 8 years, 8 months of age, Matthew presented with moderate assimilation errors and continued to have speech production problems with liquid /l, r/, and interdental voiced and voiceless /th/ sounds. His reading ability was at the 29th percentile with spelling scores at the 4th percentile. Matthew's performance on sound categorization sorting tasks were far below the mean scores for 5 1/2 year old children. Examination of his spelling errors revealed a "wide variety of phonological deviations in spelling errors" such as "omission, class deficiency, phonemic substitution, context-related/syllable-structure alterations, and assimilation" (p. 50).

6. **Language, IQ and reading problems.**

Bird, Bishop, and Freeman (1995) found that children with severe phonological disorders accompanied by poor phonological awareness and low nonverbal IQ were most at risk for reading disabilities. Stothard, Snowling, Bishop, Chipchase, and Kaplan (1998) reported findings in a longitudinal study of children identified in preschool as having language difficulties. When first examined at 4 years of age by Bishop and Edmundson (1987), the children were assigned to one of two groups: 1) impaired speech and language with nonverbal IQ of 70 or above (Specific Language Impairment, SLI) or 2) impaired speech and language with nonverbal IQ below 70 (General Delay group). At 5 1/2 years old, 30 of the 68 SLI group met criteria for satisfactory speech–language abilities (at or above the 10th percentile on language measures used), and were reclassified as resolved SLI. The other 38 SLI subjects continued to demonstrate speech–language problems and were reclassified as persistent SLI (scoring at or below the 3rd percentile on language measures). In their follow-up study of 85 of the original Bishop and Edmundson subjects, at 15 years of age, Stothard et al. included 52 control subjects. Included among their findings were the following:

The persistent SLI group scored significantly lower than the Control group on all spoken language measures. This group also scored significantly lower than the resolved SLI group on all spoken language measures except the *Test for Reception of Grammar* (TROG; Bishop, 1983) in which the subjects must select one of four pictures that best represents a phrase or sentence spoken by the examiner. Children who still have language problems at 5 1/2 years "are at high risk for long standing language impairments" (p. 416).

The resolved SLI and Control groups performed similarly on all tests except Sentence Repetition, Nonword Repetition, and Spoonerisms, on which the resolved SLI performed at a significantly lower level than the Control group. "These findings confirm that tests of phonological processing are particularly sensitive indicators of residual language difficulties" (p. 416). Furthermore, the resolved SLI group scored significantly higher than the General Delay group on all spoken language tests.

Finally, the Control group scored significantly higher than both the persistent SLI and General Delay groups on all spoken language tests. The persistent SLI and General Delay groups were most at risk for developing later academic problems. Stothard et al. (1998) concluded "it is clear that most children do not simply grow out of their early language difficulties" (p. 417). The resolved SLI were at lower risk of developing reading and spelling problems than residual SLI and General Delay. However, because the resolved SLI group obtained lower scores in reading accuracy, reading comprehension, and single word spelling scores than the Control group, Stothard et al. concluded that these children continued to have "residual, but mild, processing impairments" placing them at risk for later problems with literacy skills (p. 417). While their reading skills "were significantly poorer than those of controls, they were not generally outside of the normal range as predicted by IQ" (p. 417).

D. Students Who "Fall Through the Cracks."

Students whose language problems remain obscured until reading, writing and spelling problems surface present another challenge to educators. According to NICHD (2000) "even people with a mild reading impairment do not read for fun. For them, reading requires so much effort that they have little energy left for understanding what they have just read" (p. l).

As parents, teachers, and special educators know, it takes only a few embarrassing episodes of reading poorly in front of classroom peers before a student's self-esteem is damaged and, sadly, we have another student caught in the downward spiral of failure. Of the many stories my clients have shared with me over the years about the humiliation they suffered while reading unsuccessfully in class, Cody's and Shannon's stand out. I met Cody when he was in a regular education fourth-grade class. My testing revealed significant phonological awareness and rapid automatized naming problems with reading decoding at mid-first grade level and reading comprehension at high-third grade level. Educational testing revealed Cody's IQ level to be well within normal limits. Like many children, Cody's academic scores were not low enough to qualify him for educational services because of the number of students who scored lower than Cody. He was clearly a student who had "fallen through the cracks" of the educational system. That, in and of itself, is sad. However, Cody's story will remain with me forever because of how it was handled. During reading, Cody was made to sit in the middle of the classroom with a small group of children. This group of students was identified by the classroom teacher as the "lazy boys and girls," the ones who "don't try to learn how to read and write."

Twelve-year-old Shannon's story came to me as I was writing this book. Shannon has a moderate articulation problem with a /w/ for /r/ substitution in all positions of words. At 8 years of age she was diagnosed with significant reading problems. At 12 years of age, Shannon was enrolled in a regular education sixth-grade class and trying to read her literature book along with her classmates. A classroom aide told Shannon to signal when finished reading the passage to herself. When Shannon signaled that she had read the passage the aide said: "You couldn't have read it that fast. Read it again." Shannon read the passage silently a second time and informed the aide that she was finished. In front of the other students, the aide, becoming agitated, said: "Shannon, you can't read that fast! *Even I can't read that fast.* Either read it again and *think about every word,* or I'll give you questions you'll have to answer in writing." Shannon let the aide know when she was finished reading the passage silently for a third time. This time, quite agitated, the aide loudly said: "Shannon, if you're lying to me I'll give you a detention. Read it out loud." At this, Shannon began to cry as she read the passage aloud for the aide with her classmates listening. She made some errors as she read aloud because, as she told me, "I can't read that well while I'm crying." The appalling conclusion to this story is that the aide responded "You see Shannon. You're *still* making mistakes." And as Shannon explained, the aide, using "her very nice voice" said: "*I* can't even read that fast. Everyone reads slow."

The only way I can understand these two scenarios is through Lavoi's (2001) explanation: "The challenge is not learning disabilities. The real challenge is educating those who don't have one." Aside from the lifelong pain these episodes leave in Cody's and Shannon's memories, the tragedy is that they, like so many others, *can* learn to read and write successfully with help. Cushen-White (2000) pointed out that over 33 years of NICHD-supported research has demonstrated that "for 90% to 95% of poor readers, prevention and early intervention programs that combine instruction in phoneme awareness, phonics, fluency development, and reading comprehension strategies, provided by well-trained teachers, can increase reading skills to average reading levels" (p. 5). Adams et al. (1998) concluded "research indicates that, without direct instructional support, phonemic awareness eludes roughly 25 percent of middle-class first graders and substantially more of those who come from less literacy-rich backgrounds" (p. 19). Effective intervention programs will be discussed in detail in Chapter 5.

III. WHY EARLY INTERVENTION IS SOMETIMES NOT ENOUGH

Over the years, language intervention has included approaches that emphasize different aspects of language, for example, cognitive-semantic bases, syntactic forms, and pragmatic issues. Expanded delivery of service has resulted in more naturalistic approaches provided in individual, group, and classroom environments. However, as Snyder (1980) asked, "Do these improved and expanded services adequately prepare language disordered children for their major academic task—reading?" (p. 35).

A. Fragmentation of Approaches.

Perhaps some remedial approaches are missing the mark, because language abilities are too often divided and subdivided into receptive–expressive language units rather than treated as an oral–written language continuum, each folding into the other. Rather than assessing children's isolated receptive and expressive language, we should be examining the impact that early auditory processing and oral language problems have on later reading, writing, spelling. Stated differently, rather than identifying isolated problems in a child's ability, for instance, to name a number of members of a category (Word Association subtests), and treating this deficit as an isolated oral language problem, we should examine the impact this problem may have on the student's developing reading comprehension and written language abilities. Why work on oral language isolated from written language, except with very young children? By going beyond the impact this deficit has on isolated oral skills, would we not be better serving students by stepping back and viewing the impact of this problem on the "bigger picture," that is, oral–written language?   Damico (1988) and Kent (1990) warned against the fragmentation fallacy that arises when language is analyzed into separate modules such as phonology, semantics, syntax, and pragmatics. Damico implied that subdividing rich, interacting, human behavior into a list of discrete scores is misleading and not very useful. As educators and specialists working with children, we know we must break skills up into teachable units. However, unless these fragments are melded into bigger units and

brought to an automatic skill level, results of our labor may be tantamount to Humpty Dumpty just after the fall.

B. Other Barriers to Treatment Success.

Beyond fragmentation, Damico (1988) offered four additional reasons
why one of his clients was seen for language therapy as a first grader,
dismissed from therapy as being "remediated," and re-referred as a 12-
year-old "unable to perform most of the work required in the seventh
grade" (p. 54). The first reason was therapist bias, which occurs when
a therapist perceives a student's progress as better than it actually is.
Aquiescence, agreeing with the opinions of others, for example, teachers and administrators, without dispute, presents another barrier to
treatment success. A third barrier occurs when there is lack of follow-
up. This results when a therapist dismisses a student on the basis of
meeting criteria on standardized language tests without considering
how the student is using language in the "real world." Finally, bureau-
cratic policies and procedures, when services for students are doled
out on the basis of funding formulas with services provided being adequate, not optimal, provide additional interference with treatment success.

IV. ROLE OF SPEECH–LANGUAGE SPECIALISTS IN TREATING DEVELOPMENTAL LANGUAGE AND READING DISABILITIES

Predicting how research will improve our understanding of developmental
language disabilities, Tallal (1991) characterized the 1990s as "the decade
of integration" (p. 405). Information from two lines of research, neurosciences and cognitive sciences, began merging during that time to further
our understanding of the complexity of language disabilities.

A. Historical Perspective.

Neuroscientists study brain structure and function with noninvasive,
brain imaging procedures. Cognitive scientists utilize computational,
computer modeling of neural processes to simulate task performance
by students with speech, language, and reading disorders.
Unfortunately, developmental language disorders and specific reading
disabilities have traditionally been separated in both research and
practice. Tallal explained:

In science, "facts" as well as cherished "myths" come to hold an esteemed place in our minds. Once established, it often takes more data to alter them than were originally required for their establishment. That is, once specific concepts enter our thinking about a particular topic, they take on a life of their own in guiding future theoretical constructs, which are the basis for future research (p. 399).

Issues of territoriality become apparent when we consider that speech–language specialists traditionally have been identified as the professionals concerned with diagnosis and treatment of oral language problems, and reading teachers, learning disabilities specialists, and resource specialists traditionally have worked with written language problems. Historically, then, disorders of listening and speaking have been the domain of speech–language specialists, and disorders of reading, writing, and spelling have been the domain of written language specialists.

Although the oral and written language specialists often "share" many students on their caseloads, the oral–written dichotomy continues to dictate that the oral language specialist sees the student for oral language problems, and the written language specialist sees the same student for written language problems. The student's problem is dissected, and the practitioners teach isolated skills. Tallal (1988) observed, "Continuing to separate these developmental communication disorders ultimately fails the many children who 'progress' from language impaired to reading impaired" (p. 200).

B. Reading Disabilities as Visual Perceptual Deficits.

Traditionally, reading has been viewed as a visual–perceptual process and reading problems as resulting from deficits in the visual–spatial system. This view has persisted even though a relationship between developmental reading disabilities and underlying deficiencies in oral language development has been documented for many years. The decades-old observation that children with developmental reading disabilities often demonstrate difficulty with reversible letters and words, for example, substituting "b" for "d" and "was" for "saw," led to the erroneous conclusion that these children "see backwards" and "read backwards." This myth continues despite the fact that a decade of research on visual perceptual abilities in children with developmental reading disabilities has failed to support the "backwards" hypothesis (Tallal, 1991). Smith (1994) explained:

One thing the eyes and the brain cannot do is see backward. I mention this fact, which perhaps ought to be self-evident, because a belief does exist that a visual abnormality of this kind causes some children problems in learning to read. The basis of the myth is the indisputable evidence that many children at some point in their reading careers confuse reversible letters like b and d, p and q, and even words like was and saw or much and chum. But seeing backward is both a physical and a logical impossibility (p. 83).

C. The speech–language specialist as part of the education team.

Almost three decades have passed since Rees (1974) argued that speech–language specialists should assess and develop linguistic prerequisites for reading, as well as assist students in developing specific linguistic awareness required for reading. In recent years there has been a trend for speech–language specialists to work collaboratively with students' language across the curriculum, but many hesitate to do so because they feel unqualified.

Casby (1988) surveyed 105 public school speech–language specialists to explore their attitudes and perceptions about their training, knowledge, and competencies in treating students with developmental reading disabilities. Thirty-seven percent of the respondents worked in kindergarten through 12th grades, 35% in the primary grades, and 13% with preprimary-age children. While 90% of the respondents supported the idea that they should be part of the management of students with language and reading problems only 38% had been asked to assess written language deficits and only 37% to treat them. Other members of the educational team, apparently, referred few students with written language problems to speech–language specialists. Conner and Coover (2001) examined how speech–language specialists view their competencies to meet ASHA's position defining speech–language specialists' role in literacy and the school-based expectations in literacy. The 104 speech–language specialists included in the survey represented a cross-section of training programs across the country, and the respondents averaged 11 years public schoolwork experience. Those competencies speech–language specialists were most and least comfortable with are summarized in Table 1-3.

Table 1-3. Competencies with Which Speech–Language Specialists Were Most and Least Comfortable (Connor & Coover, 2001).

Speech–language specialists were most comfortable with:

- "Working effectively as members of a team
- "Establishing and maintaining relationships with parents and school personnel
- "Using assessment tools
- "Addressing the needs of students with speech and language disabilities
- "Facilitating IEP meetings
- "Demonstrating effective conference skills
- "Developing IEPs
- "Evaluating student progress" (p. 19)

Speech–language specialists were least comfortable with:

- "Supervising and planning for speech assistants
- "Teaching the writing process
- "Determining augmentative communication options
- "Teaching alternative reading programs and strategies
- "Understanding and integrating the general education language arts curriculum into therapy
- "Acting as a resource to other school staff
- "Participating as a member of school-based committees" (p. 19).

In her review of the history of oracy to literacy, Butler (1999) summarized the paradigm shift in the 1980s as follows:

> Perhaps it was the "persona," our vision of ourselves, as "speech" people. Our clinical perception, even for the most recent graduates, was that children's spoken language problems were our domain and our proper role . . . (p. 26).

A substantial body of research now supports the relationships among phonological awareness, reading acquisition, and developmental reading disabilities. Spoken and written language are no longer viewed as separate skills or parallel processes in different modalities (Kavanagh, 1991). Dickinson and McCabe (1991) suggested that language acquisition should be viewed as a French braid rather than a sequential process. "Like a braid, language consists of multiple strands—phonology, semantics, syntax, discourse, reading, and writing—that are picked up at various times and woven in with the other strands to create a beautiful whole" (p. 1).

All language learning, including literacy learning, is a part of a continuous process that begins at birth. It is clear that reading acquisition in preschool is a valid concern for speech–language specialists (van Kleeck, 1990). Because the speech–language specialist works most directly with children who have developmental language impairments, he or she is positioned best to identify and remediate the problems these students exhibit in phonological awareness, semantics, syntax, and metalinguistic abilities. Training in phonetics, language acquisition, language disorders, and clinical experience qualify the speech–language specialist as a member of the educational team treating language-based reading disabilities.

Koppenhaver, Coleman, Kalman, and Yoder (1991) proposed that speech–language specialists provide children with the environmental stimuli needed to enhance literacy skill acquisition. Speech–language specialists promote oral language and communication skills, and oral language development will be advanced through facilitating emerging literacy skills. These authors concluded that, if speech-language specialists "are to promote maximal communication and language development, they should incorporate written language experiences in their intervention plans" (p. 39). Kamhi and Catts (1989) stated: "the sheer volume of research and clinical data should overwhelm the few remaining holdouts who still question whether reading disability is a language-based disorder" (p. 371). In their 1999 text, Kamhi and Catts concluded "the fact that language deficits are both a cause and consequence of reading disabilities ensures that language problems will be a major component of almost all cases of reading disabilities" (p. 116). Swank (1994) noted "current theory, research results, and practices demand that speech-language specialists provide differential diagnosis of language–based reading disorders" (p. 69). Because reading becomes the primary means of acquiring new information in later grades instead of a goal itself, Boudera and Hedberg (1999) suggested that it is critical to support children at risk for reading failure. They proposed "in planning speech and language intervention, addressing language goals in the context of print and literacy-based activities may be an additional strategy to support both domains of knowledge" (p. 256). Butler (1999) explained that "SLPs and other language specialists whose training and experience prepare them to support both oral and written language prevention and intervention can play pivotal roles, particularly in school-based settings" (p. iv). Finally, the following is included among the guidelines for roles and responsibilities of speech–language pathologists in literacy by the American Speech, Language, and Hearing Association (2001):

> The practice of speech–language pathology involves: Providing prevention, screening, consultation, assessment and diagnosis, treatment, intervention, management, counseling, and follow-up services for disorders of . . . language (i.e., phonology, morphology, syntax, semantics, and pragmatic/social aspects of communication) including comprehension and expression in oral, written, graphic, and manual modalities; language processing; preliteracy and language-based literacy skills (pp. 7–8).

V. SUMMARY

The focus of this chapter has been on laying out the scope of the problem for speech–language specialists working with students who have language disabilities. Follow-up studies of children with early speech-language problems clearly reveal that virtually any child with early oral language problems may develop later written-language problems. One does not cause the other. One evolves into the other. The importance of the speech–language specialist as part of the educational team serving students with developmental reading problems was emphasized. Before turning to identification and treatment issues, we need to understand the underlying language basis of developmental reading disabilities. To that end, the emphasis in Chapter 2 is on the oral-to-written language continuum.

VI. CLINICAL COMPETENCIES

To understand the scope of language based reading disabilities, the teacher/clinician/student will demonstrate the following competencies:

A. Identify children at risk for literacy problems.

B. Understand the relationship between early speech/ language problems and later reading/writing problems.

C. Understand why early intervention is sometimes not enough.

D. Collaborate with other professionals in defining language based developmental reading disabilities.

CHAPTER

2

The Language Continuum

OUTLINE

I. Transitioning from oral to written language

II. The next phase of literacy development: learning to read and write

III. Developmental progression of written language acquisition

IV. Summary

V. Clinical Competencies

I.   TRANSITIONING FROM ORAL TO WRITTEN LANGUAGE

Throughout their early years children gradually, and usually quite easily, develop a complex linguistic system. By the time they enter school, most children are equipped with innovative, rule-governed language enabling them to verbally communicate their thoughts, feelings, and needs. "Language is so readily acquired and so universal in human affairs that it is easy to forget what a complex phenomenon it is" (Bishop, 1997, p. 1).

Learning to read does not begin at the conclusion of oral language development. Rather, oral language is the foundation from which written language will emerge. Furthermore, reading and writing are not discrete skills isolated from listening and speaking. They are integral parts of general language acquisition, and the development of each skill provides the scaffold for the other.

A.   Emergent Literacy.

While traditional definitions of literacy refer to *mastery* of written language forms (reading and writing), the notion of emergent literacy encompasses the developmental and interactional relationship between spoken and written language forms. Paul (2001) explained that emergent literacy experiences, for example, when adults read books aloud, "are those in which children begin to develop ideas about how written language works and what it is used for before they actually begin decoding print" (p. 398). Through "literacy socialization experiences" children learn about how print represents spoken words as they simultaneously learn about new words and word uses from print that they eventually will use in their speech (Snow & Dickinson, 1991).

Understanding the relationship between oral and written language has influenced the educational shift from a traditional "reading readiness" paradigm to the "emergent literacy" process and has resulted in an appreciation for language knowledge a child brings to formal reading instruction (Roberts, 1992). Koppenhaver et al. (1991) noted that emergent literacy encompasses a broader view, including the child's perspective. Rather than being preliterate and nonconventional, literacy is placed on a continuum, and children's early attempts at literacy are legitimized and considered to be protoreading and protowriting. Children bring their prior experiences and learning, including their knowledge of oral language, to bear on written language.

Reading acquisition, therefore, is viewed as an extension of oral language development. According to Strickland and Cullinan (1990) "the term 'emergent' underscores the fact that young children are in a developmental process; there is no single point when literacy begins" (p. 427). Cheek, Flippo, and Lindsey (1997) explained that the emergent literacy view "gives credence to everything that happens in a child's development, from birth on, that shapes the child's concepts about oral and written language and the use of language in all its forms" (p. 58). Supporting this, Hoffman (1990) noted "spelling has its beginning in infancy, as children learn through gesturing that the hand communicates, through scribbling that marks are meaningful, through drawing that symbols represent meaning, and through storybook reading that print corresponds to speech" (p. 239). Finally, Silliman and Wilkinson (1994) proposed that being literate confirms an individual's social identity as a "full participant in a community" (p. 27), and the integration of communicative processes including listening, reading, speaking, and writing "is the pathway to literacy" (p. 27). In order to examine the reciprocal relationship that exists between oral and written language, it will be helpful to briefly review strands of oral language development and their relationship with written language acquisition.

B. Neurolinguistic Development and Oral Language Strands.

In his theory of neurolinguistic development, Locke (1997) proposed that language develops in four fixed, overlapping, sequential phases, during which, unique functions are accomplished.

1. Phase I.

During Phase I, the infant is orienting to speech and learns the vocal characteristics of caregivers. Locke explained that the human infant's preference for listening to people talk results from being equipped with cognitive/neural supports enabling specialization in social cognition as well as prenatal exposure to maternal prosody. Learning to vocalize and say words are facilitated by "socially cognitive operations" that allow infants to "get by" in their native language through learning vocal turn-taking with partners; orienting to and mimicing prosody; gesturing communicatively; assimilating different phonetic patterns, and trying to interpret and alter mental activity of people (p. 269).

2.   **Phase II.**

Phase II, which begins as early as 5–6 months and lasts up to 20 months, is critical for utterance acquisition and storage. Locke proposed that the right cerebral hemisphere is very active in processing and storing single words and two to three word holophrases (e.g.,"shoesnsocks" "gotabed") in prosodic memory. These utterances are being stored so that during Phase III, there is abundant material to be parsed into syllables and phonemes. Thus, for the developing linguistic system, Phase II is critical to the development of the semantic domain of language.

3.   **Phase III.**

Between 18–20 months until approximately 36 months, the child discovers some regularities about language; syntax, morphology, phonology, and pragmatics.

a. **Syntax (word strings) and morphology (grammatical markers).**

The forms that were being stored during Phase II will now be decomposed into parts as the child learns about and applies grammatical rules. In fact, adequate Phase III development is dependent upon the buildup of phrases acquired during Phase II. While earlier phases depended more on outside influences, Locke maintained that in Phase III the left cerebral hemisphere becomes more involved, acting as an "internal deducer," allowing for grammatical behavior. Phrases are broken into words and words into parts as the child learns how to divide phrases into parts and meld parts back into wholes. The linguistic rules learned by children during this phase allow them to impose organization on new language heard, thus expediting acquisition of even more words.

If language is developing normally during this phase, the child acquires approximately 400 expressive words by 28–30 months, then discovers and applies morphological rules (Locke, 1997, p. 277). As the result of analytic work accomplished during Phase III, overlapping articulatory gestures lead the child to discover the phoneme, a speech sound that can stand alone. The child becomes aware of minimal pairs (words differing from each other by one sound). The discovery of phonemes leads to the child's discovery of morphological endings such as making a word plural by adding -s or -es, or changing word tenses. Kamhi and Catts (1999) explained that grammatical morphemes are "words and inflections that convey subtle meaning and serve specific grammatical and pragmatic functions . . . (they) . . . modulate meaning" (pp. 2–3).

b. Phonology (sound system).

Within the first few months of life, human infants can verbally produce almost all the auditory discriminations needed to distinguish most phonemic categories in the English language (Kuhl, 1988). Kent (1992) explained that the wavelike aspect of the speech stream results from the syllabic crests and margins that average four per second and the intonational contours of speech with its characteristic rising and falling vocal pitch. The speech stream remains continuous, and the perception of the acoustic signal of speech stays together (coheres) allowing for predictive continuity (p. 75). Adults can recognize units in the stream because certain acoustic features are consolidated and can be recognized as segments. Infants probably hear speech as a continuous stream of sounds carrying certain conspicuous spectral and temporal details that eventually are recognized as phonetic cues (p. 75). Furthermore, the characteristics of the speech stream promote the infant's attentional focus to switch from various streams, such as "mommy's talk" to "daddy's talk," and to particular aspects of the utterance such as referents (p. 76). Infants become "narrowly tuned" to their native language and are capable of making "exceptionally fine discriminations of sounds in a manner that is linguistically significant" (Freil-Patti, 1994, p. 381).

Most adults have enjoyed the delightful experience of hearing children laugh when they discover the magic of manipulating sounds in words. Children enjoy creating "a new language" through making up novel words such as "nannie, wannie, lannie," or substituting sounds in familiar nursery rhymes, for example, changing "Twinkle, Twinkle Little Star" to "Binkle, Binkle, Bittle Bar." Young children play with sounds and words, creating strings of highly inflected jargon, nonsense words, rhymes, and alliteration (repetition of initial sound in two or more words near each other in a phrase or sentence). Older children produce playground chants or ritualized insults. All these activities are often "framed with giggles of pleasure and mischief . . . In all of these cases, the children are focusing on language as an object having its own existence. Like all other objects, language is a potential item of play" (van Kleeck, 1994, p. 54).

Henderson (1992) underscored the importance of reading nursery rhymes aloud to young children, noting that two awarenesses simultaneously emerge. First, "cadence" of oral reading divides words differently than the natural flow of oral language and leads to the physical placement of phoneme strings. Second, rhyme, alliteration, and word play focus attention on the phonemic structure of words. "Meaning is not an issue when a 'dish runs away with the spoon.' The focus is verbal segment and sound" (p. 22). Cecil (1990) proposed that children initially discover the wide sound spectrum through solitary word and sound play with noise and "phonobabble," and eventually "speech play leads children to a fascination and delight with the rhyme, rhythm, and repetition of stories that they hear read aloud and soon aspire to read on their own" (p. 25). As we will see in a later section of this chapter, an alphabetic orthography, such as used in English language, represents the sound system of our language in print.

The language domain of phonology, therefore, has been a critical area researched over the past 15 years as researchers delve into the underlying language-based aspects of developmental reading disabilities. And because of the alphabetic–phonologic relationship, researchers zeroed in on the differences between good and poor readers on many aspects of phonology (see Chapter 4, section IIIA). Liberman and Shankweiler (1991) pointed out that a broad data base now exists relating reading disabilities to problems in phonological awareness "including studies of people of a wide range of ages, of many language communities, and a full range of cultural and economic backgrounds from inner city and rural poor to suburban affluent" (pp. 8–9).

c. **Pragmatics (effective use of language in social context).**

Pragmatic knowledge—knowing about the rules of language use—becomes part of communicative competence as children experience using language. It begins to develop with an infant's initial interactions with a parent or caretaker and continues to be acquired long past learning how to string words together. Through conversations with parents and/or other caretakers at home and with teachers and other children in preschool and elementary school, children acquire strategies for conversing with others.

Whereas pragmatics refers to the "practical skill of using language in a social context" (p. 54), metalinguistic skill—language awareness—refers to the "ability to reflect consciously on the nature and properties of language" (van Kleeck, 1994, p. 53). Growth in cognitive skills leads a child to understand the correspondence between sound and meaning. This symbolic function of language establishes the foundation for metalinguistic ability and facilitates the child's recognition of words as labels for objects—that words are "things" themselves and not the objects they represent. This underlies the child's ability to shift attention from the meaning of what is being said to think and talk about the language being used, that is, to reflect on language as an object.

Language awareness is essential for the child to engage in emerging literacy activities such as dividing sentences into words and words into syllables; isolating first, last, and middle sounds in words; rhyming words; and rearranging words to make grammatically correct sentences. Van Kleeck (1994) emphasized the importance of children learning to focus exclusively on the linguistic code "because it is often used in isolation from other communication channels in one critical academic activity: reading independently" (p. 57). The outcomes of metalinguistic awareness can be classified into five broad categories: word awareness, phonological awareness, syntactic awareness, pragmatic awareness, and connected discourse awareness. Menyuk (1991) proposed that "metalinguizing" is a continuous, constantly changing process in a child's linguistic maturation. Van Kleeck summarized a two-stage cognitive model of metalinguistic development based on a Piagetian framework.

i.   *Stage 1* begins with the onset of language and lasts approximately 6 years. During this time, children's thought is characterized by centration, which is the "tendency to concentrate on one aspect of a situation at a time," and by irreversibility, which refers to "their inability to shift back and forth easily between aspects of a situation" (p. 58). In Stage 1, children focus more on meaning than on linguistic form and can focus on form if meaning is less salient to them. Consequently, when asked to provide a long word, children in Stage 1 may respond with "train" (p. 59). Likewise, when asked to segment sentences into words, children in Stage 1 will not count function words such as "the" or "is," because they do not identify these as words (p. 59).

ii. *Stage 2* occurs between 7–11 years of age. During this time, the reasoning ability of children is characterized by decentration, "the ability to hold in mind and relate more than one aspect of a situation at a time," and reversibility, which "allows thought to shift back and forth between aspects of the situation" (p. 60). Decentration allows children to consider language in two ways: "They can consider language as a medium for conveying meaning and as an object in its own right" (p. 60). This transition allows children to "focus on and compare two meanings of one particular linguistic form at a time" (p. 60), allowing them to deal with word ambiguity. They can now "manipulate the linguistic form while retaining the semantic content of the message," allowing them to judge whether or not the syntactic form of a message is correct (p. 60).

4.   Phase IV.

The final phase, Phase IV, in Locke's theory of neurolinguistic development involves integration and elaboration. It is during this phase in normal language development that a child's lexicon (word storage) substantially increases. As Locke proposed, the structural analysis accomplished during Phase III "takes the pressure off a holistic type of memory, thereby enabling the creation of larger and larger vocabularies, in which each of the individual entries is merely a unique recombination of a small set of phonemes" (p. 275). During the first five years of life, then, continuity in normal language development can be seen in the critical semantic, syntactic–morphologic, pragmatic and metalinguistic skills that children acquire. Acquisition of these aspects are in place for most children when they enter school and face the next phase in the language continuum—the overlaid function of written language.

C. A Sensitive Period for Language Development.

Because of the reciprocal interaction between oral and written language acquisition, it is of interest to consider Locke's notion that the sensitive period for language development is between prenatal infancy though 6 to 8 years. As mentioned earlier, an important aspect of Locke's theory is that the four phases are fixed (must happen), overlapping sequences (one must occur before the next). In normal language development sufficient lexical material is stored in Phase II to activate an analytic mechanism during Phase III, so that vocabularies can be expanded and the developing language system can become elaborated and integrated. If, however, there is a delay in acquisition, a cascading effect occurs. A delay in the development of Phase II results in a paucity of stored utterances to move forward at the optimal biological time to be analyzed in Phase III. The result is a child whose limited utterance processing results in lexical delays. The children described by Locke as being "lexically delayed" have small vocabularies usually not attributable to hearing problems, low intelligence, brain damage, or primary affective disorder (p. 282). Locke's lexically delayed children come from linguistically stimulating environments, but they are moving through time-locked sequential phases with neurological systems incapable of taking advantage of what must occur in those phases.

The kind of higher-order cognitive loss in lexically delayed children is the result of a shortage of stored lexical items preventing utterance analytical mechanisms from fully or permanently activating, thereby restricting the development of a linguistic grammar (p. 282). The lexically delayed child who "has not realized a sizable lexical increase by about 24 months is therefore at developmental risk" because the necessary analytical–computational capability "may not turn all the way on" (p. 288). These are the at-risk children whose lexical delay evolves into later overt or subtle receptive–expressive language problems, and/or reading and writing problems. These are the children who continue to experience language problems into adulthood because "the critical phase for grammatical analysis, timed by unidentified endogenous factors, expires too soon" (p. 288). The neurolinguistic resources critical for specializing in phonological operations are rendered inadequate leading to decreased spoken language development and ultimately inadequate phonological encoding and decoding operations needed for written language. Describing spoken and written language disorders as "phonology plus" problems, Locke proposed that there may be "limits on deeply internal phonological operations that interact with other, unspecified factors" in both disorders (p. 299).

"Working in conjunction with these other factors, the phonological deficits would impair performance in one or the other modality, or in both speech and reading" (p. 299).

D. Reciprocity Between Oral/Written Language.

Asymmetries exist among primary processes underlying reading ability in children at the early stages and those at later stages of reading development. These differences were examined by Vellutino, Scanlon, Small, and Tanzman (1991) and described by Vellutino and Scanlon (1991) and Vellutino (1993). Three major questions were addressed: 1)What combination of skills, abilities, and knowledge sources is the best predictor of performance on measures of reading ability? 2) Are reading and visual abilities weighted differently as determinants of reading ability? 3) Which measures of cognitive and linguistic abilities discriminate reliably between poor and normal readers? (Vellutino, 1993).

Subjects included 297 younger (grades 2 and 3) and 171 older (grades 6 and 7) attending suburban New York schools (Vellutino et al., 1991, p. 103). Cognitive–linguistic abilities, world knowledge (as measured by the *Wechsler Intelligence Scale for Children—Revised* (WISC-R) Information subtest), and specific key prerequisite skills for successful reading acquisition were evaluated with a comprehensive battery of psychometric and experimental tests.

Data collected by Vellutino et al. strongly indicated that oral and written language are "intrinsically related." The relationship implies that "facility in processing and comprehending written language depends directly on factors that allow one to acquire competency in the different domains of oral language" (pp. 125–126). In the developing reader, oral and written language are not parallel systems. Rather, they are increasingly interactive and convergent systems. They develop in this manner, because the same linguistic competencies are necessary for successfully acquiring oral and written language. "The child does not acquire a new language when she/he learns to read, but, in essence, 'recodes' the language she/he has already acquired" (p. 126).

Various subskills for reading depend on adequate development in other language domains. Variability exists, however, in the weight assigned to competence in a particular domain "depending on the unique processes involved in acquiring a particular subskill as well as on the level at which the child has acquired that subskill" (p. 126). The researchers observed that phonologically based skills, for example phoneme segmentation and alphabetic mapping ability, "proved to be the most important determinants of facility in word identification in younger and older students, but particularly in children at the beginning stages of reading skills acquisition" (p. 126). Their data suggested two primary generalizations. First, the developing reader must successfully learn "to capitalize on orthographic redundancy rather than be overwhelmed by it" (p. 127). Second, "children who have difficulty in acquiring symbol–sound mapping rules will, in the large majority of cases, have difficulty learning to read" (p. 127). Furthermore, with increased exposure to print, semantic knowledge, particularly word meanings, becomes an "increasingly important determinant of facility in word identification" (p. 127). The "geometric" expansion in the number of new words in second-grade basal readers, coupled with uncontrolled vocabularies in text supplements, will increase the chances that some children will encounter many words that are not meaningful to them. Vellutino et al. speculated that "children whose vocabulary is less than optimal will have difficulty learning to read (and they) should become increasingly impoverished in vocabulary development, which, in turn, should add to their difficulties in reading" (p. 127). The "modest" differences found on vocabulary measures of young, poor, and normal readers became "significantly larger" at older age levels. "Sizeable differences" between all poor and normal readers on a measure of semantic concept analysis (WISC-R Similarities) suggested that some poor readers might have semantic deficits at the early stages of reading skill acquisition. "Substantially larger" differences in performance by older children supported the notion that reading difficulties may either cause semantic deficits or complicate already existing semantic deficits (p. 127).

Additional support for the influence of different linguistic competencies on reading subskills came from the evaluation of vocabulary and world knowledge. These skills were the most powerful predictors of reading comprehension when only language and verbal measures were used and of listening comprehension when reading comprehension, word identification, spelling, and pseudoword decoding were parceled out. In addition, phonological processing abilities were found to have a greater influence on word identification than on reading comprehension. Vellutino et al. hypothesized this "quite likely came by way of the strong connection between phonological coding ability and short term memory" (p. 128).

An additional conclusion was that word identification, reading comprehension, and listening comprehension are primarily language based skills. The Vellutino group observed that language measures "were more successful than the various non-verbal measures in predicting performance on the tests evaluating these skills" (p. 128). Additional support came from observation that poor readers were deficient on reading subskills, listening comprehension, and "on virtually all of the language and language dependent tests compared with good readers"(p. 128). Nonverbal tests were "not strong and reliable predictors of performance on the reading subskills and listening comprehension tests, nor did they reliably discriminate between poor and normal readers" (p. 128). The researchers concluded:

> Given that poor readers with at least average intellectual abilities were reliably distinguished from normal readers on the language and language based measures, but not on the nonverbal measures, we also feel confident in concluding that reading difficulties in otherwise normal children will, in most cases, be caused by deficiencies in one or more of the domains of language (p. 128).

II. THE NEXT PHASE OF LITERACY DEVELOPMENT: LEARNING TO READ AND WRITE

> Speech has been around for 200,000 years or more, although the idea that it could be rendered alphabetically was born no more than 4,000 years ago. Subtracting the latter number from the former, we conclude that it took our ancestors at least 196,000 years just to discover how to describe what it was they did when they spoke. Why did it take so long? Why was it so hard for our prealphabetic ancestors to make the momentous discovery, and why is it so hard for our preliterate children to understand it? (Liberman, 1997, p. 5).

A. Learning to Read Orthography.

Numerous writing systems have evolved during the course of human culture. Examination of the systems, known as orthographies, illustrates how messages have been conveyed through objects and pictures, words and syllables, and finally alphabetic letters. Regardless of the orthographic form, the reader's task is to understand the inherent relationship that exists between the orthographic symbols (objects, pictures, or letters) and the linguistic units they represent (ideas, words, syllables, or phonemes). When learning to read "the child needs to associate orthographic with phonological patterns in memory" (Stanovich, 1991a, p. 26).

In the English orthography individual speech sound units (phonemes) are visually coded in print by alphabet letters (graphemes). Liberman,

Liberman, Mattingly, and Shankweiler (1980) explained that considerable variation exists in the demands various orthographies place on beginning readers. First, the depth of an orthography refers to "its relative remoteness from the phonetic representation" (p. 146). A language with a limited phonologic system, such as that found in the Turkish or Vietnamese languages, requires the reader to decode a shallow, limited orthography. English, on the other hand, requires that the reader learn to map a deep orthography onto an internalized deep phonologic system. An orthography that uses a morphemic transcription, for instance, the Chinese system, places relatively few demands on the reader's linguistic awareness, because morphemes can be produced in isolation and, therefore, "readily available to consciousness" (p. 148).

A second variation affecting the demands of an orthography is the linguistic unit—morpheme, syllable, or phoneme—that is overtly represented. Although the alphabetic orthography used in modern English spelling is frequently abstract, it represents the internal phonological structure of spoken words through an incredibly economical set of 26 printed symbols that provide entry into the entire printed vocabulary of the language. An alphabetic orthography is, therefore, considered more flexible than logographies and syllabaries, because readers of the alphabetic system can read words they have not seen before without having to memorize associations between symbol patterns and corresponding words (Liberman, 1983).

B. Getting to the Meaning.

Whether one receives language through the visual or auditory modality, one must get to the meaning through the basic unit of the language, the word. This requires traversing linguistic units of language, including phonological segments (words) and the larger syntactic structures (sentences) they form. Some type of linguistic processing, however automatic, is necessary for handling spoken as well as written messages, because, as Liberman (1983) indicated, "in language, as in everything else, there is no free lunch" (p. 82). Bear et al. (1996) explained "the *concept* of word and the *concept* of a phoneme must be taught; both will emerge as children gradually acquire the alphabetic principle and coordinate the units of speech with the printed units on the page" (p. 96).

Learning how to read and write an alphabetic orthography requires the reader to develop two aspects of linguistic sophistication, described by Liberman, Rubin, Duques, and Carlisle (1985) as linguistic (phonological) awareness and phonological maturity.

1. **Linguistic (phonological) awareness: learning about phonetic segmentation.**

    Although an alphabetic orthography such as English offers many advantages, it poses a major obstacle for the novice reader who must come to appreciate the relations that exist between linguistic units represented by printed characters. Unlike a syllabary, a printed form of language the smallest unit of which is the syllable, an alphabetic system contains several thousand different spoken syllables which makes syllable identification considerably complex. Contrasted with the simplistic vowel alone (V) or consonant–vowel (CV) syllable types in the Japanese syllabary, English alphabetic orthography contains many syllable types, including CCV, CCVC, CCVCC, CCCV, and CCCVCCCC. Because consonants can occur at both the beginning and end of English syllables, segmenting polysyllabic words can pose a theoretical and practical problem. Thus, even when it is relatively easy to perceive two syllables in a word such as "Chester," identification of where the syllable boundaries ought to be is unclear ("Ches-ter" or "Chest-er").

    Although an alphabetic orthography is often thought of as representing speech, it is, at best, only an abstraction from speech. Because of the manner in which speech is articulated, phonetic segments overlap and merge into syllable-sized units through a complex process of coarticulation. Speakers verbally produce strings of consonants and vowels at rates averaging 10 to12 per second, and 20 to 25 per second for short periods (Liberman, 1997, p. 10). Information about the phonological and phonetic segments is represented only approximately by alphabetic letters and transmitted simultaneously on the same part of the sound. A simple one-to-one relationship cannot exist between printed letters and their articulated speech sounds. Although it is possible to separate words and syllables out of the complex speech stream, it is impossible to separate out most consonants from syllables without an accompanying "uh" sound. To map the printed three-letter word "bag" onto the spoken word "bag" successfully, for example, the reader must know that the spoken syllable only has three segments. Otherwise, the meaningful monosyllabic word "bag" is pronounced as a nonsense, three-syllable word containing five phonetic segments, "buh-a-guh" (Liberman, 1997). According to Liberman and Shankweiler (1991) neither novice nor skilled readers can work letter-by-letter to recover words from print. Every reader must group the letters together that represent "strings of consonants and vowels that are, in the normal process of speech production, collapsed, merged, coarticulated into a single, pronounceable unit. There is no simple rule by which a reader can do this" (p. 13).

2. **Phonological maturity.**

An underlying assumption in an alphabetic orthography is that readers know the phonology of their language, so the representation of words in their personal lexicon can be matched with the orthographic transcription. Practice with oral language leads native English speakers to assimilate rules and develop an implicit knowledge of how to pronounce the different forms words may take when prefixes and suffixes are added. Consider how the first vowel in the words "telegraph," "Canada," and "contract" sound different from each other because of their placement in the stressed syllable. When suffixes are added, the stress shifts to the next syllable to the right as in "telegraphy," "Canadian," and "contractual." Rather than having two entries as part of the stored pronunciation rules, the native speaker's lexicon contains one rule to mediate both instances, that is, "pronounce all vowels as 'uh' when in unstressed syllables." As a result of being phonologically mature, the speaker has internalized the rule neutralizing unstressed vowels, and the phonologic rule will be used automatically when attempting to recover the phonetic aspect (i.e., the pronunciation of printed words). Phonological maturity, then, allows the reader to relate phonological and phonetic representations of the language.

C. The Need for a Model.

Reading is an interactive process and the act of reading calls on various cognitive abilities spread across perceptual, cognitive, and linguistic domains. This interactive base is utilized in subsequent exposure to reading instruction. During the reading process, information extracted from the printed page, whether at the level of decoding and word recognition or comprehension of text, is analyzed and compared with previously stored information. If it were a simple matter of learning a set of associations between sounds of the spoken language and printed squiggles on a page, learning to read would be relatively easy, because it would involve little that is new to the would-be reader with the exception that language will now be presented through the visual modality. The process involved in reading acquisition, however, is far more complex than a simple transfer of meanings from oral to written language.

Confusion in the study of reading results from the use of different models, labels, and teaching approaches. A plethora of reading tests and materials frustrates practitioners with definitions, subtype descriptions, remedial approaches, and prepackaged programs. Organizing knowledge in a model seems useful, and models of the reading process are offered as guides to explain how the components of the process work together in a cohesive system. Knowing the components of the reading process permits tracing reading disabilities to breakdowns in one or another of the subprocesses and leads to specific, efficient remediation. Therefore, it is essential for practitioners to adopt some model, because practicing without one promotes an "I believe what I see" point of view rather than an "I see what I believe" approach. The result of practicing without a model is a reactive response to unexpected reading and writing behaviors and exacerbation of students' frustrations. Consequently, Adams' (1990) model of reading acquisition, Chall's (1983) and Frith's (1986) stage theories of reading development are presented here. Adams' model is referred to again in Chapter 4 in the discussion of practical aspects of assessment, in Chapters 5 and 6 in a discussion of practical applications for teaching and intervention, and in Chapter 7 under "possible collaboration."

Adams (1990), summarized by Stahl, Osborn, and Lehr (1990), presented an analysis of the subcomponents inherent in reading. She described the reading system as comprising four processors (see Figure 2–1). Adams explained: "As shown by the arrows between them, the four processors work together, continuously receiving information from and returning feedback to each other . . . Within each of these processors, knowledge is represented by interconnected sets of simpler units" (p. 21).

1. **The Orthographic Processor.**

   The orthographic processor "receives information directly from the printed page. When we are reading, it is visual, orthographic information that comes first and causes the system to kick in" (Stahl et al., 1990, p. 23). Orthographic processing is "the ability to form, store, and access orthographic representations" (Stanovich, West & Cunningham, 1991, p. 220.) Orthographic processing deals with the visual processing of letters (-a) and sublexical word parts (-ing) and letter patterns (-at). Speakers of a particular language come to predict and expect certain words to

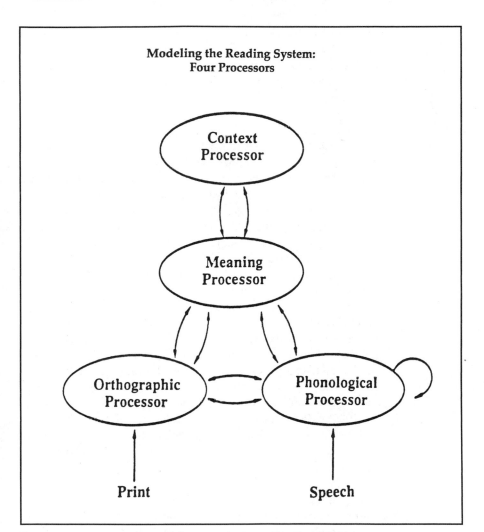

Figure 2–1. Beginning to Read. (From *Beginning to Read* by M. Adams, 1990, p. 22. Copyright 1990 The MIT Press. Reprinted with permission.)

follow other words and sounds to follow other sounds. Likewise, skilled readers and writers of English orthography "develop an implicit knowledge of such factors as what letter combinations are orthographically legitimate" (Hultquist, 1997, p. 90). Stanovich, West & Cunningham (1991) explained that the reader whose efficient phonological processes allows for accurate word decoding develops a "richer orthographic lexicon" because the phonological representations become associated with their visual forms in memory. The "amalgamated orthographic representation is what eventually enables rapid and efficient processes of direct access to the lexicon" (p. 221). Thus, these researchers concluded there is little doubt that "the development of orthographic processing skill must be somewhat dependent on phonological processing abilities" (p. 221).

Aaron (1989) explained that when reading, one's eyes fixate on points in the sentence approximately every 10 to 12 letter spaces. Skilled readers fixate their eyes approximately 1/4 of a second "on virtually every word on the printed page, even though they are entirely unaware of doing so" (Snow, Scarborough & Burns, 1999, p. 50). After this, the image decays as the eyes continue to move along in a saccadic fashion, that is, the eyes move in a rapid, involuntary way from point to point. This visual encoding is considered to be "precategorical," because the words and their meanings are not yet recognized or understood. Aaron also noted that letters in a word appear to be processed simultaneously and in parallel fashion, and letters in the beginning and end positions of words are processed at the same time and before letters in the middle. Adams added, "Given normal print, the eye can clearly resolve up to three or so letters to the left of its fixation point and about twice that many to the right during each fixation. With these letters as its basic data, the system goes to work" (Stahl et al., 1990, p. 24). Describing good readers as "efficient processors in every sense," Stanovich (2000) stated "they completely sample the visual array and use fewer resources to do so . . . (they) allocate less capacity to process this information" (p. 168).

Although the visual system is highly efficient at "extracting information necessary for letter identification, it is quite sloppy about processing letter order" (Stahl et al., 1990, p. 24). Letters in high frequency and familiar words, such as "the," are "strongly interconnected within the reader's orthographic memory . . . each will share stimulation with the others, causing them to be recognized nearly at once and to hang together in the reader's mind as a familiar, cohesive spelling pattern" (p. 24). The reader's orthographic memory will attempt to process a nonword such as "tqe" in the same manner. In this example, the "t" and "e" "will pass stimulation to each other" then to the "h." Because the "h" receives no direct visual stimulation, it cannot pass any back. And because "q" is always followed by a "u" in English, therefore the "q" passes its stimulation to a missing "u." The directly stimulated letter units "send their activation inappropriately around the letter network . . . hurting rather than helping each other's progress. Eventually the direct visual stimulation from the page will bring each of the presented letters to peak stimulation, and the reader will see the string as printed." Adams concluded "It is thus the learned associations between individual letters that are responsible for the easy, holistic manner in which we respond to familiar words" (p. 24).

2.   The Context Processor.

Adams (1990) described *the context processor* as being "in charge of constructing a coherent, ongoing interpretation of the text. As it does so, it sends excitation to units in the meaning processor according to their compatibility with its expectations" (p. 138). This relationship is reflected by the arrow from the context processor to the meaning processor in Figure 2–1. According to Adams, the amount of excitation contributed by the context processor depends on how predictable the context is. If the context is weakly predictive of the next printed word, meaning will receive "a strong and focused boost in excitation . . . (giving) it a head start toward reaching consciousness" (p. 139). Stanovich 2000) maintained that when compared with other prerequisite skills, such as phonological awareness, "variability in the ability to use context to facilitate word recognition is so relatively low that it may not be a major determinant of individual differences in reading acquisition" (p. 169).

3.   The Meaning Processor.

Adams proposed that the meaning and orthographic processors work in similar ways. "Just as the spellings of familiar words are represented in the orthographic processor as interassociated sets of letters," *the meaning processor* stores familiar word meanings "as interassociated sets of more primitive meaning elements" (Adams, 1990, p. 143). Rather than storing self-contained meaning "nodes," Adams suggested that the reader's understanding of a word, for example, "dog," would be represented as "the interassociated distribution of properties that collectively represent the person's total history, direct and vicarious, of experiences with dogs" (p. 143).

Adams explained that, when a child encounters a new word in print, the spelling of the word will be automatically sent to the meaning processor. Rather than finding any learned response, the orthographic pattern will meet "the pattern of anticipatory stimulation provoked by the context processor" (Stahl et al., 1990, p. 28). With repeated exposure to the word in a variety of contexts, the child gradually learns the word's meaning. Adams wrote "the likelihood that a child will learn the meaning of a word from a single exposure in meaningful context ranges between 5% and 20%. By implication, the extent of such incidental vocabulary acquisition depends strongly on the amount a child reads" (Stahl, et al., 1990, p. 28). Adams described text comprehension as "a hierarchically layered process," beginning with the reader retrieving the meaning of each individual word (p. 140). If the spelling of a word is only "marginally familiar," context excitation augments orthographic excitation and selects "the intended word from competitors" (p. 140). Thus, the context processor can, indirectly, speed laborious orthographic processing.

At the next level of text comprehension, readers collapse individual word meanings into a composite interpretation. Skillful readers, according to Adams, periodically interrupt word-by-word progress, usually at major syntactic boundaries, to "interpret the collective significance of the chain of words they have been reading" (p. 141). She explained that the underdeveloped syntactic sensitivities of younger and less skilled readers puts them in the "position of trying to interpret a syntactically anomalous set of words" and leads to reduced comprehension. Furthermore, the greater the time and effort invested in each individual word, "the slimmer the likelihood that preceding words of the phrase will be remembered when it is time to put them all together" (p. 141).

At the third level of comprehension, Adams explained, "readers must combine their understanding of the just-interpreted phrase or clause with their overall interpretation of the text so as to revise and update their understanding of what the text means and where it is going" (p. 142). Comprehension of written language engages the reader's prior knowledge with printed phrases and sentences. The reader maps the newly constructed representation upon pre-existing knowledge so that the hypothesized solution is congruent with what the reader knows about the topic. "Since new knowledge is gained in relation to pre-existing knowledge, comprehension is an interactive and constructive process" (Aaron, 1989, p. 75). Adams (1990) concluded that, "interpretation at this level requires active attention and thought; it is not automatic. It will be only as fruitful as the discipline and effort that the reader invests in it" (p. 142).

4. The Phonological Processor.

The fourth component is the *phonological processor*. Adams proposed that this processor is similar to the orthographic and meaning processors in that it contains "a complexly associated array of primitive units. The auditory image of any particular word, syllable, or phoneme corresponds to the activation of a particular, interconnected set of those units" (p. 157). Adams portrayed the interaction between the orthographic and phonologic processors (Figure 2–1) with arrows going to and from each other. As the visual image of letter strings is being processed in the orthographic processor, "excitatory stimulation is shipped to corresponding units in the phonological processor" (p. 157). The arrow from the phonological to the orthographic processor reflects the response to the excitatory stimulation sent from the orthographic to the phonological processor if the letter string is pronounceable. The two-way arrows between the phonological and meaning processors indicate "activation of a word's meaning results in the excitation of the phonological units underlying its pronunciation. Conversely, the activation of its pronunciation automatically arouses its meaning" (p. 158).

Adams suggested the phonological processor is different from the other components in two ways. First, like the orthographic processor, it receives information from the outside, but in the case of the phonological processor, the outside information is speech. Second, the information in this processor "can be activated or reactivated at our own volition. Not only can we speak, we can also subvocalize or generate speech images at will" (p. 158). Subvocal rehearsal allows phonological representations to be stored.

Gough and Tunmer (1986) proposed that the reader goes from print to meaning by way of speech. This involves applying orthographic rules to the contents of a character register, converting the contents to speech, and then listening while reading. Reitsma's (1984) work demonstrated that beginning readers translate print into sound prior to retrieving a word's meaning. Aaron (1989) explained that "the articulatory-rehearsal mechanism of working-memory is phonological in nature and good readers rely on phonological mediation more than poor readers do for processing written language" (p. 43). Two invaluable functions provided by the phonological processor include providing "an alphabetic backup system—a redundant processing route—that is critical for maintaining the speed as well as the accuracy of word recognition necessary for productive reading," and providing "a means of expanding the on-line memory for individual words as is essential for text comprehension" (Adams, 1990, p. 159).

III. DEVELOPMENTAL PROGRESSION OF WRITTEN LANGUAGE ACQUISITION

A developmental model is helpful in explaining how skills are sequenced and what strategies a child needs to acquire to become a proficient reader/writer. In a developmental model, strategy acquisition follows a sequence that is developmentally inevitable (i.e., a certain level of mastery must be achieved before breaking through to the next sequential step). The first steps provide the scaffolding on which later aspects will be efficiently and systematically added. Failure at any point along the continuum results in varying types of disabilities, depending on where in the sequence the failure occurs. The following description, therefore, begins with the child identifying logos and continues through sophisticated reading, writing and spelling. Spelling, unfortunately "has been the stepchild of the classroom, relegated to lists of words to be learned, often out of context, and practiced through rote memorization" (Butler, 2000, iv). Spelling is actually a complex language skill reflecting the integration of phonologic, orthographic, morphologic, and semantic knowledge bases (Kamhi and Hinton, 2000).

A. Frith's and Chall's Theories; Bear et al.'s Model.

Frith's three-stage theory, and Chall's six-stage theory describe the progression of reading acquisition and the nature of developmental reading problems. Bear et al. (1996) presented a four-stage model of reading, writing, and spelling development. In stage theories the journey to literacy can be viewed as a sequence of steps that merge cognitive interactions with other essential developmental processes. Reading competence, as judged by reading age-equivalency, increases, roughly, with chronological age and shows spurts and plateaus in growth. Frith (1985) maintained that, if failure occurs in a particular stage during the development of reading, the student will more than likely not move on to the next step. "In no way could drill in the new strategy by itself reinstate the normal progress . . . Furthermore, the

hypothesis would give a rationale for teaching compensatory strategies even though one would not expect them to be as efficient as normal strategies" (p. 310).

Frith hypothesized that certain aspects of old reading strategies might
be retained, because they facilitate emergence of, or breakthrough to,
new strategies and allow transition to the next developmental stage. A
transitional skill allows the reader to "discover" the nature of an
emerging strategy through applying it and responding to instruction in
its use (Sawyer, 1992). As Chall (1983) explained, reading in all stages
is a form of problem solving as readers adapt to their environment
through the Piagetian processes of assimilation and accomodation. "In
assimilation they use learned processes in reacting to new demands. In
accomodation they adapt by changing or restructuring the old to acco-
modate the new" (p. 11). The ability, for instance, to recognize sight
words, evolves into initial sound–symbol association. To become proficient with written language, the novice needs to master three basic
strategies, each one merging into the next as the reader's decoding
ability increases in speed and accuracy. The three kinds of strategies,
logographic, alphabetic, and orthographic, will be discussed as stages
of development. Because reading and writing strategies do not develop in unison, there is a stepwise developmental progression as illustrated in Figure 2–2.

1.   **Logographic stage: emerging recognition of printed words.**

As we saw earlier in the discussion of Locke's theory of neurolinguistic development, unless there is an interruption in their
development, children acquire speech in response to a biological-
ly determined timetable without needing formal instruction in
understanding and verbal expression. Equipped with the foundations of an oral language system, 5-year-olds enter school and
face the often arduous task of learning to read. According to
Gough and Juel (1991) "the first grade child already knows, in
their spoken or phonological form, most of the words that he will
encounter in print for the next 3 years. What he doesn't know is
their printed form" (p. 51).

a.   **Normal development at the logographic stage.**

Prior to entering the first stage, the child develops emergent
literacy symbolic skills but has only a symbolic understanding
of what print is, for example, a toy mailbox is where one
"mails" pretend letters (Sawyer, 1992). In **Chall's Stage 0:**

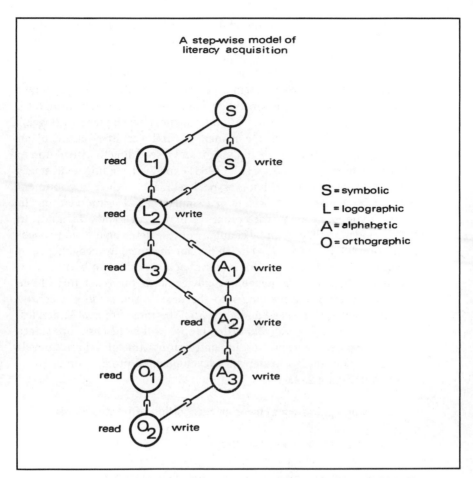

Figure 2–2. A Step-Wise Model of Literacy Acquisition. (Reprinted from U. Frith, "A Stepwise Model of Literacy Acquisition," 1986, *Annals of Dyslexia, 36,* p. 77, with permission from The Orton Dyslexia Society, Inc.)

Prereading (grades preschool–1.5; ages 6 months to 6 years), "pseudoreading" is dependent upon memory and the ability to understand pictures. "There is only a kind of global matching of story parts with pictures and other reminders of the remembered story" (Chall, 1983, p. 41). Bear et al. (1996) proposed that two forms of literacy play, pretend reading and reading from memory, during this preliterate stage are "essential practices for movement into literacy" (p. 93). Pretend reading (paraphrasing or spontaneously retelling a story while turning the pages of a familiar book) allows children to "rehearse the predictability of the text and pace their retelling to match the sequence of pictures" (p. 93). When children read from memory they recite text while moving their fingers along the line of print, thus helping them to "coordinate spoken language with its counterpart in print" (p. 94). The true beginning of literacy at this point on the language continuum is thought to occur when a child indicates that a particular printed word has a particular meaning, for example, when recognizing that a printed sequence of letters is his or her name or that the four-letter-sequence on the stop sign means the driver should stop the car.

Frith's logographic and Chall's prereading stages involve learning about and using a logographic strategy that allows for immediate visual recognition of familiar words. During this time, the beginning reader learns words as independent, visual forms similar to what occurs in learning the imageable, written form of the Chinese language. Salient graphic features, such as the length of the word and/or the first and/or last letters of the word, trigger recognition. The order of the other letters is an irrelevant and incidental detail that may or may not aid the recognition schema. Thus, a child might recognize the word "STOP" only when the letters are displayed with a red hexagon background or the name "McDonald's" when it is printed with the familiar backdrop of the Golden Arches. In fact, children will usually respond with the word "McDonald's" even when a word or nonword such as "McMania" is superimposed on the arches. Likewise, as Coltheart (1986) suggested, a child might identify the logo even though the letters are presented in different sequences or style such as "McDonalds," or "McDnolads," or "McdOnaLDs."

Although confusions between words are common initially, logographic entries increase as the reader encounters more words, "and the speed with which they can be accessed increases as a result of practice, maturation, and other factors" (Manis, Szeszulski, Holt, & Graves, 1990, p. 211). Growth during this time is contingent on the child's use of the memory skills brought to the task of learning to read. Upon visual recognition of a word, the child pronounces it without tapping phonological aspects, because these are not yet important. Although the child may refuse to respond if the word is not recognized, contextual (naming pictures), and pragmatic cues (contextual cues) facilitate guessing.

Use of the logographic strategy is assumed to prevail over the initial stage of reading acquisition, thereby allowing for development of a large sight vocabulary. Gough and Juel (1991), among others, assumed that "first words are mastered through paired-associate learning" (p. 48). Through selective association, the child selects any cue from the printed word and pairs it with the spoken word. The child searches the printed word for one particular cue from the many available, including "a character, or a matching pair of characters, or even the font in which the characters appear . . . the names of some letters . . . a property of the whole word (such as) its color, or its length, or even the resemblance of the whole to some familiar object" (p. 49). The concept of selective association helps explain why a novice reader is able to recognize words such as "Nintendo," "Pokemon," and "Tyrannosaurus," yet not be able to recognize words "and," "the," or "cat."

When the child's scribbles begin to stand for words, logographic reading is said to coexist with symbolic scribbling, and "reading leads writing." Table 2-1 lists the typical reading behaviors demonstrated by the end of Chall's Stage 0.

Table 2-1. Typical Reading Behaviors Demonstrated by the End of Chall's Stage 0 (Chall, 1983).

The reader:

- pretends to read
- retells a story when looking at pages of a book previously read to him/her
- names letters of the alphabet
- recognizes some signs
- prints own name
- plays with books, pencils, and paper (p. 92)

Sometime during Stage 1, as children build logographic vocabularies, they begin using pencils and crayons to draw and scribble. They produce lines, squiggles, and curliques, and, eventually, their scribble writing can be differentiated from their scribble drawing. Bear et al. (1996) refer to this as "pretend writing/drawing" (p. 14). Temple et al. (1993) explained that "rather than learning to write by mastering first the parts (letters) and then building up to the whole (written lines), it appears that children attend first to the whole and only much later to the parts" (p. 20). Noting the similarities between infant talk and preliterate writing, Bear et al. observed that, in both, there is a movement from gestalt to parts (see earlier section of this chapter for a discussion of Locke's Phases). During preliterate writing, "children begin to write by approximating the broader contours of our writing system; they begin with the linear arrangement of print" (p. 96). Temple et al. described the earliest stage of writing as "sort of make-believe—children make designs that look like writing but are still a long way from the real thing. Like other kinds of children's play, this make-believe writing is serious business—it is experience from which children learn" (p. 53). According to Bear et al. when emergent readers pretend to write "they may scribble or write in letter-like forms with all the seriousness and vigor of a stenographer" (p. 16). Bear et al. explained that because there is a lack of sound–symbol correspondence, this stage of writing is "preliterate," the characteristics of which are listed in Table 2-2.

Table 2-2. Typical Reading Behaviors Demonstrated During the "Preliterate Stage" (Bear et al., 1996).

- at the beginning of this stage the child produces large scribbles/drawings
- the child tells a story as he/she draws a picture
- there is little order to the direction of print, circles, and up/down lines
- through observing others, children's print begins to take the form of letters, numbers and move from top to bottom and left to right on the page
- sound–symbol correspondence emerges late in this stage
- letters that look alike, for example, b/p and d/b, are confused (pp. 16–17)

Moats (1997) also noted that at this stage "only the child can read the message back," and provided the following example: HDIAZ (interpreted as "welcome home mom") p. 21.

b. Delayed development at the logographic stage.

A delay in development prior to the logographic stage would interfere with emerging symbolic skills and, consequently, with the child's recognition of printed words as symbols for concepts or objects. Arrested development here might indicate a problem in acquiring metalinguistic awareness of the referents for "sentence" or "word," because these are developed prior to the logographic phase (De Goes & Martlew, 1983). Failure to acquire the logographic strategy is suspected when words with striking visual features are not recognized more quickly than those with unremarkable features.

2. **Alphabetic stage: learning how speech is represented by an orthography.**

Chall referred to this as **Stage 1: Initial Reading and Decoding (grades 1–2; ages 6–7 years old).** Beyond needing a general fund of knowledge about their native language and an ability to discriminate graphic symbols visually, beginning readers will need to discover how to decipher or "crack" the code that exists between spoken and written language. They need to learn the "alphabetic principle"—the relationship that exists between a spoken word and its spelling—to retrieve the spoken form of print. The ability to form links between speech and print—learning how to make connections between speech units (phonemes) and the specific letters (graphemes) representing them—is the "core subskill in learning to read" (Farnham-Diggory, 1990, p. 11).

To illustrate what the "would-be reader" experiences when learning to crack the printed code, Richardson and DiBenedetto (1991) place teachers in training in the position of not knowing how to read. Then, through a series of steps, the "novice" gradually learns to decode printed material through learning about phonemic and graphemic processing. Figure 2–3 illustrates one of the exercises.

The importance of the alphabetic principle cannot be underestimated. Stanovich (1991a) stressed that the child must learn first the general principle that spelling corresponds to sound and then learn "sufficient examples of spelling-to-sound correspondences to support efficient decoding" (p. 23). Stanovich explained that to use the alphabetic principle "the child must adopt an analytic attitude toward both written words and the spoken words they represent; that is, the child must discover and exploit the fact that the mapping takes place at the level of letters and phonemes" (p. 23).

We start by teaching you something about phonemic processing. This letter, ➤, makes a long *e* sound. If we put an /s/ sound symbolized by ▲, in front of two ➤s, we get the word, ▲➤➤. Pronounce the word, stressing the sounds, ▲▲▲➤➤➤.

Now we will add two words for graphic processing: the word *I* (☆) and the word *can* (✛●■). Now we can ask a question:

✛●■ ☆ ▲➤➤?

. . . and we can answer the question.

☆ ✛●■ ▲➤➤.

Let's add a name for fun. (The name is printed in standard orthography to simplify the demonstration.)

✛●■ Susan ▲➤➤? Susan✛●■ ▲➤➤.

✛●■ ☆ ▲➤➤ Susan? ☆ ✛●■ ▲➤➤ Susan.

Now we add another word for phonemic processing. This letter, O, makes the sound /m/, so when it comes before ➤ we get O➤. Pronounce it, stressing the sounds, OOO➤➤➤. This will help you remember it.

☆ ✛●■ ▲➤➤ Susan. ✛●■ Susan ▲➤➤ O➤?
Susan ✛●■ ▲➤➤ O➤.

Now we add another sight word for graphic processing. This word, ▢◆■, says *run*. Now you can read this:

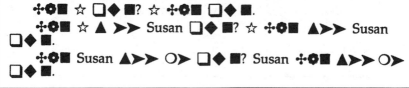

✛●■ ☆ ▢◆■? ☆ ✛●■ ▢◆■.

✛●■ ☆ ▲ ➤➤ Susan ▢◆■? ☆ ✛●■ ▲➤➤ Susan
▢◆■.

✛●■ Susan ▲➤➤ O➤ ▢◆■? Susan ✛●■ ▲➤➤ O➤
▢◆■.

Figure 2–3. Learning to Read. (Reprinted with permission from E. Richardson and B. DiBenedetto, "Acquiring the Linguistic Code for Reading" in J. K. Kavanagh, Ed., *The Language Continuum: From Infancy to Literacy*, 1991, p. 75. Timonium, MD: York Press, Inc.)

a. Normal development at the alphabetic stage.

Chall suggested that "to make the transition from Stage 0 to Stage 1, words and letters must now be recognized and matched with spoken words and sounds" (p. 41). Around 3 1/2 to 4 years of age, the child's scribbling becomes more refined, and soon the dots, lines, and loops begin to resemble letter shapes. Most children enter school with knowledge of various phonological categories and relations, and without conscious awareness, they attempt to relate these systematically to English spelling. Thus, it is through writing that children begin to learn the alphabetic principle. During this time, children engage in reading books with rhyme and predictable patterns of language. "The familiar language patterns of these materials support students as they try to make the speech–print match. They use a finger to point to words lest they get off-track and lose the speech-to-print correspondence" (Bear, et. al., 1996, p. 19).

When applying the alphabetic strategy to reading print, the child is able to use a systematic approach to analyze words into component graphemes and phonemes. Rules are generated for how phonemes map onto graphemes—sound symbol conversion or association develops into a phonological decoding mechanism. Frith (1986) emphasized the importance of a child's emerging phonemic awareness in the transition from logographic to alphabetic stage. As children become more proficient accessing their stored phonological representations of words, they begin to isolate individual phonemes within them. When first attempting to decode printed words during the alphabetic stage, the child can be heard to blend sounds together into words, as for instance, "cuh-a-tuh" reminds the child of "cat." Table 2-3 lists the typical reading behaviors demonstrated by the end of Chall's Stage 1.

Table 2–3. Typical Reading Behaviors Demonstrated by the End of Chall's Stage 1 (Chall, 1983).

Chall explained that by the end of Stage 1 the reader:

- learns relationships between letters and speech sounds and printed and spoken words
- reads simple text containing high frequency words and phonically regular words
- uses skill and insight to sound out new one-syllable words (p. 85)
- decodes/recognizes high-frequency words
- reads very simple stories
- does simple writing (p. 92)

According to Bear et al. (1996), the "beginning writing" stage occurs around 5 years of age. Like beginning reading, beginning writing is "slow and disfluent" (pp. 19-20). Children learn to write words sound-by-sound and then word-by word. As the amount of writing increases from a few words to half pages, children are able to summarize and/or retell events through writing (p. 14).

Beginning writers "invent" spelling by using the literal names of alphabet letters. Through their invented spellings, beginning spellers relay messages. For example, a 4-year-old girl was asked to write about a picture she had drawn of a person fishing. She produced, "YUTS A LADE YET GEHEG AD HE KOT FLEPR." She read this aloud as, "Once a lady went fishing and she caught Flipper" (Temple et al., 1993, p. 1). Other "spelling inventors" are not yet able to read back what they have written. For example, one of my clients, 6-year-old Jason, used a pencil to "write a note" to his mother. When asked if he would read the note, Jason responded emphatically: "Read? I can't read yet! I can only write!" A participant in one of the workshops I presented in Dallas, Texas told me about the writing of her grandson, who was diagnosed with dyslexia. He apparently wrote a paragraph and signed his name, which was the only word his grandmother could decipher. When she told her grandson this, he looked at his writing and said "Heck! I can't read it either. I must've written it in Spanish."

During this "beginning to write" stage, writing precedes reading, and practice printing eventually leads to the adoption of the alphabetic strategy for reading. Table 2-4 includes what behaviors Bear et al. (1996) considered to be characteristic of Early Letter Name stage of spelling:

Table 2-4. Characteristics Bear et al. Considered to be Characteristic of Early Letter Name Stage of Spelling

During beginning early letter name stage spelling children:

- write syllabically spelling the most salient features of syllables or words and use several letters of the alphabet
- substitute letters based on point of articulation (Y for w "when," J for dr in "drive")
- write words that lack beginnings and ends of syllables
- write words with vowels in syllables
- add some spacing between words (p. 20)

During middle early letter name stage spelling children:

- write with directionality
- use most letters of the alphabet with clear sound–letter correspondences
- continue to substitute letters based on point of articulation
- still omit vowels when writing syllables
- still write with some absence of spacing between words (p. 20)

During late early letter name stage spelling children:

- use most beginning and ending consonants
- have clear letter–sound correspondences
- continue to substitute consonants based on point of articulation
- use some vowels and may spell "bed" as BD, "when" as WN, "ship" as SP, and "drive" as JRF
- write with inconsistent use of vowels and consonant blends and digraphs (p. 20)

See Table 2-5 for many good examples presented by Moats (1997) of systematic, principled early spelling based on "awareness of what (the) mouth is doing" (p. 21).

Table 2-5. Examples of Systematic, Principled Early Spelling Based on "Awareness of What (the) Mouth Is Doing (presented by Moats, 1997)

POINTS OF ARTICULATION	EXAMPLES
	(*What student printed is in capital letters*) (*What student meant is in lower case letters*)
1. Tense (long) vowels from letter name.	DA = day; KAM = came; FEL = feel
2. Lax (short) vowels: derived from letter name closest in articulation.	a for /e/ BAD = bed e for /i/ FES = fish i for /u/ KIT = cut i for /o/ GIT = got o for /u/ SOGH = sugar
3. Preconsonantal nasals omitted.	JUP = jump; AD = and; ED = end
4. Syllabic consonants /m/ /n/ /l/ /r/.	OT = little; BIGR = bigger; OPN = open
5. Inflected endings spelled phonetically. (ed, s)	WALT = walked; DAWGZ = dogs
6. Vowel spellings show phonetic detail.	SOWN = soon; GOWT = goat; BOE = boy
7. Affrication (roof of mouth) of tr & dr.	CHRA = tray; CHRIBLS = troubles; JRAGN = dragon
8. Intervocalic flaps shown as D.	LADR = letter; WODR = water
9. Letter names Y for /w/ and H for /ch/. (pp. 21–22).	YOH = watch; YL = will; HRH = church

b. Delayed development at the alphabetic stage.

Successful movement to the alphabetic stage (Chall's Stage 1) is contingent upon the reader's accommodation to focusing attention on the words as written and on the letters within the words (Chall, 1983). Although reading skills may continue to increase gradually through overapplication of the logographic strategy, the novice reader, who continues to focus attention on pictures cues and memory, will have difficulty moving into the alphabetic stage. Frith (1985) explained that a child's difficulty in grasping and applying the alphabetic principle will become obvious when he or she attempts to print, sound out, or blend sounds when reading (decoding) unfamiliar words. Overreliance on the logographic principle will inhibit acquisition of fluent, flexible phonic recoding. Frith proposed that this reader, who will present with poor phonological and spelling-to-sound decoding skills, will have classic developmental dyslexia.

Gough and Juel (1991) hypothesized that difficulty at the alphabetic stage indicates the child is continuing to read by selective association and relies much more on word familiarity than the reader who has knowledge of the alphabetic principle. When the child, who relies on selective association makes a reading error, "it is a failure of association; either he selects the wrong cue, or he finds no cue at all. In the former case, he will produce the wrong word; in the latter case, he must guess. In either case his error must be a word" (p. 53). The child who has moved successfully into the alphabetic phase can recognize words by using the alphabetic principle, and reading errors result from misapplication of the principle. "This may result in a word error, for example, in misreading 'fate' as 'fat.' But, it can just as well result in a nonword, for example, misreading 'keep' as 'kep'" (p. 53).

3.   **Orthographic stage: learning about bigger units of print.**

It is possible that a beginning reader may initiate the process of learning to read without knowledge of the alphabetic principle. However, according to Perfetti (1991a), "the kind of reading that allows the reader to read new words—to turn reading into a productive process rather than a memorization process—requires knowledge of the alphabetic principle" (p. 215). Through what Perfetti (1991b) described as the Restricted-Interactive Model, skilled word identification is context-free and involves interactions only between multiple sources of linguistic information combined in parallel, including "letter features, letters, phonemes, and word level units . . . connected in mutual activation networks . . . (and allowing for) no influences from outside lexical data structures, no importation of knowledge, expectancies, . . . (or) beliefs" (p. 34). In a sample sentence, "John had nothing to write with so he asked the teacher for a pencil," Perfetti explained that connections between the reader's representation of the letters p-e-n-c-i-l and his representation of the word "pencil," including its pronunciation, are mutually activated . . . immediately upon encountering the printed letters. Thus, the letters pen___ activate the phonemes /p/ /e/ /n/ and the word pencil. Moreover, activation of the phonemes increase activation of the word and activation of the word increases activation of the phonemes. It is these connections among letters and words and phonemes that are the interactive part of reading (p. 34).

a. Normal development at the orthographic stage.

If the reader has been successful in moving through the logographic and alphabetic stages, instant recognition skills merge with analytic sequential skills to facilitate movement into the orthographic stage. The orthographic strategy, which appears in reading before it does in writing, allows for instant recognition of morphemes or word parts, including common prefixes, suffixes, or common intraword syllables. The orthographic strategy does not employ visual recognition, as does the logographic strategy, nor does it convert individual graphemes to phonemes, as does the alphabetic strategy. Thus, the instant recognition and fragmented analytic skills predominant during earlier stages now merge into the nonvisual and nonphonologic orthographic strategy which operates on bigger units. During this stage, attention turns to syllabic or morphemic elements within whole words. These may be phonically irregular units (e.g., "tion" as in "position") that will become recognized as whole units embedded within larger units. Others may be frequently appearing phonically regular units, and lead to efficiently synthesized phonemic elements, for example, "dis" as in "discouraged" or "be" as in "believe" (Sawyer, 1992).

During the orthographic stage, "children relinquish exclusive adherence to a linear phonetic approach in favor of letter patterns . . . (which) function as units in symbolizing sounds or word parts even though elements of the pattern are not phonetic letter by letter (e.g., -ED to symbolize /t/ as in 'stopped')" (Ehri, 1992, p. 327). See Table 2-6 for what a child faces when learning to read and moving beyond the letter–name phase of invented spelling [Temple et al. (1993)].

Table 2-6. What a Child Faces When Learning to Read Moving Beyond the Letter–Name Phase of Invented Spelling (Temple et al., 1993).

Now the task becomes one of recognizing several aspects:

- the spellings of consonant digraphs

- patterns that mark vowels as long or short, and mark some consonants as hard or soft

- that certain grammatical endings (-ed, -s, -ing) have to be spelled certain ways, though they may be pronounced variously

- there are often several likely ways to spell a given sound pattern (cream, creem, creme) but one correct way in each word

- there are some spellings that don't work the way we expect them to, because of pronunciation variations, or phonological rules

- there are other spellings that don't behave the way we expect them to because of choices made centuries ago by the first writers of modern English (we call these scribal traditions) (p. 82)

Use of the orthographic strategy allows the reader to move into **Chall's Stage 2: Confirmation, Fluency, Ungluing from Print (grades 2–3; ages 7–8 years old)**. If the reader successfully learned to decode print, reading during this stage is primarily for the reader to focus on matching what is printed to his or her knowledge and language. The purpose of reading during Stage 2, then, is to allow the reader to confirm what he/she already knows as opposed to gaining new information. See Table 2-7 for the typical reading behaviors demonstrated by the end of Chall's Stage 2.

Table 2-7. Typical Reading Behaviors Demonstrated by the End of Chall's Stage 2 (Chall, 1983).

- reads simple, familiar stories and selections with increasing fluency

- consolidates basic decoding elements, sight vocabulary, and meaning context in the reading of familiar stories and selections (p. 86)

- uses decoding and intelligent guessing to figure out new words

- pays more attention to meaning of what is read

- writes more (p. 93)

Bear et al. (1996) described a *Middle-late letter name spelling stage* in which readers can read many texts including simple chapter books. See Table 2-8 for behaviors children typically demonstrate during this stage.

Table 2-8. Typical Behaviors Demonstrated During the Middle-Late Letter Name Spelling Stage (Bear et al., 1996).

Children usually:

- begin to see differences between consonants and vowels
- realize that each syllable must contain a vowel
- grow in correct use of short vowels
- use a phonetic spelling strategy and rely less on visual patterns of letters
- begin to understand a closed syllable concept, (a syllable containing a consonant-vowel-consonant)
- learn to correctly spell words containing preconsonantal nasal sounds (/m/ and /n/)

This is one of the hallmark traits indicating the child is moving from this spelling stage to the next (pp. 21–22).

b. Delayed development at the orthographic stage.

Problems that arise during transition from the alphabetic to the orthographic strategy result from overreliance on the alphabetic principle. Automaticity, key to successful decoding and reading comprehension, is therefore not achieved, and the reader remains glued to print. (See Chapter 3 for a discussion of automaticity and reading).   Because logographic skills remain intact, the reader relies on phoneme–grapheme rules, disregards intraword structures, and tends to regularize the spelling of irregularly spelled words, for example, spelling "cough" as "coff." The reader applies the alphabetic strategy to spell regular words correctly and experiences difficulty reading irregular words. The reader who is delayed in moving from Chall's stage 1 to stages 2 to 3 is penalized again because he/she will be falling behind classmates in cognitive development (Chall, 1983, p. 30). Furthermore, many children with normal vocabulary develop vocabulary deficits as the result of their reading problems because as they fall behind in reading they are not able to read more sophisticated material (Chall, 1983; Wolf & Obregon, 1992).

While little new information about the world is learned during Chall's Stage 2, the purpose of reading during **Chall's Stage 3: Reading to Learn: A First Step (grades 4–8; ages 9–13 years)** is to learn new information and to locate information in reading material. Word meanings and prior knowledge become increasingly important during Stage 3 as the reader moves beyond reading for egocentric purposes to reading for conventional world knowledge. By the end of Stage 3 the reader can read adult length materials "but falling somewhat short of the reading difficulty of most adult popular literature" (Chall, 1983, p. 22). Stage 3 reading means "learning how to learn from reading, but essentially from only one point of view . . . essentially for facts, for concepts, for how to do things" (p. 22). See Table 2-9 for typical reading behaviors demonstrated by the end of Chall's Stage 3.

Table 2-9. Typical Reading Behaviors Demonstrated by the End of Chall's Stage 3 (Chall, 1983).

By the end of Stage 3, the reader:

• reads to learn new ideas, gains new knowledge, experiences new feelings, learns new attitudes usually from one viewpoint (p. 86)

• is using materials that now include readers, textbooks, reference works, trade books

• comprehends increasingly complex printed materials (p. 93)

Chall explained that during Stage 3 the reader must engage in "reflectiveness and the ability to accumulate facts and other details . . . (and) the reader has to know . . . when he does not know" (p. 48). If the reader uses the Stage 2 strategy of fluently reading without Stage 3 reflectiveness, recall of specific information will be poor. "The attitude toward the easy familiar stories of Stage 2, when carried over to Stage 3, may produce a rate that is too fast for the more demanding Stage 3 reading" (p. 49).

Bear et al. (1996) described this stage, lasting between 6 to 12 years, as "transitional," wherein learners approach fluency in their reading and writing. Readers "move away from a literal application of the alphabetic principle and begin to chunk elements of written language structures: Their reading changes from word-by-word to phrasal reading fluency" (p. 23). Similarly, writing becomes more fluent as "transitional readers move away from the literal application of letter names to include pattern–letter sequences which relate to sound and meaning . . . knowledge of within word patterns affords greater efficiency and speed in reading, writing, and spelling" (p. 23). See Table 2-10 for what characteristics Bear et al. included during this "Within Word Pattern" spelling stage.

Table 2-10. Characteristics Included During the "Within Word Pattern" Spelling Stage (Bear et al., 1996).

- examine vowels within syllables and patterns within words
- correctly spell most single-syllable short vowel words
- spell consonant blends and digraphs correctly
- experiment with long vowels and learn new vowel spelling patterns, for example, consonant-vowel-consonant-silent e ("name"), and consonant-vowel-vowel pattern ("hay"), or consonant-vowel-vowel-consonant patterns ("nail")
- learn that spelling patterns do not necessarily sound the same (p. 24)

Chall's Stage 4: Multiple Viewpoints (grades: high school; ages 14–18 years)

Because the reader acquired basic knowledge during Stage 3, he/she is now ready to read materials with detailed factual information, theoretical information, and multiple viewpoints. Rather than recognizing individual ideas, the successful Stage 4 reader will need to employ a strategy of recognizing patterns between differing viewpoints. Reading now becomes more global and the amount of material to be read increases significantly. See Table 2-11 for typical reading behaviors demonstrated by the end of Chall's Stage 4.

Table 2-11. Typical Reading Behaviors Demonstrated by the End of Chall's Stage 4 (Chall, 1983).

By the end of Stage 4 the reader:

- reads widely from a broad range of complex expository and narrative materials presenting a variety of viewpoints (p. 87)

- reads greater quantities (p. 94)

If the reader continues to use the Stage 3 precise detail strategy, "reading is too slow and careful, making it difficult to absorb and integrate the different viewpoints" (p. 50). The overapplication of the Stage 3 strategy becomes apparent in readers who labor over every new term and definition and who practically recopy their text when taking notes on what they read.

In their study of spelling stages, Bear et al. (1996) included an Intermediate and Specialized writing stage beginning around 10 years of age. During this time the student is acquiring a greater repertoire of reading and writing styles. Writing is more fluent as the developing writer builds expression and voice, gains experience with various writing styles and across varied genres (p. 14). Writing now reflects "personal problem solving and personal reflection" (p. 14). The spelling stages now include Syllable Juncture and Derivational Constancy stages. During Syllable Juncture stage the writer "learns how syllables fit together and studies external/inflectional junctures, prefixes and suffixes" (p. 14). Finally, during the Derivational Constancy spelling stage, the writer "studies derived forms in bases and roots, and studies the internal morphology in syllables" (p. 14).

Chall's Stage 5: Construction and Reconstruction—A World View (grades: college; ages 18 years and above) involves using acquired knowledge to decide what will be read, to understand what is read, and to construct knowlege about the information. The reader at this stage is able to utilize a faster reading rate when reading familiar subject matter and a slower rate with unfamiliar material. Using processes of analysis, synthesis, and judgment, the Stage 5 reader "has the ability to construct knowledge on a high level of abstraction and generality and to create one's own 'truth' from the 'truths' of others"

(Chall, 1983, p. 24). See Table 2-12 for typical reading behaviors demonstrated by the end of Chall's Stage 5.

Table 2-12. Typical Reading Behaviors Demonstrated by the End of Chall's Stage 5 (Chall, 1983).

By the end of Stage 5, Chall believed the reader:

* reads for one's professional and personal purposes

* reads to integrate one's knowledge with that of others

* creates new knowledge as the result of synthesizing what is read

* reads at a rapid, efficient rate (p. 87)

* reads a great variety of difficult materials, analytically, critically, and creatively (p. 94)

Because Stage 5 involves synthesis, reorganization of knowledge, and critical reaction to information presented, transitioning to it from Stage 4 is the most difficult. According to Chall, the Stage 5 reader needs a great deal of knowledge, confidence, humility, and a feeling of entitlement. "One needs to believe that one is entitled to the knowledge that exists, to think about it, use it, and to 'make knowledge' as did those whose works they read" (p. 51). The reader who relies more on the "pattern recognition" Stage 4 strategy without analyzing, synthesizing, and integrating information will be less likely to construct new knowledge. Chall concluded that at Stage 5 the reader reads and writes less but thinks and agonizes more. "In this process, many different ideas and views are fused into one's own" (p. 52).

IV. SUMMARY

The dynamic and reciprocal interaction between oral and written language acquisition has been described with an emphasis on the transition from one to the other. Written language does not suddenly begin to develop at the conclusion of oral language acquisition. Rather, written language emerges out of oral language. An interesting similarity exists among three aspects covered in this chapter; namely, Locke's neurolinguistic model of psycholinguistic development, Frith's and Chall's stages of reading development, Bear's et al. stages of spelling development, and the developmental nature of phonological awareness. In all these, the developmental transition is from gestalt to part.

According to Locke's theory, the movement toward an efficient linguistic processing-producing system is from holophrases, to parsing into discrete units, to acquiring many words. In Frith's and Chall's stages we saw how the novice reader moves from recognizing logos to learning how the alphabetic principle works, to reading to learn. In the development of writing and spelling, the trend is from whole drawings, to lines and dots, to letters and numbers. Likewise, in the development of phonological awareness abilities, children move from being able to segment the speech stream into words, then syllables, and finally phonemes. It would seem that the phoneme remains elusive to young children for some time during their development. Perhaps, as Locke explained, the phases of neurolinguistic development are time-fixed and sequential, might it not be possible that very early in the course of traversing the oral–written language continuum, many young children get left behind? These children go on to reveal language problems for years, and for some, throughout their lives.

We add to this van Kleeck's notion of metalinguistic development. Accordingly, up to approximately 6 years of age, children's thought is characterized by centration (only able to concentrate on one aspect at a time), and irreversibility (not able to shift back and forth easily between aspects of a situation). If a child's thought is still in centration mode, then this child can only focus on one or another aspect of reading, either form or meaning. To extend, if this child can only focus on word meaning, as is typical of young children, then word form, (syllables, and phonemes) cannot also be considered. If this child is sitting in a regular education classroom at six years of age, he/she is expected to focus on *meaning and form*. The educational demands placed on young children, who may still be at the earlier stage of metalinguistic development, may be too much for them to successfully develop the basics of print literacy, the ability to focus simultaneously on word meaning and word form.

The students discussed in this book struggle to get over one hurdle, "come up for air for awhile," then face more challenges as the curriculum demands change over time. I frequently explain to them and to their parents, that in the beginning, a language based problem feels like a small stone in their shoe. In the beginning the "stone" may be hardly noticeable, but continuing to walk without fixing the problem, the pain caused by the "stone" increases. The symptomatology these students present varies depending on a multitude of contributing factors. Children who move from oral to written language problems demonstrate varying degrees of semantic, syntactic, pragmatic, and phonological problems. One primary focus of this book is how the phonological code is the base to a successfully developing linguistic system. The "stone" for many language-impaired children has to do with creating and maintaining phonological representations. A second focus of this book is the role of naming speed processes in developmental reading disabilities. Wolf and Segal (1999) explained that "an extensive body of research in English and other languages now indicates that reading-impaired children differ significantly in naming speed for basic symbols from average readers and other learning-disabled children" (p. 2).

From this discussion of the developing language continuum, with its emphasis on the evolution of oral-to-written language problems, we now move to a discussion of developmental reading disabilities in which the relationship among phonological processing, visual naming speed, and reading are emphasized.

VI. CLINICAL COMPETENCIES.

To understand the oral–written language continuum, the teacher/clinician/student will demonstrate the following competencies:

A. Understand the development of oral language strands.

B. Utilize Adams' model of reading acquisition.

C. Understand Frith's, Chall's, and Bear's et al. stages of reading, writing, and spelling development.

D. Understand the dynamic and reciprocal interaction between oral and written language acquisition.

CHAPTER

3

Developmental Reading Disabilities

OUTLINE

I. COMMON COMPLAINTS

A weakness in any of the language strands described in Chapter 2, including the ability to think about and analyze language units, may appear later as a reading disorder (Dickinson & McCabe, 1991). The consequences of early oral language problems initially affect learning how to decode and, gradually, can spread across written language abilities. In time, virtually all curriculum areas become contaminated. Like a domino effect, the student experiences failure in subject after subject. Identifying early, oral language problems that may evolve into later written language problems is, therefore, critical. As the gap widens between a student's expected and actual performances, frustrations escalate.

Teachers complain: "students just can't seem to remember from day to day." Parents report that there aren't enough hours in the day to help with the student's homework and complain that their child "just doesn't seem to *get it*." No one feels the frustration more than the students themselves. Here are a few observations my students have provided.

Matt, a second grade Communicatively Handicapped Special Day Class student with specific reading disability, announced. "I just can't know what sound that letter makes."

Jeni, a regular education third grade student with specific reading disability, asked: "Why can't they just spell everything the way it sounds?"

Brad, a regular education sixth grade student with specific reading disability, lamented: "My mouth wasn't doing what my brain was telling it."

Denis, a regular education third grade student with specific reading disability, explained: "You see, I have all this information in different files in my head. Sometimes the files fall on the floor and that stuff gets all mixed up!"

Lisa, a regular education second grade student with specific reading disability, said: "It's not easy for me to remember the sounds the letters make, and then I can't put them into words."

When his sisters received more money for their good grades than he did, Robert, a fourth grade regular education student with generalized reading problems, broke into tears and asked his mother: "Why did God make my brain work the way it does?"

Scott, a regular education third grade student with specific reading disability, recalled: "I was reading just fine in the first grade, but when I got to second grade my brain just went blank."

Jose, a regular education second grade student with specific reading disability, explained: "I see the letters. I just can't hear the sounds they make."

Tyghe, an eighth grade regular education student with specific reading disability, explained "It's not that I see the letters 'b' and 'd' backwards. I just can't keep their sounds in my brain long enough to remember, so I flip them and they come back out wrong when I try saying them in the word I'm reading."

Much like Tyghe, Christopher Lee (Lee & Jackson, 1992), as an adult with lifelong reading–writing problems, wrote about his experiences "faking it" through the system.

> I am trying to write because language itself is an obstacle for me. When I am trying to spell a word, it's as if there are 26 letters spinning around in my head, each letter having its own box. The boxes contain sounds. The letters are trying to find their boxes by finding their sounds. I don't really see them but I feel like they're up there looking for a place to settle. (p. 22)

Similarly, another adult, James Evans (1983), wrote about his life as an individual with hyperactivity and dyslexia, and recalled sessions with his professional tutor.

> It was reading I feared most, and she knew it. It was her habit to concentrate on the basics, to review and review again. We would select a paragraph in a reader for students far ahead of my reading ability and wade laboriously through it. Mrs. Blake would direct me to take one word at a time, and she would correct my pronunciation as I labored. It exhausted me to attempt even one of these monsters. Each time I finished I knew what to expect: "Now, James, let us concentrate on seeing the letters"—and with a terse nod of her head would say the inevitable word: "Again!" (p. 44)

II. THREE SUBTYPES OF DEVELOPMENTAL READING DISABILITY

A vast body of literature exists on the classification of developmental reading disabilities. While some practitioners believe that subtyping various groups of poor readers is futile, others are convinced that subtypes of reading problems exist, and to accurately teach/intervene, we must carefully define and delimit the problem. Knowing that a student fits a particular subtype of reading problem helps the teacher/practitioner to consider all aspects of that subtype. Fletcher et al. (1997) explained that to "set off reading failure as an entity, disorder, diagnosis, or any partition of individuals who read poorly from those who read less poorly, a classification hypothesis has been developed" (p. 97). Although classification is not synonymous with identification, it "leads to a set of criteria that permit the identification of individuals into the subsets of the classification" (Fletcher et al., 1997, p. 98). For purposes of this book, three subtypes of developmental reading problems are examined: developmental dyslexia, generalized reading problem, and hyperlexia. Following the description of these subtypes, a conceptualization of developmental reading disabilities that focuses on the underlying core deficits, phonological processes, and visual naming speed will be presented. The reader is referred back to the discussion of Adams' model of reading processors in Chapter 2.

A. Developmental Dyslexia (a.k.a. specific reading disability).

The word "dyslexia" appeared in the literature sometime in the 1800s. Over the years, it has been defined so differently that the second edition of *Webster's Unabridged Dictionary* omitted the word altogether (Cruickshank, 1986). Confusion about what should and should not be included in the symptom complex has led many practitioners to suggest the term "dyslexia" is so ambiguous it does not exist. Others have gone to the opposite extreme. One reading authority, according to Cruickshank (1986), proposed that "children with any form of reading impairment are known as dyslexic" (p. xiii). Cruickshank cautioned that whether dyslexia is mild, moderate, or severe, it is one of the most complex, central nervous system problems that exists and demands thoughtful, interdisciplinary, diagnostic efforts. Without a proper diagnosis, dyslexia can present "insurmountable hurdles to successful life adjustment of the individual" (p. xiv).

Developmental dyslexia, or specific reading disability, as it is alternatively called, is a syndrome of characteristics, none of which would be considered symptomatic of dyslexia if it appeared in isolation. As early as 1937, Samuel T. Orton suggested the common denominator for dyslexic symptoms was difficulty repicturing or rebuilding sequences of letters, sounds, or units of movement in their order of presentation (Sawyer, 1992). Orton observed that the chief difficulty for children with dyslexia seemed to be "forming dependable, retrievable associations between sound patterns, which constitute the spoken word, and symbol patterns which represent the printed word" (Orton, 1968, p. 131).

The first description of developmental dyslexia in English was presented by Morgan (1896). He described a bright, intelligent, 14-year-old boy whose schoolmaster thought he would be the smartest boy in the school if all instruction could be presented orally. Hinshelwood

(1917) described similar students and noted three criteria that distinguished their reading disability from other learning problems: the disability affected the students' ability to handle the printed form of language without concomitant oral language or general cognitive deficits; usual instruction in reading did not ameliorate the problem; and the severity of the reading disability.

Developmental dyslexia is a lifelong language-based problem. The specificity of dyslexia has to do with a basic problem in how the brain encodes phonological features of speech. Snowling (2000), among many, believed the "core deficit is in phonological processing and stems from poorly specified phonological representations" (p. 214). The fundamental oral language problem, that is, the problem with the phonological code, does not cause a reading problem. Rather, early oral language problems involving the phonologic code *evolve into* later reading problems. "It is important to recognize that the impairment in dyslexia does not affect reading directly but affects the development of the spoken language substrate that is critical for learning to read" (Snowling, 2000, p. 214). Stanovich (1988) explained that the very nature of a specific reading disability rests on the assumption of specificity. Underlying the observable symptomatology is a brain/cognitive deficit that is restricted to the task of reading. Extension of deficits displayed by the disabled reader into other domains of cognitive functioning "would depress the constellation of abilities we call intelligence, reduce the reading/intelligence discrepancy, and the child would no longer be dyslexic!" (p. 155). Central processes, including general linguistic awareness, comprehension, strategic functioning, rule learning, active/inactive learning, and generalized metacognitive functioning are critically enmeshed with other aspects of intellectual functioning. Stanovich maintained that these processes are too global—nonspecific—and therefore the wrong place to look for the key to specific reading disability.

The following definition of dyslexia was adopted by the The Orton Dyslexia Society (now known as The International Dyslexia Association) Research Committee and the National Institutes of Health (1994):

> Dyslexia is one of several distinct learning disabilities. It is a specific language-based disorder of constitutional origin characterized by difficulties in single word decoding, usually reflecting insufficient phonological processing abilities. These difficulties in single word decoding are often unexpected in relation to age and other cognitive and academic abilities; they are not the result of generalized developmental disability or sensory impairment. Dyslexia is manifested by

variable difficulty with different forms of language, often including, in addition to problems reading, a conspicuous problem with acquiring proficiency in writing and spelling (p. 4).

In his interpretation of this definition, Lyon (1995b) explained that dyslexia is a disorder of language; is *not synonymous* with the general term *learning disabilities*; frequently co-occurs with other cognitive and academic problems; involves an impairment in phonological processing ability; aggregates in families, is heritable, and probably reflects autosomal dominant transmission; involves difficulty at single-word decoding and reading having a negative effect on reading comprehension (pp. 10–14).

Aaron and Joshi (1992) offered the following set of guidelines for parents: Developmental dyslexia refers to a condition in which an individual encounters a great deal of difficulty assigning proper sounds to the written or printed word; the dyslexic reader is not able to decode the written word easily; when encountering an unfamiliar word, the dyslexic reader must invest a great deal of effort in deciphering that word. This reader therefore forgets the part of the sentence already read. As a result, comprehension is also affected. Poor reading comprehension is, therefore, secondary to poor decoding ability. A child who fails to comprehend well both written and spoken language is not dyslexic. Dyslexic children can, invariably, comprehend the text much better than their oral reading would indicate. In fact, their listening comprehension for ordinary spoken language is almost always normal (p. 246).

Snowling (2000) hypothesized that we would expect a child's understanding of what is heard to be similar to understanding what is read. Stated differently, one's listening comprehension should be roughly equivalent to one's reading comprehension. "When reading comprehension falls short of listening skill it is reasonable to hypothesize that the child has a specific reading difficulty" (p. 25).

Denckla (1993) recognized the cognitive test battery results of dyslexia-pure, a.k.a. specific reading disability; patients reveal deficiencies in the linguistic domain, especially in the subdomain of phonology. "While semantic, syntactic, and pragmatic subdomains are relatively intact, impaired phonological awareness, analysis (segmentation), and memory are demonstrable" (p. 24).

See Table 3-1 for characteristics that frequently accompany dyslexia as reported by the International Dyslexia Association (2000).

Table 3-1. Characteristics That Frequently Accompany Dyslexia (as reported by the International Dyslexia Association, 2000).

- Lack of awareness of sounds in words, sound order, rhymes, or sequence of syllables
- Difficulty decoding words—single word identification
- Difficulty encoding words—spelling
- Poor sequencing of numbers, of letters in words, when read or written (e.g., b-d; sing-sign; left-felt; soiled-solid; 12-21)
- Problems with reading comprehension
- Difficulty expressing thoughts in written form
- Delayed spoken language
- Imprecise or incomplete interpretation of language that is heard
- Difficulty in expressing thoughts orally
- Confusion about directions in space or time (right and left, up and down, early and late, yesterday and tomorrow, months and days)
- Confusion about right or left handedness
- Similar problems among relatives
- Difficulty with handwriting
- Difficulty in mathematics—often related to sequencing of steps or directionality or the language of mathematics (pp. 1-2)

Moats (1997) summarized the symptoms associated with developmental dyslexia by grade level:

Grades K-2: trouble rhyming; doesn't know letter names and sounds or learn phonics easily; inconsistent memory for words; trouble remembering lists (days, months); mispronounces words; distracted by background noise; trouble retrieving color or object names; can't spell phonetically; demonstrates frustration and avoidance.

Grades 3-4: struggles with phonic decoding; inconsistent word recognition; poor spelling; overreliance on contextual cues and guessing; trouble learning new vocabulary; has symbolic confusion.

Grades 5-6: poor spelling continues; poor punctuation and capitalization; trouble learning cursive; overreliant on context to read; decodes poorly; usually hates to write and avoids reading.

Grades 9+: writing is poorer than reading comprehension; poor spelling and mechanics; difficulty learning a foreign language; slow, minimal or disorganized writing (pp. 106–107).

Frequently, children with dyslexia present with only subtle early language problems that remain undetected until they are faced with the task of learning to read. Denckla (1993) noted that developmental dyslexia is not typically diagnosed in "the context of a persistent concurrent language disorder" (p. 23). According to Denckla, students with discrepancy-based reading disability and students with "dyslexia-pure" symptoms fulfill the requirement that their dyslexia is specific, that is, does not occur in the context of globally/diffusely poor mental capacity. They have no emotional (psychiatric) diagnoses, no environmental disadvantages, and no educational deprivation. They have no past or present spoken language impairments noticeable to any but the professional specialist . . . having "met their milestones" for understanding and expressing language through speech. They are reasonably good athletes, often mechanically adept, quite often gifted in musical or graphic arts. They are socially well-adapted with good interpersonal perceptiveness and tact. These dyslexia-pure patients are, indeed, "unexpected reading failures" (p. 23).

Donahue (1986) explained that the subtle, oral language problems in these children are usually noticed only "on structured comprehension measures that provide few contextual cues or on tasks requiring rapid word retrieval or the use of complex sentence structures" (p. 284). With the increased verbal demands in school content areas, "the gap in academic achievement between these students and their nondisabled classmates widens rapidly" (p. 284). For this group, reading and writing problems are the first indication of a language problem. Stackhouse and Wells (1991) proposed that these children, who have intelligible speech and have never been evaluated by a speech and language specialist, are most "at risk" for remaining undetected. When these children experience difficulty with reading, they typically are referred for tutorial assistance which is often provided by resource specialists. Unfortunately, comprehensive speech and language evaluation is seldom recommended. Representative of this group is Stackhouse and Wells' (1991) presentation of 11-year, 8-month-old Richard, who had never been referred for speech and language services although his parents complained about his "unclear speech." Only when Richard showed at least a 3-year delay in literacy skills, and a wide range of problems in creative writing skills, was a comprehensive analysis of his speech and language undertaken. Although he demonstrated intelligible verbal output, age-appropriate receptive vocabulary, verbal comprehension, and use of syntax in spoken language, Richard experienced difficulty on expressive naming tests and, apparently, lacked confidence in verbal situations. Denckla (1993) wrote that specific testing unmasks the "tin ear for language" (a colloquial synonym for phonological deficit) . . . observation by a trained professional may reveal stigmata of the "tin ear for language" in the young preschooler who is "protodyslexic," but the average parent, teacher, or pediatrician may not make note of the speech–sound substitutions and missequencings of these children. Even when, after referral for their unexpectedly poor acquisition of reading skills, such children are observed to make speech–sound errors in their conversational or narrative speech, most people in their lives continue to regard them as "highly verbal" and successful communicators. Their mixing up of words ("mord-wixing") and/or malapropisms, if noted, are considered amusing but of trivial communicative consequence (p. 24).

B. Generalized Reading Problems

Generalized reading problems are referred to by several investigators as "garden variety" reading problems. This group represents the largest number of students described by labels such as "language learning-disabled (LLD)" and "slow learners." Their reading performance is generally in line with their mental ability and their reading difficulty is one manifestation of their overall poor cognitive ability (Aaron & Joshi, 1992, pp. 85–86). Most learning disabilities involve difficulty learning to read, write, and spell, although not all are language based. Factors other than language, including sensory impairment, mental retardation, social and emotional disturbance, cultural difference, insufficient or inappropriate instruction, or psychogenic factors may play causal roles in learning disabilities (Kavanagh & Truss, 1988, p. 551). While the specificity of a core weakness in encoding the phonological code defines the nature of developmental dyslexia, the scope of the language problems encountered in LLD can include any and all of the language domains discussed in Chapter 2. The core problems in learning to read for a dyslexic is in the brain's ability to form stable phonological representations to pair with the visually printed word and/or naming speed. Because decoding and/or naming speed is slow, comprehension is negatively affected. Students with LLD, on the other hand, have difficulty reading and "even when they read often fail to process and comprehend the information because of their poor mastery of semantic, syntactic, and pragmatic aspects of language" (Norris, 1991, p. 71). These students experience problems in word recognition with underlying phonological processing difficulties similar to dyslexic children (Catts & Kamhi, 2000, p. 76). However, unlike the normal listening comprehension typical of developmental dyslexic children, students with LLD present with lower listening comprehension.

The more global, pervasive nature of language problems across phonology, semantics, syntax, and/or pragmatics found in LLD results in more widespread language problems. According to Donahue (1986) many children diagnosed with LD include those who were referred for delayed speech and language development during preschool or kindergarten. Noting that this group "manifests the most severe and most general pattern of language delay within the LD population" (p. 284), Donahue described the oral language of this group as "characterized by obvious grammatical errors, simple sentence structure, and overt difficulties in expressing ideas and intentions" (p. 284). These children were enrolled in speech/language therapy and frequently discharged from these programs because they demonstrated increased receptive and expressive language skills.

Scarborough and Dobrich (1990) proposed a phenomenon that occurs in language impaired children wherein a temporary convergence of growth in language functions between the ages of 3 and 6 years appears as "recovery" from early preschool language problems. However, this may be an "illusory phenomenon" (p. 81), because it is not uncommon for some of these children to be referred back to the speech–language specialist at 7 to 8 years of age. Stackhouse and Wells (1991) speculated "the reading and spelling difficulties may well be the earlier speech problems in a different guise" (p. 187).

Paul (2001) summarized research on the language problems of LLD students based upon phonological, syntactic, semantic, and pragmatic characteristics.

1. **Phonological Characteristics:**

    About 25% of children with LLD have delayed speech development at school age, while most are intelligible. They often have difficulty with complex phonological production, that is, producing phonologically complex, multisyllabic words (aluminum) or phrases. Children with slow language development during preschool period may be at risk for LLD. They tend to have difficulty with short-term memory problems involving verbal material; difficulty rapidly naming automatized sequences such as days of the week; difficulty repeating nonwords and may have word retrieval problems (p. 389).

2. **Syntactic Characteristics:**

    LLD students may experience difficulty comprehending complex syntax particularly those with relative clauses, passive voice, or negation. Whereas normally developing children move to full comprehension of complex syntax by 7 to 8 years, LLD children continue to rely on comprehension strategies for passive sentences and those with relative and adverbial clauses. LLD students rely on word order or on when events usually happen rather than on how the word order is presented by the speaker. They have a tendency to produce "simple" or "immature" sentences with fewer complex sentences, using fewer multiple modifiers, prepositional phrases, relative clauses, and verb phrases.

    Their sentences seem longer because they do not condense through use of complex forms. They may experience difficulty with morphological markers including plurals, possessives and third-person singular, comparatives and superlatives, irregular forms, and advanced prefixes and suffixes (p. 390).

3. **Semantic Characteristics:**

    Students with LLD tend to have smaller vocabularies, restricted to high-frequency, short words. Their vocabulary problems result, in part, from reading problems. They have restricted word meanings, and poor associations among words and categorization of words into semantic classes. They typically have problems with multiple-meaning words and may rely on nonspecific terms (thing, stuff). They have difficulty with relational and abstract words; may have word-retrieval problems with many instances of substitution and circumlocution in their spontaneous speech. They may also have difficulty understanding complex oral directions, difficulty understanding and using figurative language, and problems integrating meaning across sentences (pp. 390–391).

4. **Pragmatic Characteristics:**

    LLD students typically present with limited verbal output and fluency and their speech can be characterized by dysfluencies caused by many false starts. Their verbal output tends to be less polite, persuasive, assertive, clear and complete, and is less sensitive to listeners' needs. They frequently give incomplete or inaccurate descriptions and they experience difficulty clarifying miscommunications and requesting clarification. They are likely to ignore communicative bids of others, and have poor topic maintenance. "Conversational pragmatics may be the area of the most significant deficits in the oral language of students with LLD" (p. 391).

C. Hyperlexia

Hyperlexia is a reading disability found primarily in a small set of language-impaired children who present with adequate decoding skills but poor reading comprehension. Sparks and Artzer (2000) noted that children with hyperlexia "read words spontaneously before the age of five, have impaired comprehension on both listening and reading tasks, and have word recognition skill above expectations based on cognitive and linguistic abilities" (p. 189). Aram (1997) reported that most case studies of children with hyperlexia describe "early and unusual visual recognition and recall skills, reporting unusual memories for routes traveled, product labels, program listings, and so forth" (p. 7). The majority of children with hyperlexia "demonstrate word recognition, with a striking uniformity, between 2 1/2 and 3 1/2 years of age" (p. 6). The mother of one of my hyperlexic clients, Nicco, recalled a phenomenon that occurred repeatedly when Nicco was 6 months old. When his mother carried Nicco around the house and passed a hanging picture with print on it, he tugged on her neck, looking at that picture more than the others, seemingly attempting to get her to return it. She commented that "it was as if he 'gravitated' toward print."

Aram (1997) included the following language problems that have been found in children with hyperlexia. Their difficulty understanding connected language impairs aural and written comprehension essentially the same. Their histories usually reflect late development of single words, marked delays in using word combinations, disordered expressive syntax and use of semantic information, echolalia, restricted initiation of spontaneous language, and limited interpersonal communication. They demonstrate printed word recognition prior to or coincident with talking (pp. 4–5).

The American Hyperlexia Association (AHA) described hyperlexia as a syndrome observed in children who have the following characteristics. They typically present with a precocious ability to read words, far above what would be expected at their chronological age, or an intense fascination with letters or numbers. They have significant difficulty in understanding verbal language, and abnormal social skills, difficulty in socializing and interacting appropriately with people (p. 1).

AHA also listed the following characteristics found in some children who are hyperlexic: They learn expressive language in a peculiar way; echo or memorize the sentence structure without understanding the meaning (echolalia); reverse pronouns; and rarely initiate conversations. They present with an intense need to keep routines, difficulty with transitions, ritualistic behavior, and have auditory, olfactory and/or tactile sensitivity. Many present with self-stimulatory behavior, and have specific, unusual fears. Usually, their parents report these children have normal development until 18 to 24 months, then regress. They have strong auditory and visual memories. They usually have difficulty answering Wh- questions, such as "what," "where," "who," and "why;" think in concrete and literal terms having difficulty with abstract concepts, and listen selectively, even appearing to be deaf (p. 1).

Aaron and Joshi (1992) cautioned that many hyperlexic children present additional symptoms including "autistic tendencies and social aloofness; they also have a unique childhood history of having started 'reading' in a compulsive, ritualistic manner at a very early age" (p. 98). Richman (1995) identified two subtypes of hyperlexia. Subjects in the first group, with a strong *language* disorder component, were characterized by lower verbal IQ, higher performance IQ, and superior visual memory. Subjects in the second group, with a *visual–spatial* disorder, typically had a lower performance or nonverbal IQ with higher verbal IQ (p. 1).

Richman's hyperlexia *language* disorder group is defined as an expressive language deficit with good rote memory skills. "Language is delayed, echolalic and perseverative. Problems in understanding overall meaning beyond rote recall; (there are) autistic-like symptoms" including: tangential associations and offbeat responses; immature and unaware of other's reactions; does not consider consequences of behavior; distractible and impulsive, but this may be related to a language deficit; processing speed problems; and autistic symptoms drop off as language improves. When these students read they tend to make more phonic type errors than the visual–spatial group (p. 1–2).

The hyperlexic *visual–spatial* disorder may or may not have a motor delay. In this subtype, children present with a "language pragmatic deficit in expressing and interpreting experiential aspects of language and environment; (there are) Asperger-like symptoms." Included among the symptoms are: possible letter/ word reversals, reading with few phonic errors, and tend to have good reading comprehension; difficulty with worksheets and copying problems from the blackboard or book; unorganized and impulsive behavior; social imperceptions with problems reading nonverbal cues; does not learn from experience but continues to make same mistakes; superior auditory memory but impaired cognitive organization (Richman, 1995, pp. 1–2).

Finally, the findings of her study led Aram (1997) to offer the following suggestions as to the nature of reading in a group of 12 children with hyperlexia ranging in age from 7 years, 11 months to 13 years, 7 months. They tended to read words that adhered to regular phonologic rules significantly better than reading exception words. This was interpreted to mean that this group relied more on phonologic strategies, rather than orthographic strategies, to assist word recognition. A dissociation between word decoding and meaningful comprehension was apparent in two trends observed in the subjects' reading: only a few of them tried to correct their reading errors on exception words read incorrectly in sentence contexts, and meaningful context had little effect in facilitating word decoding (pp. 10–11). Aram concluded the underlying disorder in hyperlexia is one of language comprehension, and that decoding is a splinter skill at least in part dissociated from meaning (p. 11).

The focus in the remaining section of this chapter is on the underlying core deficits in two of the developmental reading disabilities described above, dyslexia and generalized reading problems. For more information on hyperlexia, the reader is referred to the research in the following areas: hyperlexia, Asperger's, autism, pervasive developmental disorder, semantic–pragmatic disorder, and the American Hyperlexia Association which can be accessed on the internet: *http://www.hyperlexia.org*

III. UNDERLYING CORE DEFICITS IN DEVELOPMENTAL READING DISABILITIES

Investigating the relationship between speech–language impairments and reading disabilities, Catts (1993) found that receptive and expressive language abilities, phonological awareness, and rapid automatized naming were associated with reading achievement, but the nature of the relationships depended on how reading was measured. Phonological awareness and rapid naming were the best predictors of word recognition in isolation and context. A large body of research reveals that problems with phonological awareness and rapid automatized naming often precede and are integrally associated with learning to recognize printed words. In fact, "it has been proposed that phonological awareness and rapid-naming deficits lie near the core of reading disabilities in young children" (Catts, 1993, pp. 955–956).

A. Phonological processing and reading problems.

Reading and writing problems demonstrated by students with developmental reading disabilities are obvious, but these symptoms may be manifestations of underlying language deficits. We saw in the earlier discussion of reading disability subtypes, that phonological processing problems are evident in both developmental reading disability and generalized reading problems.

The term *phonological* (relating to speech sounds), became widely used in the 1990s. Because some of the "phonological" terms overlap, there has been considerable confusion and **misuse of terms, the worst of which is referring to "phonological awareness" and "phonics" as synonymous.** Problems students present with along the phonological continuum can range from those involving the motoric aspects of oral–motor sequencing to those involving cognitive aspects, namely, phonological awareness. In order to understand the important relationship of phonological processing and reading, the following eleven terms are defined here: phonological processing, phonological processing difficulties, phonological representation, phonetic coding, phonological encoding, phonological memory (coding), phonological recoding, phonological awareness, phonemic awareness, phonological retrieval, and phonological production.

1. Phonological Processing.

Phonological processing is "using phonological information to process oral and written language" (Hodson & Edwards, 1997, p. 230). The ability to form and hold strong phonological representations in our brains while we process and/or verbally produce language, decode the printed form of our language, and/or encode to produce the written form of our language is critical. Torgesen, Wagner, and Rashotte (1999) defined phonological processing as "the kind of auditory processing that is most strongly related to mastery of written language, and is clearly implicated as the most common cause of reading disabilities or dyslexia" (p. 2). Phonological processing is a general ability or compilation of independent abilities, but Wagner and Torgesen (1987) recommended separating awareness from coding/retrieval. Those studying reading acquisition use the term phonological processing to refer to "an individual's mental operations that make use of the phonological or sound structure of oral language when he or she is learning how to decode written language" (Torgesen, Wagner, & Rashotte 1994, p. 276). The important role of phonological processing in the earliest stages of reading acquisition has been deemed "one of the more notable scientific success stories of the last decade" (Stanovich, 1991b, p. 78).

As a child practices producing speech, articulatory gestures become integrated into automatic phonetic routines (Stackhouse, 1997). The phonologic code, therefore, becomes a more efficient code for encoding and retrieving structures in verbal working memory. As phonemes begin to emerge as definite forms, the child becomes aware of them as structures in and of themselves. Becoming aware of these structures is critical for the language learner to develop strong, efficient phonological representations. The child comes to appreciate that phonemes can be "played with" as if they were mental toys. Words can be broken into parts, and syllables and sounds within syllables can be added, deleted, and/or substituted. Becoming aware of phonemes as structures provides a solid foundation upon which the language learner can build, that is, add another layer of language, namely, a visual representation. A strongly stored phonological system allows the novice reader to have a much easier time mapping a visual, graphemic system onto it. Stated differently, the phonological code forms the foundation onto which the graphemic system will be laid. Phonological processing should naturally lead the way to phonological awareness; then the child's exposure to print facilitates phonological awareness development. Kamhi and Catts (1989) explained that "phonological processing abilities account for the majority of individual variation in early reading performance, whereas other kinds of language, conceptual, and metacognitive knowledge/processes account for a greater portion of reading ability in more proficient readers" (p. xiii). Kamhi et al. (1990) explained that differences in phonological processing tasks and early reading lie in the ability to form accurate phonologically-based memory codes, which is a basic cognitive process.

2.   **Phonological Processing Difficulties.**

Phonological processing difficulties are "problems with phonological input (auditory processing), lexical representation, and/or phonological output (speech)" (Hodson & Edwards, 1997, p. 230).

3.   **Phonological Representation.**

Phonological representation refers to stored knowledge about what
a word sounds like (sufficient to recognize it when heard) and
how to discriminate it from similar sounding words (Hodson &
Edwards, 1997, p. 230). Torgesen et al. (1999) differentiated
among three levels of phonological representation: *acoustic level*:
acoustic energy represents spoken words; *phonetic level*: one step
removed from the actual acoustic signal, "speech is represented
by strings of phones or basic sounds of a language" (p. 3); *phonological level*: one step removed from the phonetic level where
related phones (allophones) combine into phonemes, representing "differences in speech sounds that signal differences in meaning—they are differences listeners hear when attending to speech
in everyday conversation" (p. 3).

4.   **Phonetic Coding.**

Phonetic coding is the translation of the acoustic signal into
speech sounds and involves speech perception and storage in
short term memory. Brady (1997) summarized why speech perception, which is the initial encoding of linguistic input, is a plau-
sible correlate with reading achievement. First, the quality of
speech perception may directly affect how successful children
will be acquiring phoneme awareness. Discovering the phonemic
elements in words might be more difficult if phonemic categories
are not clearly defined (Fowler, 1991). Second, the quality of
speech perception may directly affect vocabulary acquisition and
confrontation naming. Third, if speech is not fully perceived at
this level, inaccurate phonological representations will result that
can lead to verbal short-term memory problems. "Inaccurate formation of phonological representations might limit resources
available for recall or might result in a less durable memory trace"
(Brady, p. 22). Inaccurate phonological representations may, in
turn, interfere with reading decoding and comprehension. If the
phonological form of a new word is imprecise, more exposure
might be needed to retain accurate representations. "Likewise,
the problems reported on productive naming tasks for poor readers could be a by-product of the same difficulty establishing fully
specified phonemic representations of words" (p. 22). Catts
(1989) noted that students with specific reading disabilities typically need multiple presentations of new words before they can
verbally produce them accurately and consistently. Although
good and poor readers perform similarly on nonverbal, visual

memory tasks, poor readers perform significantly worse than good readers on auditory memory span tasks.

Brady (1991) explained that, "although deficiency in metaphonological awareness is certainly the language factor most strongly implicated in reading disability" (p. 130), the cause is "more basic problems in language use" (p. 130). Brady continued: "At the level of underlying language processes, perhaps the most striking characteristic of poor readers is the common occurrence of verbal memory problems" (p. 130). In reading, phonetic recoding occurs when print is translated to speech. Spoken words are automatically registered in the phonological store, but printed information becomes registered in the phonological store by way of an articulatory loop that is activated when the reader subvocalizes the information. Stein (2001) explained that unfamiliar printed words, which includes most or all words for novice readers, "have to be sounded out using the letter sound correspondences, that have to be learned. This sounding out engages more anterior parts of the articulatory loop." Even when the reader sounds out printed words entirely mentally, "using 'inner speech,' the whole articulatory loop is engaged" (p. 5). Poor readers have been found to have major memory problems in phonetic coding and that it is a specific auditory working memory rather than a general memory problem (Wagner & Torgesen, 1987).

5.   **Phonological Encoding.**

Swank (1994) defined *phonological encoding* as "the ability to process rapidly paced human speech that requires the listener to impose a phonemic identity on incoming speech sounds" (p. 60). That 8-year-old children with poor reading abilities made "more errors identifying speech stimuli degraded by noise . . . (than) nonlinguistic sounds masked by noise" (p. 61) was interpreted by Swank to mean the subtle deficit may be impaired ability to encode phonological information rather than impaired general perception (p. 62).

6.   **Phonological Memory.**

Catts and Kamhi (1999) defined *phonological memory,* also called *phonological coding,* as "the encoding and storage of phonological information in memory" (p. 113). Torgesen et al. (1994) explained that *phonological memory* refers to the representations, or codes, we use when storing verbal material such as digits, letters, words, or pronounceable nonwords. Phonological memory is assessed when one is asked to recall information immediately, verbatim, and in the correct order (p. 276). Rate of access for phonological information refers to "children's ability to easily and rapidly access phonological information that is stored in long-term memory" (p. 277). In the reading literature this typically has been assessed by rapid automatic naming tasks. "Presumably, the efficiency with which children can access phonological codes associated with letters, word segments, and whole words influences the extent to which phonological information is useful in decoding" (p. 277). Although reading problems do not seem to cause phonological memory problems, the difficulty poor readers have with phonological memory and phonological awareness tasks "stem from a common cause, namely, deficiencies in the quality of phonological representations" (Catts & Kamhi, 1999, p. 114). What may be of relevance here is the notion that when learning new words, normally developing children "pick and choose," that is, learn new words phonologically similar to those already stored in their expressive vocabulary (Schwartz & Leonard, 1982). It would seem likely that children with impoverished phonological representations would also "pick and choose" new words phonologically similar to those already stored. These newly acquired, fragile phonological representations would further compound the developing oral and written language systems.

7.   **Phonological Recoding.**

Phonological recoding refers to the translation from either oral or written representation into a sound-based system to arrive at the meaning of words in the lexicon (stored vocabulary) in long-term memory (Wagner & Torgesen, 1987).

8.   **Phonological Awareness.**

Stackhouse (1997) defined *phonological awareness* as "the ability to reflect on and manipulate the structure of an utterance (e.g., into words, syllables, or sounds) as distinct from its meaning" (p. 157). Phonological awareness is usually defined as "one's sensitivity to, or explicit awareness of, the phonological structure of the words in one's language . . . it involves the ability to notice, think about, or manipulate the individual sounds in words" (Torgesen & Mathes, 2000, p. 2). It taps the organization of the phonological system (Gombert, 1992). The terms linguistic awareness, phonological awareness, auditory analysis, phoneme segmentation, and phonemic analysis are used interchangeably in the literature. They refer to the metalinguistic ability that allows a language user to perceive spoken words as consisting of a series of individual speech sounds. Lance et al. (1997) concluded phonological awareness is not one-dimensional but is "considered to be a constellation of cognitive abilities that are related to the child's understanding of the segmental nature of English" (p. 1002). Most children enter kindergarten with well developed listening and speaking vocabularies but have not yet had to attend to specific sounds within the words consciously.

A reciprocal relationship exists between phonological awareness and reading. Yopp (1992) proposed that, to benefit from formal reading instruction, students must have developed a certain level of phonemic awareness and that specific reading instruction facilitates language awareness. "Phonemic awareness is both a prerequisite for and a consequence of learning to read" (p. 697). Lyon (1995a) noted "some degree of awareness in the phonological structure of words helps to make learning to read a more understandable task. Without such awareness, the alphabetic system that our written language is based on is not comprehensible." Emphasizing the importance of phonological awareness skills in learning to read, Adams (1990) wrote:

> It is because we have so thoroughly automated, so thoroughly mechanized and sublimated our processing of phonemes that we have attention and capacity for the higher order meaning and nuances of spoken language . . . having learned the phonemes so well, there is almost no reason whatsoever for us to lend them conscious attention—no reason, that is, unless we need to learn to read an alphabetic script. And there is the rub. To learn an alphabetic script, we must learn to attend to that which we have learned not to attend to (p. 66).

According to Lyon (1995a), approximately 80% of children develop phonological awareness without much difficulty, while the remaining 20% are confused by the system. Because the phonological component is involved in phonological awareness tasks and in reading, limitations in creating and using phonological representations might impede discovery of the phonological structure of words and delay mastery of an alphabetic writing system (Brady, 1991). Working from this theoretical framework, Shankweiler and Liberman (cited by Shankweiler, 1991) believed the basis of specific reading disabilities to lie within the cognitive domain at the intersection of oral and written language rather than in the perceptual or motor domains. Liberman believed that becoming phonologically aware is essential for discovering the alphabetic principle and that phonologic awareness is the acid test of reading an alphabetic orthography. "Subsequent research here and in other countries has borne her out: The degree to which phoneme awareness exists is the best single predictor of reading success" (Shankweiler, 1991, p. xvi).

Finally, in answer to the question "what does phonological awareness have to do with oral language?" the answer is: *"phonological awareness has everything to do with oral language."* When engaged in a phonological awareness task, a student is utilizing receptive language abilities in a bottom-up mode. The student is being asked to break wholes into parts, that is, words into syllables, and syllables into sounds. In answer to the question: "Is phonological awareness the same thing as phonics?" the answer is a resounding "No." While phonological awareness has to do with explicit manipulation of words, word parts, and sounds, phonics is a method of teaching reading by associating sounds with letters.

9.   **Phonemic Awareness.**

Phonemic awareness refers specifically to segmenting the sounds of the speech stream. Stanovich (1991a) noted that phonological sensitivity tasks relate to reading acquisition "because they predict the ease or difficulty with which a child will learn to segment spoken words at levels below the syllable" (p. 23). Phonemic awareness can be considered to be at the highest end of a hierarchy of metalinguistic skills "that begins with the conscious awareness that sentences are made up of words and culminates in an awareness that words are made up of phonemes, those small units of sound that roughly correspond to individual letters" (Snider, 1997, p. 203). Adams (1990) wrote:

> It turns out that it is not working knowledge of phonemes that is so important but conscious analytic knowledge. It is neither the ability to hear the difference between two phonemes nor the ability to distinctly produce them that is significant. What is important is the awareness that they exist as abstractable and manipulable components of the language. Developmentally, this awareness seems to depend upon the child's inclination or encouragement to lend conscious attention to the sounds (as distinct from the meanings) of words (p. 65).

See Table 3-2 for Adams' summary of five different levels of phonemic awareness.

Table 3-2. Adams' (1990) Summary of Five Different Levels of Phonemic Awareness.

1. Knowledge of nursery rhymes—"the most primitive level"—refers merely to "an ear for the sounds of words" (p. 80).

2. Oddity tasks, which require that the child methodically "compare and contrast the sounds of words for rhyme or alliteration," necessitates "sensitivity to similarities and differences in the overall sounds of words," (and) the ability to focus attention on the components of their sounds that make them similar or different" (p. 80).

3. Blending and syllable-splitting—tasks at the third level—"seem to require . . . a comfortable familiarity with the notion that words can be subdivided into those small meaningless sounds corresponding to phonemes" and that the child be "comfortably familiar with the way phonemes sound when produced 'in isolation' and, better yet, with the act of producing them that way by oneself" (p. 80).

4. Phonemic segmentation requires that the child has "a thorough understanding that words can be completely analyzed into a series of phonemes" and be able to perform such an analysis "completely and on demand" (p. 80).

5. Phoneme manipulation tasks require the child have "sufficient proficiency with the phonemic structure of words" leading to the ability "to add, delete, or move any designated phoneme and regenerate a word (or a nonword) from the result" (p. 80).

Perfetti (1991b), Goldsworthy (1996), Stackhouse (1997), and Moats (personal communication, 1997) among others, have presented developmental perspectives for the emergence of phonological awareness skills in children. The following sections provide current information about developmental progression of phonological awareness.

a. At 3 years of age, children are usually able to

Recite known rhymes, for example, Jack and Jill.
Produce rhyme by pattern, for example, give the word "cat" as a rhyming word for "hat."
Recognize alliteration (words beginning with the same first sound), for example, "Mommy, Michele, they're the same."

b. At 4 years of age, children are usually able to

Segment syllables, for example, know there are two parts to the word "cowboy."

Count the number of syllables in words (50% of 4-year olds can do this).

c. At 5 years of age, children are usually able to

Count syllables in words (90% of 5-year olds can do this).
Count phonemes within words (fewer than 50% of 5 year olds can do this).

d. At 6 years of age, children are usually able to

Match initial consonants in words, for example, able to recognize that "shoe" and "sheep" begin with the same first sound.
Blend two-three phonemes, for example, recognize that the sounds /d/ /o/ /g/ form the word "dog."
Count phonemes within words (70% of six-year olds can do this).
Identify rhyming words, for example, "pit" rhymes with "mit."
Divide words by onset (first consonant or blend) and rime (rest of the word), for example, can divide the word "stop" into /st/ /op/.

e. At 7 years of age, children are usually able to

Blend phonemes to form words.
Segment three- to- four phonemes within words.
Spell phonetically.
Delete phonemes from words, for example, omit the /t/ sound in the word "cat."

f. At 8 years of age, children are usually able to

Segment consonant clusters /bl/.
Delete consonant clusters.

10. Phonological Retrieval.

German (2001) explained that *phonological retrieval* is involved when a student is asked to complete tasks requiring verbal responses such as naming pictures, answering questions, and reading aloud. These tasks assume phonological processing, which is observed when tasks do not require oral responses (e.g., "point to picture that begins with /d/" cow, dog, goat) German's model for child word finding is an adaptation of Levelt's (1989) adult speech production model and includes four stages of single word retrieval, that is, the order of what happens when a single word is retrieved from the lexicon:

Stage I: eliciting the target word's conceptual structure (category, function, location, and perceptual attributes); *Stage II*: eliciting the corresponding lemma (semantic and syntactic features); *Stage III*: eliciting the target word's phonological features (number of syllables and sounds); *Stage IV*: constructing a corresponding motor plan and movements to complete the articulatory process.

German (2001b) explained that word finding errors can occur because of disruptions at one of the above four stages in the lexical process. The causes and resulting errors include:

Lemma-related error (Slip of the Tongue) in which the conceptual structure (picture in a naming task or question asked verbally) is unsuccessful in accessing the word's lemma. When this involves a meaning error, a semantic substitution ("orange" for "apple") results. When this involves a sound-form error, a close approximation of the target word will be produced ("continuous" for "continuum"), that is, the produced word shares some of the same sounds as the target word.

Word-form-related error (Tip of the Tongue) resulting in one of two outcomes. If the lemma cannot find the word form (syllabic or phonological) the resulting responses will be: no response (blank stare), or "I don't know." If the phonological form of the word cannot be accessed, the resulting responses will be: a semantic substitution ("dog" for "cat") or the speaker accesses the first sound or number of syllables of the word, but is not yet able to retrieve the complete word entry.

Word-form segment-related error (Twist of the Tongue) in which partial access of the target word's syllables or sounds results in phonemic approximations of the word, including any of the following errors as examples when trying to name "octopus": -phoneme shift: "octucus"; -substitution: "octobus"; -addition: "octgopus"; -omission: "ocpus"; -malapropism: "octagon"; -real word rhymes (p. 6).

When accessing the meaning of a printed word while reading, the word is translated into its phonological form and mapped onto its lexical entry. Phonological recoding of print, then, involves converting the printed features of words into corresponding sound or phonological equivalents through application of the alphabetic principle or grapheme–phoneme conversion. The printed form of the word is converted (recoded) into sound, allowing for subvocal rehearsal and access to its lexical referent. The beginning reader must learn to decode a series of visually presented letters, temporarily store the sounds the letters make, and blend the contents of the temporary store to form words (Wagner & Torgesen, 1987). Vellutino (1993) described children who read well as having "good mental tape recorders"—good phonological recoding abilities. Although the direct visual route is used by skilled readers for high frequency words, phonological recoding is used to some extent by all readers depending on how familiar the words are.

A vast body of research exists documenting word retrieval problems in poor readers. "Studies have consistently found that poor readers perform less well than good readers on tasks involving confrontation picture naming" (Catts & Kamhi, 1999, p. 112). Poor readers have problems naming common objects, learning nonsense words, learning automatized sequences such as the alphabet, and recalling numbers, letters, words, and sentences presented visually or verbally. "Whether these difficulties are the result of poor lexical retrieval processes, more domain-general factors such as timing processes, or weak vocabulary knowledge" is a complex issue (Wolf & Segal, 1999). The literature also strongly indicates that many individuals with reading disabilities have problems when naming tasks are timed, as in rapid automatized naming tasks (RAN). During a RAN task the subject is asked to name a series of pictured items (for example, colors, numbers, letters, or objects) as quickly as possible. Wolf (1997) explained early naming speed is most predictive of later word recognition (regularly and irregularly spelled words, and made-up or nonsense words), "whereas early confrontation naming, which places heavy emphasis on semantic processes and expressive vocabulary development, is more highly predictive of later reading comprehension" (p. 72). (See the section on naming speed and reading problems in this chapter for further considerations.)

11. Phonological Production.

Phonological production is the ability to fluently and flexibly articulate spoken language incuding multisyllabic words and phrases. A phonological production problem is a frequent concomitant of developmental reading disabilities. In their review of studies on phonological production and subjects with reading disabilities (RD), Catts and Kamhi (1999) found that the RD group had more problems with: repeating complex phonological sequences (e.g., "Swiss wristwatch) and repetition of nonwords, which may be related to "formation and storage of accurate phonological memory codes" (pp. 115–116); and rapidly repeating complex phrases, which may be related to deficits in speech planning (p. 116).

Catts (1989) concurred with observations that subjects with specific reading disabilities perform more slowly and/or less accurately than normally achieving subjects in the rapid, continuous repetition of complex speech sound sequences. This suggests that phonological coding deficits may disrupt phonological programming during the speech production planning stages. In speech planning, abstract lexical units are converted into a serial order of phonological segments. During this conversion, errors may occur and result in segments being misordered or misproduced. The observation that dyslexics produced significantly more of these errors than normal subjects suggests that they may be slower and less accurate than normal individuals in converting lexical information into a sequential sound based code (p. 117).

B. Verbal Naming Speed and Reading Problems.

Wolf (2001) summarized three converging factors that lead many researchers to look beyond the phonological-core deficit as the sole contributor to developmental reading disabilities, namely time- and fluency-related issues. First, researchers have been searching for contributions beyond the phonological core deficit (discussed in the previous section of this chapter) to explain the "heterogeneity of reading disabilities and the complexity of reading breakdown—especially in the area of fluency" (p. xii). Second, there is an increased awareness of the "multiple, underlying sources that can contribute to or impede fluency development" (p. xiii). (See the discussion of rapid automatized naming later in this chapter.) And third, the growing body of research demonstrating children's reading problems may be related to phonological processing problems, or naming speed problems, or both (p. xiii).

1.   Need for Fluency in Reading.

The authors of the Primary Literacy Standards for kindergarten through third grade (1999) likened the task children face learning to read to putting together a jigsaw puzzle. Like successful puzzle solving, learning to read involves many trials, and "beginning readers actually work puzzle after puzzle on their way to mastery" (p. 20). Beyond cracking the print–sound code, children must achieve the other half of the successful reading formula, grasping the author's intended meaning. The Standards Committee underscored how important it is for readers to recognize words. Because of limited attention spans, readers are only able to consciously attend to a few things at a time. If a reader's attention is focused too much on sounding out word for word, he/she will not be able to allot the attention needed to arrive at the meaning of the passage. Wolf, Miller, and Donnelly (2000) defined "automaticity" as a "continuum" wherein processes are only considered automatic "when they are fast, obligatory, and autonomous and require only limited use of cognitive resources" (p. 377). They defined "fluency" as the "acquisition of smooth rates of processing speed in reading outcomes (e.g., word identification, word attack, and comprehension)" (p. 377). (See further discussion of modified RAVE-O in Chapter 6.)

Fluency requires "automaticity, or the ability to recognize individual words quickly and without much conscious attention" (New Standards Primary Literacy Committee, p. 20). Fluency was defined by the committee as "the ability to read aloud with appropriate intonations and pauses indicating that students understand the meaning, with only an occasional need to stop to figure out words or sentence structures" (p. 21). Torgesen, Rashotte, and Alexander (2001) identified the following five components that may potentially result in lower reading fluency: 1) The passage contains too few known sight words for the reader; 2) The reader has not seen the sight words enough times, or constitutional differences in the reader leads to slower word processing; 3) Slow speed in identification of "novel" words. Words not recognized as orthographic units must be identified through conscious analysis: "The most common of these methods involve phonetic decoding, recognition by analogy to known words, and guessing from the context or meaning of the passage" (p. 337); 4) Inefficient use of contextual cues. "Children who are more adept at constructing meaning because of a larger knowledge base may experience a stronger beneficial effect of context on reading fluency than those who are less able to construct the meaning of a passage"; 5) Slow identification of word meaning.

2.   **Rapid Automatized Naming.**

Because naming speed and reading both require the student to automatically retrieve a verbal match for an abstract visual form, Wolf (1999) described naming speed as a "mini, multicomponential version of reading" (p. 12). In this view, naming speed uses the same visual, auditory, and motor processes used in reading but in a less complex fashion. Naming and reading, therefore, represent "two levels of rapid, precise integration of cognitive systems, a basic level and a more complex level" (Wolf, 1997, p. 85). Problems in the more basic system, naming speed, warn us of potential weaknesses in the later developing system, reading, possibly even causing the reading problem (p. 86). "Thus, naming speed provides us with a deceptively simple, extraordinarily useful, early window on some developing disabilities in the reading systems" (p. 86)

Wolf and Segal (1992) addressed the issue of a specific naming deficit in children with dyslexia. They found significant differences in naming speed on all rapid automatized naming (RAN) and rapid alternating sequences (RAS) tests in first through third grade subjects with dyslexia. These investigators concluded that RAN tasks require the subject to name "highly familiar visual stimuli (i.e., letters, digits, colors, or common objects) rapidly in a serial format" (p. 53). In a RAS task, "two or three differing stimulus sets are presented serially (letter–number–letter–number)" (p. 53). Second through fourth grade subjects demonstrated significant differences in all RAS tasks and RAN letter and digit naming tasks but not RAN color and object tasks. A "developmental, differential pattern of prediction between particular naming and reading tasks" was found and "of particular importance . . . is the evolving specificity of the prediction ability over time" (p. 56). From Grade 2 on, for example, retrieval tasks measuring rapid recognition and naming speed (e.g., of letters and numbers) predicted word-recognition skills in Grades 3 and 4. Both retrieval and word-recognition skills emphasize basic or lower level cognitive processes. On the other hand, confrontation naming, which requires more complex forms of retrieval, predicted the more complex third and fourth grade abilities of oral reading and reading comprehension. According to Wolf (1997) the primary conclusions that emerged from this 8-year longitudinal study are: "naming-speed deficits are a powerful, predictive, and diagnostic indicator of severe reading disabilities; and they should be considered a specific core deficit in the dyslexias" (p. 73).

Wolf (2001) wrote "there is considerable evidence and consensus that at least one type of time-related problem, naming-speed deficit (NSD), represents a very strong predictor of reading disabilities across every language tested to date" (p. xiv).

To differentiate between vocabulary knowledge and word retrieval, Wolf and Segal (1992) designed a multiple-choice, receptive component for the *Boston Naming Test* (Kaplan, Goodglass, & Weintraub, 1983). Comparing test results with a standardized receptive vocabulary test, the researchers concluded: "garden-variety poor readers" experienced problems in vocabulary knowledge, contrasted with dyslexic subjects who had "quite dramatic problems" in retrieval of lexical knowledge (p. 57).

Snyder (1994) summarized six explanatory hypotheses for rapid naming problems in students with dyslexia: 1) Storage elaboration deficit. These students are delayed in acquiring first words and words in the lexicon are not as well connected; 2) Retrieval deficit. Strategies for organizing words in the lexicon are not as fast; 3) Phonological specification deficit. The representation of the phonetic word shape may be "fuzzy." The student tries to access a word but because the shape is not well defined, the system is hunting around for a vague entry; 4) Oral motor inefficiency. This student may be inefficient in planning, organizing or executing responses; 5) Generalized response slowing. This student may be "slower at everything"; 6) Temporal precision performance deficit. This student may have problems with the automatized, precise responses needed in reading, naming, and motor tasks.

In her discussion of the nature of naming-speed deficits, Wolf (1997) maintained that what happens within the temporal gap between seeing a stimulus on a RAN task and naming the stimulus is important. Obregon and Wolf (1995) found no differences in articulation speed of verbal labels or the line-to-line scanning by dyslexic readers. "Rather, there were large significant differences across all categories of the RAN stimuli during the interstimulus intervals, or the gap in time it takes to process each stimulus and move on to the next" (p. 83). (See discussion of "nervous system timing problems" later in this chapter.) As the result of an 8-year longitudinal study on the predictive relationships between word-retrieval problems and reading operations, Wolf concluded: "I am convinced that naming-speed deficits are a second core deficit in reading disabilities and that their conjunction with phonological deficits represents a formula for the most impaired readers" (p. 86).

C. The Double-Deficit Hypothesis.

As mentioned in an earlier section of this chapter, a core phonological processing problem inhibits word recognition skills in reading acquisition resulting in developmental dyslexia or generalized reading problems.   Viewing phonological processing as the primary deficit in developmental reading problems is considered a single-deficit hypothesis. In this unitary causation hypothesis, naming speed is considered to be subsumed within phonological processing, that is, naming speed is a member of the "phonological family" (Torgesen et al., 1997). Torgesen, Wagner, and Rashotte (1999) considered rapid naming to be one of three kinds of phonological processing, along with phonological awareness and phonological memory, to be especially relevant for mastery of written language. The degree to which the reader can efficiently retrieve phonemes corresponding with the printed letters (graphemes), coupled with efficiency of word and word-part pronunciations, will affect how phonological information facilitates decoding print (p. 6). In this unitary cause hypothesis dyslexic readers are considered to possess adequate semantic representations of words they know, but "their representations of the phonological forms of words are impoverished" (Snowling, 2000, p. 44). Why look further? Indeed, Wolf (1999) answered the question "Why does the field of dyslexia need a second-core deficit?"

Despite some of the best work in the field on phonological-based explanations and interventions, there remain aspects of dyslexia unexplained by our theories; there remain reading-impaired children who slip through our diagnostic batteries with adequate decoding and phonological awareness skills but poor comprehension; and there remain dyslexic children who resist our best phonological-based treatments, children whom Blachman (1994) and Torgesen (1998) call the "treatment resisters" (pp. 4–5).

Work by Bowers et al. (1988) and Bowers and Swanson (1991) contributed significantly to our understanding that phonology and naming speed are two independent contributors to developmental reading problems. Their work revealed "that phonological awareness contributed significantly to word attack skills in reading, whereas naming speed contributed more to the orthographic aspects in word identification" (Wolf, 1999, p. 12). If the two factors contribute independently to reading development, "then two dissociated single-deficit subgroups and one combined deficit subgroup would be hypothesized" (Wolf, 1997, p. 68). The double-deficit hypothesis, which considers rapid naming problems to result from a faulty timing mechanism, includes four reading groups (see Wolf et al., 2000; Bowers & Wolf, 1993).

1. The *average reader* presents with intact naming speed, phonological decoding, and reading comprehension.

2. The reader with intact naming speed and impaired reading comprehension caused by *diminished phonological awareness* has a single deficit problem.

3. Likewise, the reader with intact phonological awareness and impaired reading comprehension caused by *slower naming speed* has a single deficit problem.

4. The reader whose reading comprehension is impaired because of *both impaired phonological awareness and naming speed* has a double-deficit and is the most severely impaired reader ("treatment resister"). (Figure 3–1 summarizes these groups.)

	Naming Speed	Phonological Awareness	Reading Comprehension
1. Average Reader:	Intact	Intact	Intact
SINGLE DEFICITS			
2. Rate Problem	Problem	Intact	Problem
3. Phonological Awareness (P.A.) Problem	Intact	Problem	Problem
DOUBLE DEFICIT			
4. Rate & P.A. Problems	Problem	Problem	Problem

Figure 3–1. Four Reading Groups. *Source:* Bowers and Wolf (1993); Wolf (1998)

Wolf (1997) concluded that the double-deficit hypothesis offers a way to examine the heterogenity of developmental reading problems and is particularly important because of the potential for new treatment directions (see Chapters 4 through 6 for discussions of assessment and intervention). "By directing our attention to dual emphases on phonological processes and automaticity/fluency skills, we may well increase our effectiveness for a greater number of our at-risk children" (p. 86).

IV. CAUSES AND CONSEQUENCES OF DEVELOPMENTAL READING DISABILITIES

The causes of developmental reading disabilities have received considerable attention. Some of the most frequently explored causes are reviewed here. Like Nelson's (1993) view of factors contributing to developmental language problems, factors contributing to developmental reading disabilities are not limited to a single influence that appears at a specific time and then disappears. They are "vectors that may assume different levels of strength at different times" (Nelson, 1993, p. 79). The following eight causal factors are reviewed in this book: oral language problems, heredity, neural basis, nervous system timing problems, selective attention and attention deficit disorder, middle ear problems, limited print exposure, and cognitive rigidity and learned helplessness.

A. Oral Language Problems (see Chapters 1 and 2).

B. Heredity.

Converging evidence indicates deficient phonological awareness skills and subsequent problems with deficient phonological coding of written language are genetically influenced. Shaywitz (1998) summarized some of the relevant information as to the heritability of dyslexia:

> Dyslexia is both familial and heritable. Family history is one of the most important risk facors, with 23 percent to as much as 65 percent of children who have a parent with dyslexia reported to have the disorder. A rate among siblings of affected persons of approximately 40 percent and among parents ranging from 27 to 49 percent provides opportunity for early identification of affected siblings and often for delayed but helpful identification of affected adults. Linkage studies implicate loci on chromosomes 6 and 15 in reading disability (p. 307).

Results of a 10-year study of 14 families with a three-generation history of relatively pure dyslexia were reported by Lubs et al. (1991). The researchers determined "a significant subgroup of children and adults with autosomal dominant inheritance of dyslexia" (p. 115). Lubs et al. recognized an interaction between a gene(s) for "dyslexia, sex hormones, and possibly even concomitantly caused immunologic responses in the development of brains in dyslexia" (p. 115). Findings from two linkage studies suggested that there are genes that lead to dyslexia associated with chromosomes 15 and 6. Lubs et al. observed that: "these variant genes must have been present 10,000 years ago, long before reading and writing began" (p. 115). Stein (2001) explained that linkages to "a site on the short arm of chromosome 6 near the Tumour Necrosis Factor and Major Histocompatibility Complex immunological sites" (p. 16) have been found for both phonological and orthographic problems. Stein added that "people with dyslexia and their families very often have a higher incidence of asthma, eczema, hay fever, and other immune conditions than controls" (p. 17). Pennington (1991) explained that genetic differences may result in alterations or constriction of the range of neurological development and produce "hardwired" aberrations in neural tissue, which, in turn, influence reading acquisition.

The etiology of reading disability is one facet of an ongoing research project initiated in 1979 at the University of Colorado. Data from the Twin/Family Study component of the Colorado Reading Project, involving over 400 families, has provided compelling evidence for a genetic cause of specific reading disability. DeFries, Olson, Pennington, and Smith (1991) reported the following findings:

> The correlation between phonological coding and word recognition is largely due to heritable influences, whereas the relationship between orthographic coding and word recognition is due primarily to environmental influences . . . About 20% of families (have) . . . apparent autosomal dominant transmission for reading disability with manifest linkage to chromosome 15, but not to chromosome 6. Some evidence for linkage to chromosome 6, but not to 15, was obtained from data on other families (p. 83).

C. Neural Basis.

A large body of research has accumulated on the neurophysiological substrates of reading ability and disability. Research is now revealing that children with developmental dyslexia present with brain-based processing difficulties. According to Galaburda (1991) the overabundance of tree-like connections—synapses—produced during the development of the human brain, are usually pruned—weeded out—

by a natural process of selection resulting from chemical and experiential influences. Galaburda found that the right hemisphere in brains of dyslexics have an abundance of brain cells, suggesting that something interfered with the normal pruning process. According to Galaburda, an optimal match is needed between the number of neurons and their connections in a neural net so that a particular behavior can be achieved. Too many or too few neuron match-ups can be deleterious for the developing skill. Galaburda hypothesized "that the neurons in question are not only misplaced, but the affected cortex is different in terms of its cellular and connectional architecture, hence its functional architecture as well" (p. 127). (See discussion in Chapter 2 on Locke's theory of the neurolinguistic development.).Denckla (1987) explained:

> With too many cells, the right side will have grabbed up the lion's share of the connections. So the poor old left side of the brain comes along ten days later and there is no place to connect, and so you get a reorganized brain. This is a much more subtle kind of pathology—the underpruned right side of the brain may have grabbed up all the connectivity sites, all the places to get plugged in, and then the left side of the brain . . . will experience a shut-out, a relative shut out (p. 3)

A number of developmental neuropathologic malformations have been identified in microscopic studies of human dyslexic brains according to Rosen, Fitch, Clark, LoTurco, Sherman, and Galaburda (2001). These researchers concluded that "these abnormalities range in number from 30 to 150 focal lesions per brain, tend to be located in perisylvian regions, affect the anterior vascular border-zone, and usually involve the left more than the right hemisphere" (p. 131). Rumsey and Eden (1998) explained that "these congenital lesions might impair reading by rendering dysfunctional those brain regions which are critical to reading and/or by disconnecting them from other brain regions involved in language and visual processing" (p. 41).

Brain activity studies have provided insights into the physiological processes involved in reading and the differences in such activity between individuals with normal and disordered reading abilities. Functional neuroimaging in positron emission tomography (PET) and functional magnetic resonance imaging (fMRI) offer noninvasive techniques for determining task-related changes in regional cerebral blood flow providing "a window through which to capture a glimpse of brain activity" (Rumsey & Eden, 1998, p. 35). Zeffiro and Eden (2000) summarized some current findings.

1. In developmental dyslexia, neuronal abnormalities have been found at the microscopic level in the visual system. And in the perisylvian cortical structures, "abnormalities including foci of myelinated glial scarring and molecular layer ectopias in the perisylvian neocortex . . . have been interpreted as evidence supporting intrauterine damage resulting from an autoimmune process" (p. 7).

2. Interhemispheric communication between the left and right cerebral hemispheres through the corpus callosum may be reduced because of callosal structural anomalies in developmental dyslexia.

3. Various types of structural anomalies have been located in the temporal and parietal banks of the sylvian fissure as well as macrostructural abnormalities including the insula in developmental dyslexia. In roughly 70 to 80% of people, the left planum temporale is larger than the corresponding region in the right cerebral hemisphere, but this leftward asymmetry is reduced in people with developmental dyslexia.

4. The normal neuronal asymmetry is absent in the primary visual cortex in developmental dyslexia with control brains having larger left hemisphere neurons. Cortical connections in left hemisphere perisylvian white matter tracts were abnormal in individuals with below-average reading problems, that is, not dyslexia (pp. 7–8).

5. Poor readers (adults or children) performed more poorly on phonological awareness tasks. Functional brain imaging revealed "less activity is identified in certain temporal, occipital, and parietal areas than in good readers" (p. 9).

Shaywitz et al. (1998) reported their findings with 29 dyslexic adult readers and 32 adult normal readers. The researchers used fMRI, which produces computer-generated images of the brain while performing various intellectual tasks. Subjects were asked to read nonsense rhyming words, such as "lete" and "jeat," which is a far more difficult task for dyslexic readers than rhyming actual words that may have previously been memorized. Results indicated that brains of dyslexic readers showed reduced activity in neural areas linking visual cortex and visual association areas (angular gyrus) to language regions in the superior temporal gyrus (Wernicke's area). While normal readers did not show increased activity in the frontal cerebral area

(Broca's area) while performing the rhyming task, the dyslexic readers showed activation in this region, possibly compensating for impairments in Wernicke's area normally used for phonological tasks.

D. Nervous System Timing Problems.

Wolf (2001) explained that "there is a convergence of evidence across several perceptual, motor, and linguistic areas and several orthographies that many dyslexic children have rate of processing differences, particularly in naming speed tasks, but also on tasks well beyond the linguistic domain" (p. xv). Rosen et al. (2001) summarized three interesting hypotheses as to the linguistic and nonlinguistic cognitive problems in developmental dyslexia.

Hypothesis 1: Low-level processing problems. The "correct type" of lower level processing of information is needed by language processing centers during development. Higher level processing problems are the consequence of impaired low-level processing. Research into "anatomical, psycho-physiological, and neurophysiological substrates underlying developmental dyslexia and other language disorders" indicates some dyslexics present with a "disruption of cellular architecture at the thalamic level" which would interfere with processing at lower levels (p. 133).

Hypothesis 2: High-level processing problems. Underdeveloped high-level processing centers are not able to reinforce developing low-level processing areas for functions such as fast temporal processing "because they are incapable of processing those stimuli further." Studies of the neural basis of dyslexia have found that in some people with dyslexia there are "fundamental structural disturbances at the cortical level" located primarily in the perisylvian regions that affect high-level processing of information (pp. 129–133).

Hypothesis 3: High- and low-level processing problems. Pathology can be acquired at many neural levels simultaneously causing both high- and low-level processing problems (p. 133).

Nicolson and Fawcett (1995) believed there are two deficits at work in dyslexic subjects: a phonological deficit and a nonphonological deficit involving slower reaction time when classifying stimuli. Stein's (2001) overall conclusion is that there are two reading mechanisms that are strongly interconnected, and "at least conceptually separable" with the faster whole word semantic route drawing heavily on the visual system, and the "slower phonological route, which probably depends more on auditory mediation" (p. 5). See Table 3-3 for a summary of Stein's work in this area over the past 30 years.

Table 3-3. Summary of Stein's (2001) Hypotheses on Two Reading Mechanisms.

- Reading requires "a highly sensitive visual magnocellular system to acquire good orthographic skills" (p. 4).

- Reading requires a sensitive "auditory transient system to parse the phonological structure of words" (p. 4).

- The two strongly interconnected reading mechanisms include "the faster whole word semantic route, which draws heavily on the visual system," and a slower phonological system more dependent on "auditory mediation" (p. 5).

- Magnocells (large, heavily myelinated cells) which carry visual signals from the retina to the rest of the brain (along with many more parvocells), are crucial for timing events visually (p. 5).

- Impaired magnocells have been found throughout the brains of dyslexics leading Stein and others to speculate that dyslexia is "part of a much more generalized neurodevelopmental syndrome," and that "it results from genetically mediated, disordered immunological regulation of their development in utero" (p. 17).

- "People with dyslexia seem to have impaired processing of both visual and auditory transients, because they tend to have impaired development of magnocellular neurons in both the visual and auditory systems." Consequently they fail to develop "adequate orthographic and phonological skills, respectively" (p. 15).

- The cerebellum, which functions as the brain's primary timing device, receiving "dense inputs from all the magnocellulary sytems," has been found to be deficient in dyslexia (p. 17).

- Reduced sequencing and timing ability in dyslexics "may be attributed partly to impaired cerebellar function, particularly on the right side, which connects to the left (language) hemisphere" (p. 17).

- The left hemisphere should receive more magnocellular input than the right for mediating "precise timing of auditory and visual transients required for literacy," but in fact, Rae et al. (1998) found "evidence to support reduced magnocellular input to the left hemisphere in dyslexics" (p. 17).

Wolf (1997) cited work by Galaburda, Menard, and Rosen (1994) on the variation in cellular differences in "size, structure, myelination, and organization in the magnocellular systems in thalamic regions responsible for vision and audition" (p. 84). These systems may explain the slower reaction times in dyslexic readers because the systems "have critical roles in rapid processing and in *inhibiting* previous information" (p. 84). Wolf also highlighted Ojemann's (1990) findings revealing "common brain mechanisms in the thalamus and left peri-sylvian cortex for some language and motor functions" (p. 85). Ojemann believed that within the cortical areas responsible for sequential motor movements and speech sound identification, which is critical to phonology, "there may be a precise timing mechanism that operates for both production and decoding." A deficit in this timing mechanism "offers one explanation for the conjunction of naming speed and motoric deficits" in dyslexic readers (p. 85). Summarizing several studies of visual system abnormalities, Zeffiro and Eden (2000) explained that the deficits found in dyslexic readers are most obvious during rapid processing, and "may well involve processes where functions are localized in cortical parietal areas and also receive strong projections from the magnocellular system" (p. 19). These researchers concluded that the findings provide evidence for a rate-related *visual processing deficit* lending further support to the "theory of abnormal magnocellular processing in dyslexia" (p. 19).

The central tenet of an *auditory processing limitation* in children with language and reading problems is that neural temporal mechnisms play a critical role in aspects of information processing and production, "and may be especially critical for the normal development and maintenance of sensory motor integration systems as well as phonological systems" (Tallal, 1993, p. ix). Results from a series of studies beginning in the 1970s led Tallal and colleagues to believe that some students with developmental language and reading problems have a "severe developmental deficit in processing brief components of information that enter the nervous system in rapid succession, and a concomitant motor deficit in organizing rapid sequential motor output" (Tallal, Miller, & Fitch, 1993, p. 36). They described this deficit as "highly specific, impinging primarily on neural mechanisms underlying the organization of information within the tens of millisecond range" (p. 36).

Tallal et al. (1993) also reported the results of testing students with language impairment and two groups of students with dyslexia—one with concomitant oral language problems and one without overt, oral language problems. A significant deficit in both nonsense word reading and nonverbal temporal processing was found in the students with dyslexia and concomitant oral language disabilities. "These deficits were highly correlated ($r = 0.81$; $p < 0.001$) in this subgroup" (p. 35). The students with dyslexia without concomitant oral language problems "had neither phonological decoding nor temporal processing deficits in any sensory modality" (p. 35). The research group suggested the underlying temporal deficits cause a cascade of effects, starting with disruption of the normal development of an otherwise effective and efficient phonological system . . . (and) that these phonological processing deficits result in subsequent failure to learn to speak and read normally . . . both the language and reading problems have their basis in deficiently established phonological processing and decoding (p. 27).

Llinas (1993) suggested that an "intrinsic clock"—responsible for controlling the rate of neuronal firing patterns or oscillations—might be impaired in some subjects with language impairment and some with dyslexia. According to Tallal et al. (1993), such neuronal oscillations are hypothesized to be essential for "gating or 'binding' sensory information in cortico–thalamo–cortical networks" (p. 36). A functional result of slowing in these intrinsic oscillation rates of neural firing would be an "inability to process either sensory and/or motor information presented in rapid succession within tens of milliseconds" (p. 36). This is "precisely the deficit" the Tallal group described earlier "for language and reading impaired children having concomitant phonological disorders" (p. 36). Further studies (see Bedi, 1994; and Watson & Miller, 1993) found associations between reading achievement performance in studies of temporal order judgment (TOJ) for brief tones (Brady, 1997, p. 34). Interestingly, Reed's (1989) findings revealed difficulty in reading-disabled students on TOJ involving stop consonants (/ba/-/da/) but not for steady-state vowel (/E/ as in "bed" and /ae/ as in "bat"). This finding was interpreted as "an indication of a general auditory deficit, not one specific to speech" because the processing difficulty affected rapidly changing consonants and tones "but not longer, steady-state items such as vowels" (Brady, 1997, p. 34). Furthermore, work by Mody et al. (1997) revealed difficulties identifying /ba/ and /da/ rapidly result "because of their close phonetic similarity rather than from a deficit in judgments of temporal order itself" (Brady, 1997, p. 34).

Relating her findings to phonological processing, Tallal (1996) hypothesized that the basic deficit in neural processing of brief, transient sensory information leads first to the infant's decreased ability to set up distinctive phonological representations for the sounds of their native language, and secondarily to delayed overall language acquisition. Their difficulty getting to the more finite structures of language, namely syllables, phonemes, and unstressed morphological endings, results in bottom-up processing deficits, and they learn to rely on top-down information processing strategies (pp. 10–11). Merzinich (1996) explained that his research group's studies have convinced them that approximately 15% of children acquire language constructs by "simply taking in integrated sound chunks that extend over the entire period of syllables and storing information about speech using an integrated-based representation, as contrasted with a normal, phoneme-based schema" (p. 3). Because these children develop their alternate schema through "many hundreds of thousands or millions of 'practice events,'" they become "experts at a language representational system that lacks the symbolic representational power of normal, fully competent phonologically-based language" (pp. 3–4). Llinas (1993) concluded:

> Ultimately, dyslexia is a nervous system dysfunction, and as such, must be reducible to problems at a level more basic than that at which it is expressed (behavior), that is, to the realm of neuronal or synaptic malfunction. In addition, the dyschronicity of dyslexia may interfere with rapid processing and could lead to problems with the ability to learn associatively and, therefore, with phonologically learned skills (p. 48).

E.   Selective Attention and Attention Deficit Disorder.

The primary purpose of reading is to obtain the author's intended meaning. To do this, one must proceed through a series of reading skills. The most fundamental of these is the ability to attend selectively to relevant features while ignoring irrelevant stimuli. Selective attention develops with maturation and learning. A lag in its development can contribute to difficulties in reading, writing, and spelling.

Keller (1992) explained that children diagnosed with attention deficit disorder with hyperactivity (ADHD) have difficulty remaining on task and focusing attention. "It is believed that they are distractible both auditorally as well as visually; however, their inability to remain attentive might also cause them to seek out distractions" (p. 108). According to the DSM-IV (1994), the essential feature of ADHD is "a persistent amount of inattention and/or hyperactivity–impulsivity that is more frequent and severe than typically observed in individuals at a comparable level of development" (p. 78).

Attention deficit hyperactivity disorder has been implicated as a contributing factor to specific reading disability and, in many cases, co-occurs with it. Denckla (1993) described subclinical aspects of ADHD as the major contributor to, and the developmental disorder category frequently co-morbid with, cases of "dyslexia-plus." Denckla noted "some aspects of ADHD add to the cognitive profile the deficits of inattention, impulsivity, disorganization, and output-inefficiency" (p. 23). Zentall (1993) found that students with ADHD are more likely to receive lower grades in academic subjects and on standardized reading and math tests than their normally achieving peers. Zentall reported that "more than 80% of 11-year-olds with ADHD were reported behind at least 2 years in reading, spelling, math, or written language . . . (and that) over one-third will fail to finish high school" (p. 143). Moreover, students with ADHD who are in regular classrooms "risk school failure two to three times greater than other children without disabilities but with equivalent intelligence" (Zentall, 1993, p. 143).

F. **Middle Ear Problems.**

Roberts and Medley (1995) defined otitis media as "inflammation of the middle ear" (p. 15). Otitis media with effusion (OME), or serous otitis media, is "when there is fluid in the middle ear that is not infected . . . When there is an infection in the middle ear, the condition is called acute otitis media (AOM)" (p. 15). Klein (1986) noted that most children experience at least one episode of acute otitis media, and some experience severe and recurrent disease (p. 45). Menyuk (1992) reported that otitis media results in a variety of differences in language acquisition during different periods of development and causes consistent delays in acquisition across-the-board between 2 and 3 years of age. Menyuk explained that the following complex aspects of language processing result from early otitis media: attention problems and distractibility affecting the ability to process narratives, problems retrieving morphological endings as distinct from word stems, and deficient confrontation naming and rapid retrieval of lexical items. Roberts and Medley (1995) proposed hearing loss associated with persistent and/or recurrent OME causes the child to receive a partial or inconsistent auditory signal. Auditory information is consequently encoded incompletely and inaccurately into the database from which language develops. "A child may then be at a disadvantage for learning speech and language. This, in turn, may negatively influence later academic achievement, particularly in reading and other language-based subjects. Additionally, a child who hears a decreased or inconsistent auditory signal may tune sound out and become inattentive" (p. 16).

G. **Limited Print Exposure.**

Unfortunately, many children are reared in homes where little emphasis is placed on literacy. In these homes, reading materials are limited or even absent. In many homes that do contain books, families are so rushed with the ever-increasing fast pace of life, there does not seem to be enough hours in the day to incorporate literacy experiences. Add to this the burgeoning number of hours children spend playing video games, "clicking away" on the Internet, and hours spent watching television rather than engaged in reading. For multiple reasons, when looking for causal factors for reading problems, we cannot overlook the consequences of young children being reared in low print or low-print expectation environments. Without early print exposure, children are at a disadvantage when required to learn to read. Catts and Kamhi (1999) suggested the absence of joint book reading during preschool may play a role in reading problems. "A lack of early literacy experience may be particularly detrimental to children with other risk factors. Children from low socioeconomic status backgrounds and/or those with language impairments may be at increased risk for reading disabilities if they have not had home literacy experiences" (p. 97).

1.   **Lower socioeconomic status and literacy.**

Nicholson (1997) summarized a number of studies indicating that children from low-income homes are less likely to do well in school when compared with children from middle-class homes. Factors working against success for low-income students are summarized in Table 3-4.

Table 3-4. A Summary of Factors Working Against Success for Low-Income Students (Nicholson, 1997).

- Needing to help out more at home
- Lack of study facilities
- Attendance at schools that are made up primarily of other students from low-income homes
- Stress and feelings of inadequacy dealing with school is more frequently experienced by low-income parents
- Children from low-income homes tend to start school with less knowledge of rhyme and alliteration
- Middle class families tend to have more books at home
- Parents in middle class homes tend to become more involved in helping their children learn to read than parents in low-income homes (pp. 388–389).

2.   Distractions.

Children spending too much time at computers, playing video games, and watching television represent another group of students who may develop reading problems because they may not be actively engaged in reading. Commenting on the "atmosphere of hysteria " in the rush to "connect even preschoolers to electronic brains" Healy (1998) found that "of the ten best-selling children's CD-ROM titles sold in 1996, four are marketed for children beginning at age three. Furthermore, computer program advertisements range as low as eighteen months" (p. 20). Some of the interesting points contained in Healy's text are summarized below.

Learning on the computer is "far less brain-building" than are spontaneous play or board games with adults or older children. "'Connecting' alone has yet to demonstrate academic value, and some of the most popular 'educational' software may even be damaging to creativity, attention, and motivation" (p. 20).

When interacting with "computer games, programmed learning software, and computer camps," children are "working with external symbols (pictures on a screen) rather than with internal ones (language, mental images)." Contrasting this with the need for interacting with others in developing oral language, Healy warned "cybertots with too much screen time" and too little talking time may develop good thoughts and vocabulary, "but they lack practice in formulating ideas into succinct and meaningful sentences." Healy underscored the pervasiveness of language problems as they affect social relationships, reading, and writing, and "inner speech or self-talk—by which the brain regulates behavior, attention, metacognition, and understanding" (p. 231).

Citing deKerckhove and Lumsden (1987) and Logan (1986), Healy also commented on the resulting changes in brain organization that will occur as the result of computers. "Scientists have observed that even differences between pictorial languages (one form of Japanese writing, for example) and alphabetic scripts of European languages cause physical alterations during brain development" (p. 32). Healy continued "fast-paced, nonlinguistic, and visually distracting television may literally have changed children's minds, making sustained attention to verbal input, such as reading or listening, far less appealing than faster-paced visual stimuli" (p. 32).

Referring to the computer as "edutainment" rather than "educational" Healy also warned about the decreased demands on writing ability. Stoll (1995) cautioned "The computer requires almost no physical interaction or dexterity, beyond the ability to type . . . and demands rote memorization of nonobvious rules. You subjugate your own thinking patterns to those of the computer. Using this 'tool' alters our thinking processes." Furthermore, Stoll pointed out that "learning to depend on a computer when confronted with a problem, we will limit our ability to recognize other solutions, and ultimately degrade our own thinking powers" (as cited by Healy, p. 33).

Noting that reading involves so much more than reciting words or alphabet sounds, Healy explained that it "consists much more of a person's 'habits of mind'—e.g., sustained concentration, language, imagery, (and) questioning strategies" (p. 234). Finally, older students apparently can perform better on the mechanics of reading (not comprehension) after using computer "drill-and-practice software." Younger children, however, do not fare as well. "In one study children using very popular reading software drill-and-practice (disguised as games with reward screens) demonstrated a *50 percent drop in their creativity scores*" (p. 234).

H. Cognitive Rigidity and Learned Helplessness.

Possibly as the result of one or more of the above factors, many students with developmental reading disabilities display cognitive rigidity that slows information retrieval. Clay (1984) suggested that students with reading disabilities have stopped making appropriate responses, and instead, rigidly specialize in particular types of responses, many of which, are ineffective.

Because any of the contributing factors discussed may interfere with the normal, developmental progression of reading acquisition, a child may enter school unprepared for the materials and approaches used in the regular curriculum. Coles (1987) cautioned that children get caught in a web of unwarranted expectations. He maintained that learning and reading disabilities may result when the school's erroneous expectations and teaching methods are out of sync with the child's acquisition of prerequisite abilities. Failure in the classroom can lead students to become passive learners, and soon they are unengaged in the learning process. It is easy, then, to see why students increase their dependency on learned helplessness. In a vicious cycle of failure, how frequently our students answer questions with the same one or two ways they usually answer, and if these do not work, there is always the roll of the shoulders with a grunt indicating "I don't know." Bransford, Delclas and Bristow (1985) proposed that the passivity observed in poor readers is tied to inappropriate materials that frustrate students and repeated failure leads to learned helplessness. Stanovich (1994) explored the effects of early educational success on reading achievement. He coined the term "Matthew Effect," relating to the biblical passage in the Book of Matthew: "For unto every one that hath shall be given, and he shall have abundance; but from him that hath not shall be taken away even that which he hath" (XXXV:29) (p. 281). Stanovich explained that, because children with minimal phonological awareness ability have trouble learning the alphabetic principle, their word recognition skills are slow and hinder reading comprehension. Unrewarding reading experiences lead to fewer reading-related activities. Limited exposure and practice then further delay the speed and accuracy of word recognition. Reading for meaning is reduced and as negative reading experiences multiply, "practice is avoided or merely tolerated without real cognitive involvement, and the negative spiral of cumulative disadvantage and failure continues. Troublesome emotional side effects begin to be associated with school experiences, and these become a further hindrance to school achievement" (p. 281). Furthermore, Stanovich (2000) explained how Matthew effects can eventually lead to a pattern where poor readers develop increasingly global cognitive deficits. "The existence of Matthew effects raises the startling possibility that a young dyslexic might actually develop into a garden-variety poor reader!" (p. 118).

Gerber (1993) described factors contributing to students' learning problems. These turn into a "vicious spiral with cumulative negative impact on the individual with learning disabilities" (p. 268). Whether one specific cause can be pinpointed or a combination of contributing factors lead to a student's academic problems, it is likely that children with language-related learning disabilities "enter the educational experience ill-equipped to meet the language and learning demands of the classroom" (p. 268). See Table 3-5 for Gerber's "Failure cycle"

V. SUMMARY

This chapter has included information on three types of developmental reading disabilities: dyslexia, generalized reading problems, and hyperlexia. Current research was presented as to the recognized phonological processing and naming speed problems characteristic of dyslexia and generalized reading problems. The increasingly popular description of

Table 3-5. Gerber's (1993) "Failure Cycle."

I. Linguistic deficits are important determinants of reading disability and auditory verbal learning problems in education.

2. Difficulties in processing the linguistically encoded information transmitted in education are major causes of academic failure.

3. Academic failure reflects and contributes to a reduced knowledge base in both semantic and general information.

4. Academic failure results in low self-esteem and fear of further failure.

5. An impoverished knowledge base, possible constraints on information processing capacity, and a sensed inadequacy, individually or in combination, interfere with the development and efficient use of effective learning strategies. The inactive or inefficient learner is more subject to distractibility and response impulsivity.

6. Failure to actively employ effective information processing strategies reduces the probability of academic success.

7. Repeated experiences of academic failure and persistent reading disability are attributed by the student to an intrinsic inability to succeed.

8. Learned helplessness reduces motivation and effort, with a resultant decreased probability of present and future academic success, continued impoverishment of the knowledge base, and failure to master basic skills (pp. 268-269).

developmental reading problems as having single deficits (phonological awareness or rapid naming speed problems) or double deficits (both phonological awareness and rapid naming speed problems) were included to provide readers with another way of conceptualizing and classifying developmental reading problems. The common causes and consequences of developmental reading disabilities were discussed under the following headings: oral language problems (see Chapters 1 and 2); heredity; neural basis; nervous system timing problems; selective attention and attention deficit disorder; middle ear problems, and limited print exposure. Consequences of developmental reading disabilities including cognitive rigidity, learned helplessness, and the downward spiral of failure were briefly considered. Chapter 4 will examine the important issues surrounding assessment of development reading disabilities. Assessing to probe the phonological processing and naming speed cores will be discussed with suggested tasks and tests to use.

VI. CLINICAL COMPETENCIES.

To understand the nature of developmental reading disabilities the teacher/clinician/student will demonstrate the following competencies:

A. **Identify three subtypes of developmental reading disability: developmental dyslexia, garden variety reading problem, and hyperlexia.**

B. **Understand the relationship between phonological processing and reading.**

C. **Understand the relationship between verbal naming speed and reading.**

D. **Identify single- and double-deficit reading problems.**

E. **Know about the causes and consequences of developmental reading disabilities.**

CHAPTER

4

Assessment of Developmental Reading Disabilities

OUTLINE

I.   INTRODUCTION

In their guidelines for the "roles and responsibilities of speech–language pathologists with respect to reading and writing in children and adolescents," the American Speech–Language–Hearing Association (2001) stated:

> Speech–language pathologists "have a primary role in both early identification of literacy problems and in the identification of literacy difficulties among older students . . . Early identification may take place during the preschool years or after formal reading instruction has begun, but before children become discouraged and enter the cycle of failure" (p. 6).

Because of the heterogeneity of symptoms presented by children with developmental reading disabilities, it is simply *not possible* to generate *the* perfect assessment battery to be used in all cases. In Chapter 3 a myriad of oral and written language problems commonly observed in children diagnosed with developmental dyslexia or generalized reading problems was presented, as well as what typifies core deficits in single and double-deficit reading problems. Traditionally, reading ability is assessed after reading instruction has begun, and typically a referral for assessment of reading performance in a student *suspected* of having problems is not done until the problem is fairly noticeable (See Cody's and Shannon's stories in Chapter 1). The problem with this approach, beyond how it negatively influences developing self-esteem, is that it *totally ignores* the oral–written language continuum. As explained in Chapter 2, learning to read does not begin when oral language development ends. Oral language must be considered the foundation from which written language emerges. Reading and writing are integral parts of general language acquisition wherein the developing skill provides the scaffold for the other. To adequately define the nature of a written language problem, the underlying oral language must also be evaluated. Before turning to symptoms and assessment tools, let us look at four typical scenarios surrounding referrals of children with possible oral–written language problems.

Scenario #1: The referring teacher, parent or other concerned individual states: "No, this student doesn't really have a reading problem per se. She's just not following what's going on in the classroom." (See the discussion later in this chapter on "assessment of the phonological processor.") While this student may not present with blatant problems, an underlying phonological processing problem may be causing confusion in following classroom discourse. If this is the case, there may be other subtle language problems with which this student presents, for instance in taking messages, repeating sequences of words, verbally producing or repeating multisyllabic words, immature syntax, word finding problems, circumlocution, nonspecific word use, and/or decreased vocabulary. **This student *needs* language assessment. She may be *at-risk* for oral and written language problems.**

Scenario #2: The referring teacher, parent or other concerned individual states: "No, this student doesn't really have a reading problem. He is just reading slower than the other students in the class. And you know, boys are just slower. He'll surely outgrow this." (See the discussion in Chapter 3 about "the need for fluency in reading.") While this student may not present with blatant reading problems, an underlying problem in the phonological processor may be causing him to have problems holding words in short-term memory long enough to access their meaning from long-term memory, or, difficulty with phonological awareness may be hampering this student's ability to manipulate words, syllables, onset-rimes, and/or sounds. Difficulty with orthographic processing may reveal itself as a timing problem in reading, so this student is not able to "name" the printed words or sublexical word parts as rapidly as needed for print to make sense to him. A reading comprehension problem may be growing. **This student *needs* a language assessment.** Slow reading rate may have a domino effect, and **this student is *at-risk* for reading comprehension problems.**

Scenario #3: The referring teacher, parent or other concerned individual states: "Yes this student is showing some reading problems. She isn't decoding well and relies on contextual cues way too much. But it's only second grade and I think with extra homework in reading every night she'll pick up the pace. Maybe the third grade teacher will refer her for help." **This student *needs* a language assessment.** (See the discussion in Chapter 3 under "downward spiral of failure.") Sitting in the classroom day after day struggling with reading aloud in front of peers is, at the very least, humiliating. And "more of the same" won't help the problem. If there is an underlying language problem, this student's reading performance will not improve significantly enough with "just more practice reading."

Scenario #4: The referring teacher, parent or other concerned individual states: "Oh yes indeed! This student has fallen hopelessly behind and now it's the fourth grade! It's probably just too late. Let's just teach him survival reading skills. It's too bad everyone waited so long to refer him." **This student** *needs* **a language assessment.** Yes, it is too bad this student was not referred for help before the fourth grade. By now he probably has major academic problems because reading across the curriculum has suffered, and vocabulary has not grown at the rate it should. Unfortunately, this student may dislike reading so much by now he may never read for pleasure. But there's good news. If the various aspects of the underlying oral language problem are correctly identified, the written language problem can be defined, delimited, and treated. This student will more than likely still need some fundamental work in phonological awareness and naming speed. It will then be necessary to select books of high interest and low readability to build his reading skills, vocabulary level, writing skills, and confidence.

II. ASSESSING FOUR PROCESSORS INVOLVED IN READING

Assessing the many aspects of developmental reading disabilities can seem daunting. To impose an overall structure to the many components that must be considered, Adams' (1990) model is revisited here. (See Chapter 2 to review the analysis of subcomponents of reading.) According to Adams' model, we can consider four broad areas, or processors, that must work together efficiently to be successful in reading: phonological, orthographic, meaning, and context. As Adams explained "the four processors work together, continuously receiving information from and returning feedback to each other . . . Within each of these processors, knowledge is represented by interconnected sets of simpler units" (p. 21). A brief review of these processors follows.

A. The Phonological Processor.

The phonological processor contains "a complexly associated array of primitive units. The auditory image of any particular word, syllable, or phoneme corresponds to the activation of a particular, interconnected set of those units" (p. 157). As noted in the definitions presented in Chapter 3, the ability to form and mentally hold strong phonological representations while we process and/or verbally produce language, decode the printed form of our language, and/or encode to produce the written form of our language is critical.

B. The Orthographic Processor.

The orthographic processor involves the visual information from the printed page. Orthographic processing is "the ability to form, store, and access orthographic representations" (Stanovich, West & Cunningham, 1991, p. 220.) This processor is important for the reader to store individual letters as well as sublexical word parts (-ing) and letter patterns (-at).

C. The Meaning Processor.

The meaning processor stores familiar word meanings "as interassociated sets of more primitive meaning elements" (Adams, 1990, p. 143). Rather than storing self-contained meaning "nodes," Adams suggested that the reader's understanding of a word, for example, "dog," would be represented as "the interassociated distribution of properties that collectively represent the person's total history, direct and vicarious, of experiences with dogs" (p. 143).

D. The Context Processor.

The context processor, as described by Adams, is "in charge of constructing a coherent, ongoing interpretation of the text. As it does so, it sends excitation to units in the meaning processor according to their compatibility with its expectations" (p. 138). While the ability to use context to facilitate word recognition is considered "relatively low" (Stanovich 2000), it must be considered in the assessment formula. Each of the four processors will be considered in the next four sections.

As we found in Chapter 3, at least two core deficits underly language-based reading problems: phonological processing and verbal naming speed. To assess the phonological core, we must assess the many areas that can affect a student's ability to: 1) use the phonological code to hold sounds and words in memory; 2) use the phonological code in phonological awareness; 3) use the phonological code in verbal output; 4) use the phonological code in word retrieval. To assess the verbal naming speed core, we must assess the areas that can affect a student's: 5) verbal naming speed.

These five areas are critical to the assessment of developmental reading disabilities. However, as oral and written language skills develop, their scaffolding produces a network of intertwining abilities. How do we go about unraveling this network? To delineate the many vectors of a language-based reading problem, numerous areas will be presented. Stated differently, the oral language base of a reading problem can contaminate many areas. To assess only the most visible aspects of a student's problem, for instance, word attack, letter-word identification, and spelling, would be short-sighted. To fully remediate a language-based reading problem, the true nature of the underlying causes must be defined. Like a French braid, the strands of phonological, orthographic, meaning, and context processors become part of the developing problem at different times during reading acquisition. To illustrate how processor problems will impact reading and writing, Figure 4-1 depicts how the phonological and orthographic processors are the first to become involved, followed by the impact that all four processors have on reading and writing.

To more fully understand the impact that each processor has on reading acquisition, the following four sections present language domains affected by each processor.

PHONOLOGICAL PROCESSOR	ORTHOGRAPHIC PROCESSOR	MEANING PROCESSOR	CONTEXT PROCESSOR
To assess student's ability to use the phonetic code to hold sounds and words in memory, assess: • auditory discrimination • auditory temporal pattern recognition/use • auditory figure ground selection • auditory selective attention • auditory memory • auditory integration (closure, synthesis) • simple receptive language • listening comprehension • verbal repetition	To assess student's ability to use the orthographic processor, assess: • visual-perceptual-motor • verbal naming speed		

Figure 4-1. Areas to Assess Under the Four Processors of Reading.

PHONOLOGICAL PROCESSOR	ORTHOGRAPHIC PROCESSOR	MEANING PROCESSOR	CONTEXT PROCESSOR
To assess student's ability to use the phonological code in phonological awareness, assess: • phonological awareness at the word level • phonological awareness at the syllable level • phonological awareness at the onset-rime level • phonological awareness at the phoneme level			
To assess student's ability to use the phonological code in oral language (verbal output), assess: • oral vocabulary • syntax/morphology • oral narrative skills • saying complex words • phonological processes			
To assess student's ability to use the phonological code in word retrieval, assess: • word finding • word finding in discourse			
To assess student's ability to use the phonological code in reading, assess: • phonological awareness • word attack (decoding)	To assess student's ability to use the orthographic processor in reading, assess: • letter-word identification • verbal naming speed	To assess student's ability to use the meaning processor in reading, assess: • reading comprehension: word level • reading comprehension: sentence/paragraph level	To assess student's ability to use the context processor in reading, assess: • use of contextual cues

Figure 4–1. Areas to Assess Under the Four Processors of Reading (continued).

PHONOLOGICAL PROCESSOR	ORTHOGRAPHIC PROCESSOR	MEANING PROCESSOR	CONTEXT PROCESSOR
To assess student's ability to use the phonologic, orthographic, meaning and context processors in reading, assess: • word attack (decoding) • letter-word identification • reading fluency: accuracy, rate, prosody			
To assess student's ability to use the phonologic, orthographic, meaning and context processors in writing, assess: • written narrative skills • vocabulary used in writing • written syntax/morphology • spelling • capitalization/punctuation • writing fluency • proofing			

Figure 4-1. Areas to Assess Under the Four Processors of Reading (continued).

III. PHONOLOGICAL PROCESSING AND ORAL–WRITTEN LANGUAGE

The relationship among phonological processing, oral language, and written language was discussed in Chapter 2. Phonological processing is a general ability or compilation of independent abilities. To impose some order onto the vast array of vectors emanating from the umbrella term "phonological processing," I chose to follow the description by Wagner and Torgesen (1987) separating coding/retrieval from phonological awareness (Figure 4–2).

A. Description of Coding/Retrieval Levels and Phonological Awareness in Oral–Written Language with Corresponding Symptoms of Problems.

Think of the umbrella term as "phonological processing" and its relation to oral-written language. Follow first its many vectors through **coding/retrieval**.

1. Level 1: Phonetic coding/recoding.
In oral language, this refers to translating the acoustic signal to speech; saying letters, numbers, sounds, and words to oneself; and holding speech in short-term memory. To better understand

the discussion of assessment of the phonological processor, some thoughts as to how auditory processing and phonological awareness relate will help clarify the division of suggested goals below.

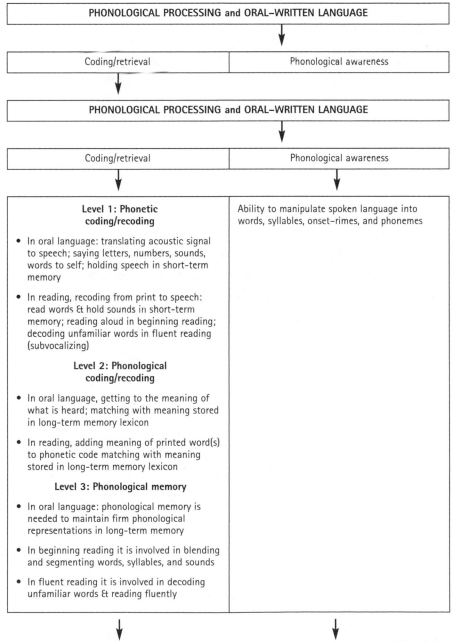

Figure 4-2. Phonological Processing and Oral-Written Language.

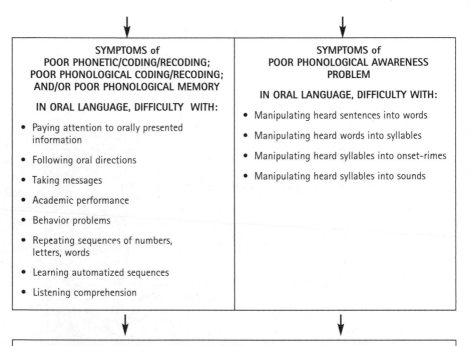

SYMPTOMS of
POOR PHONETIC/CODING/RECODING;
POOR PHONOLOGICAL CODING/RECODING;
AND/OR POOR PHONOLOGICAL MEMORY

IN ORAL LANGUAGE, DIFFICULTY WITH:

- Paying attention to orally presented information
- Following oral directions
- Taking messages
- Academic performance
- Behavior problems
- Repeating sequences of numbers, letters, words
- Learning automatized sequences
- Listening comprehension

SYMPTOMS of
POOR PHONOLOGICAL AWARENESS
PROBLEM

IN ORAL LANGUAGE, DIFFICULTY WITH:

- Manipulating heard sentences into words
- Manipulating heard words into syllables
- Manipulating heard syllables into onset-rimes
- Manipulating heard syllables into sounds

SYMPTOMS OF THE COMBINED EFFECT OF POOR PHONETIC/CODING/RECODING;
POOR PHONOLOGICAL CODING/RECODING;
POOR PHONOLOGICAL MEMORY, AND POOR PHONOLOGICAL AWARENESS

IN ORAL LANGUAGE, DIFFICULTY WITH:

- Using a variety of vocabulary
- Using mature syntax & morphology
- Cohesive story formulation/retell
- Word finding
- Firm lexical representations. Produces some words differently even within same sentence (curious, curis: petified, pretified, petrified)
- Saying complex words (bingle jells, besketti, evelator, renember)
- Phonological processes

IN READING, DIFFICULTY WITH:

- Decoding
- Letter-word identification
- Holding read words in short-term memory
- Getting to the meaning of printed words through matching phonologically recoded forms with meanings stored in long-term memory lexicon
- Holding onto accessed word meanings (the word's meaning was accessed but faded)
- Reading comprehension
- Reading fluency

Figure 4–2. Phonological Processing and Oral–Written Language.

**SYMPTOMS OF THE COMBINED EFFECT OF POOR PHONETIC/CODING/RECODING;
POOR PHONOLOGICAL CODING/RECODING;
POOR PHONOLOGICAL MEMORY, AND POOR PHONOLOGICAL AWARENESS**

IN WRITING, DIFFICULTY WITH:

- Written narrative abilities
- Range of words used in written formulation
- Syntax and morphology
- Spelling
- Capitalization/punctuation
- Writing fluency
- Proofing

Figure 4-2. Phonological Processing and Oral-Written Language.

In his discussion of thinking and cognition, Benson (1994) explained that thinking "represents the activities of a number of diverse, precisely interrelated nervous system functions that process thought contents" (p. 5). While thought content represents "data received and accumulated by the individual, thought processing involves "acts of receiving, perceiving, comprehending, storing, manipulating, monitoring, controlling, and responding to the steady stream of data" (p. 5). Benson pointed out that thought processing "demands interrelationships" among the following nine functional systems, many of which are involved in responding to the steady stream of input data: sensory (visual, auditory, tactile), motor, basic mental control, emotion/autonomic, memory, visual imagery, language, cognition, and higher mental control (p. 25). Auditory processing abilities comprise one of the functional systems engaged in *ongoing activity* during thought processing. In essence, it is always occurring as the brain recognizes and interprets heard sounds, and it functions at a lower level than phonological awareness. Central auditory processing is "what we do with what we hear" (Katz, Stecker, & Henderson, 1992, p. 4).

Benson further explained that cognition, which is one step in the process of thinking, "is the process by which information is manipulated in the brain" (p. 5). Phonological awareness is *not an ongoing activity*. Phonological awareness is a cognitive, metalinguistic activity, which Gombert (1992) described as comprising: 1) "activities of reflection on language and its use," and 2) "subjects' ability intentionally to monitor and plan their own methods of linguistic processing in both comprehension and production" (p. 13). Auditory processing is ongoing and, for the most part, nonintentional. The higher level phonological awareness occurs when the subject intentionally reflects upon language and language parts as if they were physical objects to be manipulated. To decipher the fundamental phonetic/phonological nature of a developmental reading disability, it may be necessary to assess the auditory processing abilities including auditory discrimination, auditory temporal/time processing, auditory figure ground selection, auditory selective attention, auditory memory, and auditory integration.

In reading, the reader recodes print into speech. Stated differently, the reader sees print, converts this to speech sounds, and holds these sounds in short-term memory.

2.   **Level 2: Phonological coding/recoding.**

In oral language, this refers to getting to the meaning of what is heard by matching the heard message with meanings stored in one's long-term memory lexicon.

In reading, the reader gets to the meaning of the phonetic code (the word or words the reader has decoded from print and is temporarily storing in short-term memory) by matching the sounds with word meanings stored in one's long-term memory lexicon.

3.   **Level 3: Phonological memory.**

In oral language phonological memory is needed to maintain firm phonological representations in long-term memory. *In beginning reading* phonological memory is needed for blending and segmenting words. *In fluent reading* it is involved in decoding unfamiliar words and reading fluency.

4.   **Symptoms of poor phonetic coding/recoding; phonological coding/recoding; and/or phonological memory in oral language.**

   a. **Difficulty paying attention to information presented orally**

   b. **Difficulty processing information presented orally**

   c. **Difficulty following oral directions**

   d. **Difficulty taking messages**

e. Low academic performance

f. Behavior problems

g. Difficulty repeating sequences of numbers, letters, or words

h. Difficulty learning automatized sequences

i. Decreased listening comprehension

B. Description of Phonological Awareness.

Now, recall the umbrella term "phonologcal processing" and its relation to oral–written language. See Figure 4–3 to follow its many vectors through *phonological awareness*.

1. **Level 1: Phonological awareness at the word level.**
   In oral language, phonological awareness at this level is the ability to segment/break a sentence heard into words. *In reading*, phonological awareness at this level is the ability to segment/break a printed sentence into words.

2. **Level 2: Phonological awareness at the syllable level.**
   In oral language, phonological awareness at this level is the ability to segment words heard into syllables. *In reading*, phonological awareness at this level is the ability to segment printed words into syllables.

3. **Level 3: Phonological awareness at the onset–rime level.**
   Researchers including Treiman and Zukowski (1991) found that "syllable awareness is easier than onset–rime awareness and that onset–rime awareness is in turn easier than phoneme awareness" (p. 76).

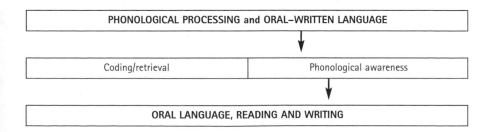

Figure 4-3. Phonological Processing and Oral-Written Language: Phonological Awareness.

In oral language, phonological awareness at this level is the ability to segment syllables heard into sublexical units: initial sound or sounds, that is, onset, and the remaining part of the word, that is, rime. Onsets can consist of one or more sounds: "pl" is the onset and "ay" is the rime in "play;" "c" is the onset and "at" is the rime in "cat."

In reading, phonological awareness at this level is the ability to segment printed syllables into initial letter or letters (graphemes) and the remaining sublexical word part, then associate them with corresponding sounds (phonemes).

4. **Level 4: Phonological awareness at the phoneme level.**

    In oral language, phonological awareness at this level is the ability to segment syllables heard into individual sounds. *In reading*, phonological awareness at this level is the ability to segment printed syllables into individual letters (graphemes) and associate them with corresponding sounds (phonemes).

5. **Symptoms of poor phonological awareness in oral language.**

    a. **Poor at tasks manipulating heard sentences into words.**

    b. **Poor at tasks manipulating heard words into syllables.**

    c. **Poor at tasks manipulating heard syllables into onset and rime.**

    d. **Poor at tasks manipulating heard syllables into individual sounds.**

C. The Combined Effect

Recall again the umbrella term "phonological processing" and its relation to oral–written language. Follow Figure 4-4 now to see the *combined effect* that coding/retrieval *and* phonological awareness has on oral language, reading, and writing.

1. **Oral Language Difficulty.** Symptoms of poor phonetic coding/retrieval, poor phonological coding/recoding, poor phonological memory, and poor phonological awareness on oral language.

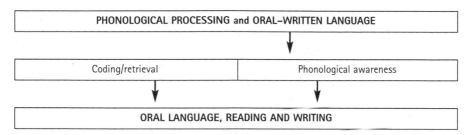

Figure 4-4 Phonological Processing and Oral-Written Language: The Combined Effect of Coding/Retrieval and Phonological Awareness.

a. Decreased variety of vocabulary

b. Immature syntax and morphology

c. Stories lack cohesiveness; difficulty with story formulation and retell

d. Word finding problems

e. Underspecified lexical representation. Produces some words differently even within same sentence (curious, curis, petified, pretified, petrified)

f. Reverses sounds in words (bingle jells, besketti, evelator, renember)

g. Phonological processes/deviations, a.k.a. expressive phonological disorder

2. Reading Difficulty.

Symptoms of poor phonetic coding/recoding, poor phonological coding/recoding, poor phonological memory, and poor phonological awareness in reading.

a. Poor decoding or word attack abilities

b. Poor letter–word identification abilities

c. Difficulty holding read words in short-term memory

d. Difficulty getting to the meaning of printed words through matching phonologically recoded forms with meanings stored in long-term memory lexicon

e. Difficulty holding onto accessed word meanings, that is, the word's meaning was accessed but faded

f. Poor reading comprehension caused either by one or both of the above two symptoms

g. Poor reading fluency

3. Writing Difficulty.

Symptoms of poor phonetic coding/recoding, poor phonological coding/recoding, poor phonological memory, and poor phonological awareness in writing.

a. Decreased oral narrative abilities

b. Decreased range of words to use in written formulation

c. Immature syntax in writing

d. Poor spelling

e. Poor capitalization and punctuation

f. Decreased writing fluency

g. Decreased proofing

IV. ASSESSMENT OF THE PHONOLOGICAL PROCESSOR

Published assessment tools are only named under the various sections. Specific information about the tests can be found at the end of this chapter.

A. Poor phonetic coding/recoding, poor phonological coding/recoding, and/or poor phonological memory in oral language

If student demonstrates any of the following:
Difficulty paying attention to information presented orally
Difficulty processing information presented orally
Difficulty following oral directions
Difficulty taking messages
Low academic performance
Behavior problems
Difficulty repeating sequences of numbers, letters, or words
Difficulty learning automatized sequences
Decreased listening comprehension

Domains to consider assessing: phonetic coding/recoding, receptive language, and verbal repetition

1. Phonetic Coding/Recoding (Auditory Processing)

a. Auditory discrimination:

to determine if an underlying auditory processing problem results in a student's confusing similar sounds or words spoken. See Table 4-1 for some suggested tests for assessing auditory discrimination.

Table 4-1. Some Suggested Tests for Assessing Auditory Discrimination.

- *Wepman Auditory Discrimination Test—Second Edition*
- *Carrow Auditory–Visual Abilities Test: Auditory Discrimination in Quiet and Auditory Discrimination in Noise* subtests (CAVAT)
- *Goldman–Fristoe–Woodcock Test of Auditory Discrimination*
- *Lindamood Auditory Conceptualization Test* (LAC)
- *Test of Auditory–Perceptual Skills Revised* (TAPS-R) and *Test of Auditory–Perceptual Skills Upper Level* (TAPS-UL): Auditory Word Discrimination subtest
- *Test of Language Development—P:3* (TOLD-P:3): Word Discrimination subtest

b. Auditory temporal patterning:

to determine if an underlying auditory temporal/timing problem in pattern recognition and use affects the student's ability to follow a list of directions/instructions, confuses number sequences (hears "forty-nine for "ninety four"), misarticulates words such as deleting sounds (says "pay" for "play'), substitutes sounds (says "goodnitch" for "goodness," or not sure where one word ends and the next one begins, for instance: "jabe nimbe jabe quick jajumoer canletick" (Lucker & Wood, 2000). See Table 4-2 for some suggested tests for assessing auditory temporal patterning.

Table 4-2. Some Suggested Tests for Assessing Auditory Temporal Patterning.

- *Lindamood Auditory Conceptualization Test* (LAC)
- *Test of Auditory–Perceptual Skills—Revised* (TAPS-R)
- *Test of Auditory–Perceptual Skills—Upper Level* (TAPS-UL)
- Ask the student to tell you or to repeat nursery rhymes or tongue twisters
- Ask the student to repeat increasingly complex words

c. Auditory figure–ground:

to determine if an underlying auditory processing problem involving the ability to correctly select what is said orally from a background of competing sounds. See Table 4-3 for some suggested tests for assessing auditory figure–ground.

Table 4-3. Some Suggested Tests for Assessing Auditory Figure–Ground.

Administer any test and check student's performance when items are administered without background noise compared with performance on items administered in the presence of background noise.

d. Auditory selective attention:

to determine if an underlying auditory processing problem affects the student's ability to select relevant information and filtering out irrelevant information presented orally. See Table 4-4 for some suggested tests for assessing selective attention.

Table 4-4. Some Suggested Tests for Assessing Auditory Selective Attention.

Informal assessment of whether the student is able to recognize relevant auditory stimuli against a background of competing sounds. Ask the student to answer questions or follow increasingly complex directions while playing audiotaped cafeteria noise, for instance, in the background.

e. **Auditory memory:**

to determine if an underlying auditory processing problem affects the student's ability to remember what was heard such as following directions or the important points presented by the teacher during class. See Table 4-5 for some suggested tests for assessing auditory memory.

Table 4-5. Some Suggested Tests for Assessing Auditory Memory.

- *Carrow Auditory–Visual Abilities Test:* (CAVAT): Picture Memory, Picture Sequence Selection, Digits Forward, and Digits Backward, Sentence Repetition, and Word Repetition subtests

- *Clinical Evaluation of Language Fundamentals—3:* (CELF-3): Oral Commands subtest

- *Detroit Test of Learning Aptitude—4:* (DTLA-4): Reversed Letters and Word Sequences subtests

- *Lindamood Auditory Conceptualization Test* (LAC)

- *Language Processing Test—Revised* (LPT-R)

- Repeating nursery rhymes or automatized lists such as the days of the week, months of the year, alphabet

- *Test of Auditory Perceptual Skills—Revised* (TAPS-R) and *Test of Auditory–Perceptual Skills—Upper Level:* (TAPS-UL): Auditory Number Memory–Forward, Auditory Number Memory–Reversed, Auditory Sentence Memory, Auditory Word Memory, and Auditory Interpretation of Directions subtests

- *Test of Language Development—P:3* (TOLD-P:3): Sentence Imitation subtest

- *Test of Language Development—Intermediate* (TOLD-I:3): Sentence Combining subtest

- *Test of Memory and Learning:* Memory-for-Stories, Objects Recall, Digits Forward/Backward subtests

- *Ross Information Processing Assessment—Primary* (RIPA-P)

- *Token Test for Children*

- *Woodcock–Johnson III Tests of Cognitive Abilities:* Subtests of Working Memory

f. Auditory integration (auditory closure, binaural integration, or auditory synthesis)

to determine if an underlying auditory processing problem affects the student's ability to combine pieces of information and form a whole message. See Table 4-6 for some suggested tests for assessing auditory integration.

Table 4-6. Some Suggested Tests for Assessing Auditory Integration.

- Present the student with only pieces of a message, for instance, some words of a known nursery rhyme, and see if the student can put the pieces together to form the whole.

- Possible referral to physician to determine if the student has ADD or ADHD

- Possible referral to audiologist to determine if the student has a central auditory processing problem

2. Receptive Language Abilities

a. Simple Receptive Language:

to determine if an underlying phonological processing problem affects the student's ability to understand at the simple single-word level. See Table 4-7 for some suggested tests for assessing simple receptive language.

Table 4-7. Some Suggested Tests for Assessing Simple Receptive Language.

- *Assessing Semantic Skills Through Everyday Themes* (ASSET): Identifying Labels, Identifying Categories, Identifying Attributes, Identifying Functions, Identifying Definitions subtests
- *Boehm Test of Basic Concepts—3* (BOEHM-3)
- *Boehm Test of Basic Concepts—3: Preschool* (BOEHM-P:3)
- *Comprehensive Receptive and Expressive Vocabulary Test—2* (CREVT-2)
- *Fluharty—2:* Following directives and answering questions
- *Peabody Picture Vocabulary Test—3rd Edition* (PPVT-3)
- *Peabody Individual Achievement Test* (PIAT-R/NU): General Information
- *Preschool Language Scale—3* (PLS-3)
- *Receptive One-Word Vocabulary Test—2000 Edition* (ROWVT)

Table 4-7. Some Suggested Tests for Assessing Simple Receptive Language (continued).

- *Test of Early Language Development—3* (TELD-3)
- *Test of Language Development—Primary:3* (TOLD-P:3): Picture Vocabulary subtest
- *Test of Language Development—Intermediate:3* (TOLD-I:3): Picture Vocabulary subtest
- *Woodcock Language Proficiency Battery—Revised* (WLPB-R): Picture Vocabulary subtest

b. Listening Comprehension:

to determine if an underlying phonological processing problem affects the student's ability to understand more complex language. See Table 4-8 for some suggested tests for assessing listening comprehension.

Table 4-8. Some Suggested Tests for Assessing Listening Comprehension.

- *Basic Reading Inventory*
- *Burns—Roe Informal Reading Inventory:* Listening Comprehension subtest
- *Clinical Evaluation of Language Fundamentals—Preschool* (CELF-P)
- *Clinical Evaluation of Language Fundamentals—3* (CELF-3): Concepts and Directions, Semantic Relationships, and Listening to Paragraph subtests
- *Comprehensive Assessment of Spoken Language* (CASL): Nonliteral Language, Meaning from Context, Inference, Ambiguous Sentences, and Pragmatic Judgment subtests
- *Oral—Written—Listening Language Scales* (OWLS): Listening Comprehension Scales
- *Peabody Individual Achievement Test* (PIAT-R/NU): General Information
- *Test for Auditory Comprehension of Language—3rd Edition* (TACL-3)
- *Test of Auditory—Perceptual Skills—Revised* (TAPS-R) and *Test of Auditory—Perceptual Skills—Upper Level* (TAPS-UL): Interpretation of Directions and Auditory Processing (Thinking and Reasoning) subtests
- *Test of Auditory Reasoning and Processing Skills* (TARPS)
- *Test of Early Language Development—3rd Edition* (TELD-3)
- *Test of Language Development—Intermediate:3* (TOLD-I:3): Malapropisms subtest
- *Token Test for Children*
- *Woodcock Diagnostic Reading Battery:* Listening Comprehension subtest

Table 4–8. Some Suggested Tests for Assessing Listening Comprehension (continued).

- *Woodcock–Johnson III Tests of Cognitive Abilities* (WJIII): Verbal Comprehension, General Information, Concept Formation, Analysis–Synthesis, and Planning subtests

- *Woodcock Language Proficiency Battery–Revised* (WLPB-R): Listening Comprehension subtest

3. Verbal Repetition:

to determine the student's ability to use the phonological code to store information presented auditorally. See Table 4-9 for some suggested tests for assessing verbal repetition.

Table 4–9. Some Suggested Tests for Assessing Verbal Repetition.

- *Clinical Evaluation of Language Fundamentals–3* (CELF-3): Recalling Sentences subtest

- *Fluharty–2:* Repeating Sentences

- *Detroit Tests of Learning Aptitude–4* (DTLA-4): Sentence Imitation and Word Sequences subtests

- *Test of Language Development–Primary:3* (TOLD-P:3): Primary: Sentence Imitation subtest

- *Test of Auditory Perceptual Skills–Revised* (TAPS-R): Auditory Number Memory–Forward, Auditory Number Memory–Reversed, Auditory Sentence Memory, and Auditory Word Memory subtests

- *Woodcock Language Proficiency Battery–Revised* (WLPB-R): Memory for Sentences subtest

- *Woodcock Diagnostic Reading Battery:* Memory for Sentences

B. Poor phonological awareness in oral language

If student demonstrates any of the following:
Difficulty manipulating sentences into words
Difficulty manipulating words into syllables
Difficulty manipulating syllables into onsets and rimes
Difficulty manipulating syllables into sounds

Domains to consider assessing: the areas listed in A above (poor phonetic coding/recoding: auditory processing), *and* phonological awareness at the word, syllable, onset–rime, and phoneme levels.

1. **Phonological Awareness at the Word Level:**
   to determine the student's ability to use the phonological code to manipulate words in the speech stream.

2. **Phonological Awareness at the Syllable Level:**
   to determine the student's ability to use the phonological code to manipulate words at the syllable level.

3. **Phonological Awareness at the Onset–Rime Level:**
   to determine the student's ability to use the phonological code to manipulate words at the onset and sublexical unit level.

4. **Phonological Awareness at the Sound Level:**
   to determine the student's ability to use the phonological code to manipulate syllables at the sound level. See Table 4-10 for some suggested tests for assessing phonological awareness.

Table 4-10. Some Suggested Tests for Assessing Phonological Awareness.

- *Comprehensive Test of Phonological Processing* (CTOPP): Phonological awareness and Phonological memory subtests
- *Illinois Test of Psycholinguistic Abilities–3* (ITPA:3): Sound Deletion and Rhyming subtests
- *Lindamood Auditory Conceptualization Test* (LAC)
- *Phonological Awareness Test* (PAT)
- *Phonological Awareness Skills Program* (PASP)
- *Pre-Literacy Skills Screening* (PLSS): Phonological Awareness
- *Test of Auditory Analysis Skills* (TAAS): See Appendix A
- *Woodcock Diagnostic Reading Battery:* Incomplete Words and Sound Blending subtests

C. **Poor phonetic coding/recoding; poor phonological coding/recoding; poor phonological memory, and poor phonological awareness in oral language**

If student demonstrates any of the following:
Decreased variety of vocabulary
Immature syntax and morphology
Stories lack cohesiveness; difficulty with story formulation and retell
Word finding problems
Underspecified lexical representation. Produces some words differently even within same sentence (curious, curis, petified, pretified, petrified)
Reverses sounds in words (bingle jells, besketti, evelator, renember)
Phonological processes/deviations, aka expressive phonological disorder

Domains to consider assessing: the areas listed in A (poor phonetic coding/recoding: auditory processing) and B (poor phonological awareness) above, *and* oral vocabulary, syntax and morphology, oral narrative ability, word finding, saying complex words, and phonological processes

1.   **Oral Vocabulary:**

to determine if the student's use of the phonological code results in adequate vocabulary development. See Table 4-11 for some suggested tests for assessing oral vocabulary.

Table 4-11. Some Suggested Tests for Assessing Oral Vocabulary.

* *Assessing Semantic Skills through Everyday Themes* (ASSET): Stating Labels, Stating Categories, Stating Attributes, Stating Functions, Stating Definitions subtests

* *Clinical Evaluation of Language Fundamentals—3* (CELF-3): Semantic Relationships and Word Associations subtests

* *Comprehensive Assessment of Spoken Language* (CASL): Comprehension of Basic Concepts, Antonyms, Synonyms, Sentence Completion, and Idiomatic Language subtests

* *Comprehensive Receptive and Expressive Vocabulary Test—2* (CREVT-2)

* *Detroit Tests of Learning Aptitude—4* (DTLA-4): Word Opposites and Basic Information subtests

* *Expressive One-Word Picture Vocabulary Test—2000 Edition* (EOWPVT)

* *Fluharty—2:* Describing Actions

* *Illinois Test of Psycholinguistic Abilities—3* (ITPA-3): Spoken Vocabulary subtest

Table 4-11. Some Suggested Tests for Assessing Oral Vocabulary (continued).

- *Pre-Literacy Skills Screening:* Naming

- *Test for Auditory Comprehension of Language—3rd Edition* (TACL-3): Vocabulary subtest

- *Test of Language Development—Primary:3* (TOLD-P:3): Picture Vocabulary, Relational Vocabulary, and Oral Vocabulary subtests

- *Test of Language Development—Intermediate:3* (TOLD-I:3): Generals, Malapropisms, Relational Vocabulary, and Oral Vocabulary subtests

- *Woodcock Language Proficiency Battery—Revised* (WLPB-R): Oral Vocabulary and Verbal Analogies subtests

- *Word Test—Elementary:R*

- *Word Test—Adolescent*

2. Syntax and Morphology:

to determine if the student uses the phonological code to understand and verbally produce sentences with correct order and grammatic markers. See Table 4-12 for some suggested tests for assessing syntax and morphology.

Table 4-12. Some Suggested Tests for Assessing Syntax and Morphology.

- *Clinical Evaluation of Language Fundamentals—3* (CELF-3): Word Structure, Formulated Sentences, and Sentence Assembly subtests

- *Comprehensive Assessment of Spoken Language* (CASL): Syntax Construction, Paragraph Comprehension of Syntax, Grammatical Morphemes, Sentence Comprehension of Syntax, and Grammaticality Judgment subtests

- *Fluharty—2:* Sequencing Events

- *Illinois Test of Psycholinguistic Abilities—3* (ITPA-3): Morphological Closure, Syntactic Sentences, and Story Sequences subtests

- *Structured Photographic Expressive Language Test—II* (SPELT-II)

- *Structured Photographic Expressive Language Test—II:* Primary (SPELT-II:P)

- *Test for Auditory Comprehension of Language—3rd Edition* (TACL-3): Grammatical Morphemes and Elaborated Phrases and Sentences subtests

- *Test for Examining Expressive Morphology* (TEEM)

- *Test of Adolescent & Adult Language—3* (TOAL-3)

Table 4-12. Some Suggested Tests for Assessing Syntax and Morphology (continued).

- *Test of Early Language Development—3* (TELD-3)

- *Test of Language Development—Primary:3* (TOLD-P:3): Grammatic Understanding subtest

- *Test of Language Development—Intermediate:3* (TOLD-I:3): Word Ordering, Grammatic Comprehension, Grammatic Understanding, and Grammatic Completion subtests

3. Oral Narrative Skills:

to determine if the student uses the phonological code to produce a cohesive story with essential elements and in sequence. See Table 4-13 for some suggested tests for assessing oral narrative skills.

Table 4-13. Some Suggested Tests for Assessing Oral Narrative Skills.

- *Dynamic Assessment and Intervention; Improving Children's Narrative Abilities*

- *Detroit Tests of Learning Aptitude—4* (DTLA-4): Story Construction subtest

- Informal assessment of narrative abilities. Ask the student to retell a story, TV program, movie or to give directions to make something or directions to a geographical location known to both of you

- *Test of Pragmatic Language* (TOPL)

4. Word Finding Abilities:

to determine if the student uses the phonological code to store and retrieve verbal labels. See Table 4-14 for some suggested tests for assessing word finding abilities.

Table 4-14. Some Suggested Tests for Assessing Word Finding Abilities.

- *Comprehensive Assessment of Spoken Language* (CASL): Antonyms, Sentence Completion, and Idiomatic Language subtests

- *Test of Adolescent Adult Word Finding* (TAWF)

- *Test of Word Finding—Second Edition* (TWF-2)

- *Test of Word Finding in Discourse* (TWFD)

5. **Saying Complex Words:**

to determine the student's use of the phonological code in verbal output of complex words. See Table 4-15 for some suggested tests for assessing verbal production of complex words.

Table 4-15. Some Suggested Tests for Assessing Verbal Production of Complex Words.

* Naming pictures of objects with complex names, for example, "aluminum."
  Possible source: *Adapting 40,000 Selected Words* or sources on apraxia with lists of complex words

* *Pre-Literacy Skills Screening: Multisyllabic Word Repetition*

* Reading words with complex names

* *Assessment of Phonological Processes—Revised* (APP-R): naming multisyllabic pictures

6. **Phonological Processes:**

to determine if the student uses the phonological code to reduce the use of phonological processes at age-appropriate times. See Table 4-16 for some suggested tests for assessing phonological processes.

Table 4-16. Some Suggested Tests for Assessing Phonological Processes.

* *Assessment Link Between Phonology and Articulation* (ALPA)

* *Assessment of Phonological Processes—Revised* (APP-R)

* *Khan–Lewis Phonological Analysis* (KLPA)

* *Bankson–Bernthal Test of Phonology*

D. **Poor phonetic coding/recoding, poor phonological coding/recoding, poor phonological memory and poor phonological awareness in reading**

If student demonstrates any of the following:
  Poor decoding or word attack abilities
  Poor letter–word identification abilities

Difficulty holding read words in short-term memory

Difficulty getting to the meaning of printed words through matching phonologically recoded forms with meanings stored in long-term memory lexicon

Difficulty holding onto accessed word meanings, that is, the word's meaning was accessed but faded

Poor reading comprehension caused either by one or both of the above two symptoms

Poor reading fluency

Domains to consider assessing: the areas listed in A, B, C above *and* word attack (decoding), letter–word identification, reading comprehension, reading fluency

1.   **Word Attack (Decoding):**

to determine if the student uses the phonological code to make sound–symbol associations. See Table 4-17 for some suggested tests for assessing word attack.

Table 4-17. Some Suggested Tests for Assessing Word Attack.

- *Decoding Skills Test* (DST)

- *Illinois Test of Psycholinguistic Abilities–3* (ITPA-3): Sight Decoding and Sound Decoding subtests

- *Woodcock Language Proficiency Battery–Revised* (WLPB-R): Word Attack subtest

- *Woodcock Reading Diagnostic Battery:* Word Attack subtest

- *Woodcock Reading Mastery Tests–Revised:* Word Attack subtest

2.   **Letter–Word Identification:**

to determine if the student uses the phonological code to facilitate recognition of printed letters and words. See Table 4-18 for some suggested tests for assessing letter-word identification.

Table 4-18. Some Suggested Tests for Assessing Letter–Word Identification.

- *Basic Reading Inventory*
- *Burns-Roe Informal Reading Inventory:* Word Recognition subtest
- *Peabody Individual Achievement Test:R* (PIAT-R/NU): Reading Recognition
- *Slosson Oral Reading Test—Revised* (SORT-R)
- *Woodcock Language Proficiency Battery—Revised* (WLPB-R): Letter–Word Identification subtest
- *Woodcock Diagnostic Reading Diagnostic Battery:* Letter–Word Identification subtest
- *Woodcock Reading Mastery—R/NU:* Letter Identification and Word Identification subtests

3. **Reading Comprehension:**

to determine if the student uses the phonological code to facilitate understanding what is read. See Table 4-19 for some suggested tests for assessing reading comprehension.

Table 4-19. Some Suggested Tests for Assessing Reading Comprehension.

- *Basic Reading Inventory*
- *Burns Roe Informal Reading Inventory*
- *Gray Oral Reading Tests—Fourth Edition* (GORT-4)
- *Nelson–Denny Reading Test CD-ROM:* Vocabulary and Reading Comprehension
- *Peabody Individual Achievement Test R/NU* (PIAT-R/NU): Reading Comprehension
- *Qualitative Reading Inventory* (QRI)
- *Test of Early Reading Ability: 3rd Edition* (TERA-3)
- *Test of Reading Comprehension—Third Edition* (TORC-3)
- *Woodcock Language Proficiency Battery—Revised* (WLPB-R): Reading Vocabulary and Passage Comprehension subtests
- *Woodcock Reading Diagnostic Battery:* Reading Vocabulary and Passage Comprehension subtests
- *Woodcock Reading Mastery Tests—Revised:* Passage Comprehension subtest

4. **Reading Fluency:**

to determine if the student uses the phonological code to facilitate reading accurately, with adequate speed and prosody. See Table 4-20 for some suggested tests for assessing reading fluency.

Table 4–20. Some Suggested Tests for Assessing Reading Fluency.

- *Gray Oral Reading Tests—Fourth Edition* (GORT-4)

- *Gray Silent Reading Tests* (GSRT)

- Informal assessment of student's reading rate: available through school district

- Informal assessment of student's prosody when reading, that is, how words are appropriately chunked together to facilitate comprehension

- *Nelson–Denny Reading Test* CD–ROM: Reading Rate

- *Qualitative Reading Inventory* (QRI)

- *Test of Word Reading Efficiency* (TOWRE)

- *Verbal Naming Speed:* (see section VI.A.2 under Orthographic processor)

- *Informal Testing:*
  To determine a student's reading accuracy, divide the number of words read correctly by the total number of words in the passage. As a rule of thumb, the following headings and percent accuracy are helpful in determining the relationship between reading fluency and reading comprehension.

  Independent reading: 97–100% accuracy = good/excellent comprehension

  Instructional: 96–94% accuracy = good/satisfactory comprehension

  Frustrational: 93% accuracy and below =unsatisfactory/poor comprehension

Meyer and Felton (1999) explained that the most common way to assess fluency is to measure oral reading rate per minute. They noted that satisfactory fluency in first graders is 30–50 words per minute. Hasbrouck and Tindal (1992) presented the following range of fluency standards that can be used to help evaluate students' reading for placement into reading groups and for appropriate selection of reading materials:

Grade	Fall word count per minute	Winter word count per minute	Spring word count per minute
2	53–82	78–106	94–124
3	79–107	93–123	114–142
4	99–125	112–133	118–143
5	105–126	118–143	128–151

Meyer and Felton (1999) described two additional ways to assess fluency: 1) Counting the number and length of pauses; and 2) Rating phrasing, fluency, and expression of oral reading.

Finally, these researchers suggested that "given the escalating demands for reading skills in our technological society, it is critical that researchers and practitioners focus on fluency as an important component of reading instruction" (p. 284).

E. **Poor phonetic coding/recoding; poor phonological coding/recoding, poor phonological memory, and poor phonological awareness in writing**

If student demonstrates any of the following:
   Decreased written narrative skills
   Decreased range of words to use in written formulation
   Immature syntax and morphology in writing
   Poor spelling
   Poor capitalization/punctuation
   Decreased writing fluency
   Decreased proofreading abilities

Domains to consider assessing: the areas listed in A, B, C, D above, *and* written narrative, vocabulary, syntax/morphology in writing, spelling, capitalization/punctuation, writing fluency, and proofing.

1. **Written Narrative Skills:**

   to determine if the student uses the phonological code to produce a cohesive story with essential elements and in sequence in writing. See Table 4-21 for some suggested tests for assessing written narrative skills.

Table 4-21. Some Suggested Tests for Assessing Written Narrative Skills.

- see section IVC.3 above for oral narrative assessment
- *Burns–Roe Informal Reading Inventory*
- *Dynamic Assessment & Intervention:* Improving Children's Narrative Abilities
- *Oral and Written Language Scales* (OWLS): Written Expression
- *Peabody Individual Achievement Tests—R/NU* (PIAT-R/NU): Written Expression
- *Slosson Written Expression Test:* Composition for sentence length and type–token ratio
- *Test of Early Written Language—2* (TEWL-2): Contextual Writing subtest for story format, cohesion, thematic maturity, ideation, and story structure
- *Test of Written Language—3:* Story Construction
- *Woodcock Language Proficiency Battery–Revised* (WLPB-R): Writing Samples subtest
- *Woodcock–Johnson Tests of Achievement—R:* Writing Sample

2.   Vocabulary:

to determine if the student uses the phonological code to develop adequate vocabulary skills to facilitate reading comprehension. See Table 4-22 for some suggested tests for assessing written vocabulary skills.

Table 4-22. Some Suggested Tests for Assessing Written Vocabulary Skills.

- *Oral and Written Language Scales* (OWLS): Written Expression
- *Test of Written Language—3* (TOWL-3): Contrived format: Vocabulary and Sentence Combining subtests
- *Test of Adolescent & Adult Language—3:* Writing/Vocabulary subtest

3.   Syntax and Morphology:

to determine if the student uses the phonological code to develop adequate grammatical strings and markers for written language formulation. See Table 4-23 for some suggested tests for assessing written syntax and morphology skills.

Table 4-23. Some Suggested Tests for Assessing Written Syntax and Morphology Skills.

- *Oral and Written Language Scales* (OWLS): Written Expression

- *Test of Early Written Language—2nd edition* (TEWL-2): Basic Writing subtest for sentence construction and metacognitive knowledge

- *Test of Adolescent & Adult Language—3:* Writing/Grammar subtest

- *Test of Written Language—3* (TOWL-3): Contrived formats: Sentence Combining

- *Woodcock Language Proficiency Battery—Revised* (WLPB-R): Writing Samples subtest

- *Woodcock—Johnson Tests of Achievement—R:* Usage

4. **Spelling:**

to determine if the student uses the phonological code to facilitate spelling during written language formulation. See Table 4-24 for some suggested tests for assessing spelling skills.

Table 4-24. Some Suggested Tests for Assessing Spelling.

- See Ball: Appendix A

- *Illinois Test of Psycholinguistic Abilities—3* (ITPA-3): Sight Spelling and Sound Spelling subtests

- *Oral and Written Language Scales* (OWLS): Written Expression Scale

- *Peabody Individual Achievement Test—R/NU* (PIAT-R/NU): Spelling

- *Slosson Written Expression Test* (SWET): Spelling

- *Test of Early Written Language—2nd edition* (TEWL-2): Basic Writing subtest for spelling

- *Test of Written Language—3* (TOWL-3): Contrived format: Spelling

- *Test of Written Spelling—4th Edition* (TWS-4)

- *Woodcock—Johnson Tests of Achievement—R* (WLPB-R): Spelling

- *Woodcock Language Proficiency Battery—Revised* (WLPB-R): Dictation subtest

5. **Capitalization/Punctuation:**

to determine if the student uses the phonological code to use correct capitalization and punctuation in written language formulation. See Table 4-25 for some suggested tests for assessing capitalization/punctuation.

Table 4-25. Some Suggested Tests for Assessing Capitalization/Punctuation.

- *Oral and Written Language Scales* (OWLS): Written Expression
- *Slosson Written Expression Test* (SWET): Capitalization/Punctuation
- *Test of Early Written Language—2nd Edition* (TEWL-2): Basic Writing subtest for capitalization and punctuation
- *Test of Written Language—3* (TOWL-3): Style
- *Woodcock—Johnson Tests of Achievement—R:* Dictation and Punctuation & Capitalization subtests

6. Writing Fluency:

to determine if the student uses the phonological code to facilitate fluency during written language formulation. See Table 4-26 for some suggested tests for assessing writing fluency.

Table 4-26. Some Suggested Tests for Assessing Writing Fluency.

- *Woodcock Language Proficiency Battery—R:* Writing Fluency subtest
- *Woodcock—Johnson Tests of Achievement—R:* Writing Fluency subtest

7. Proofing:

to determine if the student uses the phonological code to facilitate proofing during written language formulation. See Table 4-27 for some suggested tests for assessing proofing skills.

Table 4-27. Some Suggested Tests for Assessing Proofing Skills.

- *Test of Written Language—3:* Logical Sentences
- *Woodcock Language Proficiency Battery—Revised* (WLPB-R): Proofing subtest
- *Woodcock—Johnson Tests of Achievement—R:* Proofing subtest

V. SUMMARY OF DOMAINS TO ASSESS UNDER PHONOLOGICAL PROCESSOR

A. **Poor phonetic coding/recoding, poor phonological coding/recoding, and poor phonological memory in oral language**

1. Phonetic coding/recoding (auditory processing)

   a. Auditory discrimination

   b. Auditory temporal patterning

   c. Auditory figure-ground

   d. Auditory selective attention

   e. Auditory memory

   f. Auditory integration (closure, synthesis)

2. Receptive Language Abilities

   a. Simple receptive language

   b. Listening comprehension

3. Verbal repetition

B. **Poor phonological awareness in oral language**

1. Phonological awareness at the word level

2. Phonological awareness at the syllable level

3. Phonological awareness at the onset–rime level

4. Phonological awareness at the phoneme level

C. Poor phonetic coding/recoding; poor phonological coding/recoding; poor phonological memory, and poor phonological awareness in oral language

1. Oral vocabulary

2. Syntax and morphology

3. Oral narrative skills

4. Word finding abilities

5. Saying complex words

6. Phonological processes

D. Poor phonetic coding/recoding; poor phonological coding/recoding; poor phonological memory, and poor phonological awareness in reading

1. Word attack (decoding)

2. Letter–word identification

3. Reading comprehension

4. Reading fluency

E. Poor phonetic coding/recoding; poor phonological coding/recoding; poor phonological memory, and poor phonological awareness in writing

1. Written narrative skills

2. Vocabulary

3. Syntax and morphology

4. Spelling

5. Capitalization/punctuation

6. Writing fluency

7. Proofing

VI. ASSESSMENT OF THE ORTHOGRAPHIC PROCESSOR

Recalling that the orthographic processor deals with visual print, we turn from phonological processing to consider the visual aspects of assessment. At this point, we are assuming an intact visual system, that is to say, adequate visual acuity, even if glasses are worn for reading. We are now interested in knowing how well the student uses the print on the page. How adept is the reader at seeing/naming letters, at grouping sublexical word parts, for example, "-at" or "-og?" How is the reader able to focus his/her vision on the printed line being read? Mather (2001) defined orthographic awareness as the "rapid and accurate formation of letter images, letter strings, or word images in memory."

Furthermore, we learned in Chapter 3, that because naming speed and reading both require the student to automatically retrieve a verbal match for an abstract visual form, Wolf (1999) described naming speed as a "mini, multicomponential version of reading" (p. 12). In this view, naming speed uses the same visual, auditory, and motor processes used in reading but in a less complex fashion. Naming and reading, therefore, represent "two levels of rapid, precise integration of cognitive systems, a basic level and a more complex level" (Wolf, 1997, p. 85). Problems in the more basic system, naming speed, warn us of future weaknesses in the later developing system, reading, possibly even causing the reading problem (p. 86). "Thus, naming speed provides us with a deceptively simple, extraordinarily useful, early window on some developing disabilities in the reading systems" (p. 86). Slow naming speed will necessarily have an impact on reading rate, reading fluency, and, therefore, reading comprehension.

Think of the umbrella term as "visual–verbal naming speed" and its relation with written language. See Figure 4-3 to follow its vectors through naming speed, reading rate, reading prosody, and reading fluency.

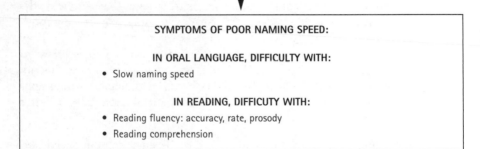

VISUAL-VERBAL NAMING SPEED and WRITTEN LANGUAGE

Level 1: Naming speed
- In oral language: the ability to rapidly name objects or pictured stimuli
- In reading: the ability to rapidly "name" printed words and to recognize sublexical word parts (e.g., "at" in "cat)

Level 2: Reading fluency:
includes reading accuracy, speed and prosody (grouping words during reading)

SYMPTOMS OF POOR NAMING SPEED:

IN ORAL LANGUAGE, DIFFICULTY WITH:
- Slow naming speed

IN READING, DIFFICUTY WITH:
- Reading fluency: accuracy, rate, prosody
- Reading comprehension

Figure 4-5. Visual-Verbal Naming Speed and Written Language.

A. Slow visual–verbal naming speed

If student demonstrates any of the following:
Slow naming object and pictures
Slow reading fluency
Poor reading comprehension

Domains to consider assessing: visual perceptual/motor skills, verbal naming speed, reading fluency, and reading comprehension

1. Visual/Perceptual/Motor Abilities:

to determine if the student has adequate visual–motor skills for reading and writing. See Table 4-28 for some suggested tests for assessing visual/perceptual/motor abilities.

Table 4-28. Some Suggested Tests for Assessing Visual/Perceptual/Motor Abilities.

- *Carrow Auditory–Visual Abilities Test* (CAVAT): Visual Discrimination Matching, Visual Discrimination Memory, Visual–Motor Copying, and Visual–Motor Memory subtests

- *Detroit Tests of Learning Aptitude–4* (DTLA-4): Design Sequences, Reversed Letters, and Design Reproduction subtests

- *Developmental Test of Visual–Motor Integration*

- *Developmental Test of Visual Perception–2nd Edition* (DTVP:2)

- *Test of Visual-Perceptual Skills–Revised* (TVPS-R)

- *Test of Visual–Motor Skills–Revised* (TVMS-R)

- *Woodcock–Johnson III Tests of Cognitive Abilities* (WJIII): Visual Matching, Decision Speed, Pair Cancellation, Spatial Relations, Picture Recognition, and Planning subtests

2. **Verbal Naming Speed:**

to determine if the student has adequate naming speed to facilitate reading and written language formulation. See Table 4-29 for some suggested tests for assessing verbal naming speed.

Table 4-29. Some Suggested Tests for Assessing Verbal Naming Speed.

- *Clinical Evaluation of Language Fundamentals–3* (CELF-3): Word Associations and Rapid Automatic Naming subtests

- *Comprehensive Test of Phonological Processing* (CTOPP): Rapid Automatized Naming subtests

- *Woodcock–Johnson III Tests of Cognitive Abilities* (WJIII): Rapid Picture Naming subtest

3. **Reading Fluency:**

to determine if the student's verbal naming speed facilitates reading accurately, with adequate speed and prosody. See Table 4-30 for some suggested tests for assessing reading fluency.

Table 4-30. Some Suggested Tests for Assessing Reading Fluency.

• see section IV.D.4 under phonological processor section: Reading Fluency
• see section VI.A.2 under orthographic processor section: Verbal Naming Speed

4. **Reading Comprehension:**

to determine if the student naming speed problem contributes to understanding what is read. See Table 4-31 for some suggested tests for assessing reading comprehension.

Table 4-31. Some Suggested Tests for Assessing Reading Comprehension.

• see section IV.D.3 under phonological processor section: Reading Comprehension.

VII. SUMMARY OF DOMAINS TO ASSESS UNDER ORTHOGRAPHIC PROCESSOR

A. Slow visual-verbal naming speed

1. **Visual perceptual/motor abilities**

2. **Verbal naming speed**

3. **Reading fluency**

4. **Reading comprehension**

VIII. ASSESSMENT OF THE MEANING PROCESSOR

We learned in Chapter 2 that Adams' proposed meaning processor is responsible for storing familiar word meanings. Repeated exposure to printed words in various contexts facilitates the student's ability to learn and store the word's meaning. Adams wrote "the likelihood that a child will learn the meaning of a word from a single exposure in meaningful context ranges between 5% and 20%. By implication, the extent of such incidental vocabulary acquisition depends strongly on the amount a child reads" (Stahl, et al., 1990, p. 28).

A. Combined effect of poor phonetic/coding/recoding; poor phonological coding/recoding; poor phonological memory, and poor phonological awareness

If student has difficulty with any of the following:
Poor reading comprehension
Slow reading rate

Domains to consider assessing: vocabulary, prior knowledge, and reading fluency

1. Vocabulary:

to determine if the student's vocabulary facilitates reading comprehension and written language formulation. See Table 4-32 for some suggested tests for assessing vocabulary.

Table 4-32. Some Suggested Tests for Assessing Vocabulary.

* see section IV.C.1 under phonological processor above: Oral Vocabulary

2. Prior knowledge:

to determine if the student's prior knowledge of the topic facilitates reading comprehension. See Table 4-33 for some suggested tests for assessing prior knowledge.

Table 4-33. Some Suggested Tests for Assessing Prior Knowledge.

* ask the student questions about the passage to be read

* *Qualitative Reading Inventory:* Oral Free Association task

3. **Reading fluency:**

to determine if the student's verbal naming speed facilitates reading accurately, with adequate speed and prosody. See Table 4-34 for some suggested tests for assessing reading fluency.

Table 4–34. Some Suggested Tests for Assessing Reading Fluency.

• see phonological processor section IV.D.4 above: Reading fluency

IX. SUMMARY OF DOMAINS TO ASSESS UNDER MEANING PROCESSOR

A. Vocabulary

B. Prior knowledge

C. Reading fluency

X. ASSESSMENT OF THE CONTEXT PROCESSOR

Adams (1990) described the *context processor* as being "in charge of constructing a coherent, ongoing interpretation of the text. As it does so, it sends excitation to units in the meaning processor according to their compatibility with its expectations" (p. 138). Adams suggested that highly predictable context increases the amount of excitation contributed by the context processor, while weakly predictive context does not.

A. **Combined effect of poor phonetic/coding/recoding; poor phonological coding/recoding; poor phonological memory, and poor phonological awareness**

If student has difficulty with any of the following:
    Poor reading comprehension
    Slow reading rate
Domains to consider assessing: use of context

1. **Use of Context:**

    to determine if the student's use of context facilitates reading comprehension. See Table 4-35 for some suggested tests for assessing use of context.

Table 4-35. Some Suggested Tests for Assessing Use of Context.

*   *Basic Reading Inventory*

*   *Burns-Roe Informal Reading Inventory*

*   *Decoding Skills Test* (DST)

*   *Qualitative Reading Inventory* (QRI)

XI. SUMMARY OF DOMAINS TO ASSESS UNDER CONTEXT PROCESSOR

A. Use of context

XII. PUTTING IT TOGETHER: PRACTICAL ASPECTS

When I first outlined topics for this book, a section on "Subtypes of Reading Disability" was included to facilitate the reader's understanding of the various characteristics of reading disability. When a myriad of subtypes emanating from various classification systems emerged in the literature (see, for example, Hooper & Willis, 1989), I realized the futility of this endeavor. Furthermore, factors such as when the problem was diagnosed, resources available for help, differences in teaching methods, and so on contribute to a "patchwork quilt" profile that is as unique as each student. Although there are similarities in performance profiles among students with reading disabilities, no two profiles will ever be identical.

Thus, I believe that efficient assessment and smooth transition into teaching is expedited by general guidelines that assist the practitioner in navigating the course of decision-making. To that end, the approach presented here is a clinical–inferential classification system that groups individuals into homogeneous clusters based on similarities in their performance profiles.

The procedure I recommend for assessing developmental reading disabilities combines static and dynamic assessment. Rather than identifying a single test battery, I suggest using components of both standardized and nonstandardized tests. These components were selected according to the following rationale: recommended in published research; my experience with them; and the relative ease with which they can be administered, scored, and interpreted. As mentioned previously, standardized tests may be used to determine qualification or entry criteria needed in various work settings. For further evaluation of specific skills, I suggest that test batteries be taken apart and selected subtests be administered when appropriate. In settings that require rigid qualification scores, it may not be necessary or useful to administer complete static test batteries.

A. Performance profiles suggesting dyslexia.

In Chapter 3, two different approaches to describing/categorizing developmental reading disabilties were presented. The first approach is to differentiate between developmental dyslexia and garden variety reading problems. According to this schema, a reader with the following characteristics would be described as having *developmental dyslexia.*

> May be average or poor in the following: auditory sequencing, auditory discrimination, auditory memory, verbal repetition, oral vocabulary, syntax and morphology, phonological awareness, oral narrative, word finding, saying complex words, phonological processes, verbal naming, letter–word identification, word attack (decoding), reading comprehension at the sentence/paragraph level, reading fluency, visual/perceptual/motor, written narrative skills, written syntax and morphology, spelling, capitalization/ punctuation, and proofing.

> May be average or above in the following: simple receptive language and listening comprehension.

B. Performance profiles suggesting generalized reading problems.

A student who demonstrates the following characteristics suggests a *generalized reading problem* that caused deficits in decoding and reading comprehension.

May be average or poor in the following: auditory sequencing, auditory discrimination, auditory memory, simple receptive language, listening comprehension, verbal repetition, oral vocabulary, syntax and morphology, phonological awareness, oral narrative, word finding, saying complex words, phonological processes, verbal naming, letter–word identification, word attack (decoding), reading comprehension at the sentence/paragraph level, reading fluency, visual/perceptual/motor, written narrative skills, written syntax and morphology, spelling, capitalization/punctuation, and proofing.

When first comparing the two profiles, one is struck with the similarity in the number of areas affected by the underlying oral language problem. Unlike the student with dyslexia, however, the student with generalized reading problems presents with more pervasive language problems. These may include more receptive and expressive language problems typical of students with language-learning problems (see discussion of language characteristics of language-learning disabled students in Chapter 3.) The student with developmental dyslexia typically demonstrates average to above-average abilities in listening comprehension reflecting good knowledge of the world and good use of cognitive/linguistic schema. Is the profile of a student with generalized reading problems more severe than that of the dyslexic student presented above? Not necessarily. The student with a phonological core problem may present with a more severe reading problem than the student with generalized reading problems. Because the student's reading is limited, vocabulary development slows, which thwarts the dyslexic student's expanding vocabulary. It is, therefore, helpful to consider the second system for classifying developmental reading problems, namely, single versus double-deficit problems.

C. **Performance profiles that suggest single or double-deficit core(s) underlying developmental disabilities.**

The double-deficit hypothesis, which considers rapid naming problems to result from faulty timing mechanism, includes four reading groups (Figure 4-6) (see Wolf et al., 1999; Wolf 1998; Bowers & Wolf, 1993).

1. The *average reader* presents with intact naming speed, phonological decoding and reading comprehension.

2. The reader with intact naming speed and impaired reading comprehension caused by *diminished phonological awareness* has a single deficit problem.

	Naming Speed	Phonological Awareness	Reading Comprehension
1. Average Reader:	Intact	Intact	Intact
SINGLE DEFICITS			
2. Rate Problem	Problem	Intact	Problem
3. Phonological Awareness (P.A.) Problem	Intact	Problem	Problem
DOUBLE DEFICIT			
4. Rate & P.A. Problems	Problem	Problem	Problem

Figure 4–6. Four Reading Groups. *Source:* Bowers and Wolf (1993); Wolf (1998)

3. Likewise, the reader with intact phonological awareness and impaired reading comprehension caused by *slower naming speed* has a single-deficit problem.

4. The reader whose reading comprehension is impaired because of *both impaired phonological awareness and naming speed* has a double-deficit and is the most severely impaired reader ("treatment resister").

Wolf (1997) concluded that the double-deficit hypothesis offers a way to examine the heterogenity of developmental reading problems and is particularly important because of the potential for new treatment directions (see Chapters 4 and 5 for discussion of intervention). "By directing our attention to dual emphases on phonological processes and automaticity/fluency skills, we may well increase our effectiveness for a greater number of our at-risk children" (p. 86).

Finally, I find the "short-cut" characteristic differences between the two reading groups in Table 4-36 to be helpful.

Table 4-36. Characteristic Differences Between Developmental Dyslexia and Generalized Reading Problem Types.

Profile: Developmental Dyslexia

- Listening comprehension: at or above grade level
- Word identification: poor
- Word attack and spelling: poor
- Poor phonological awareness or slow naming speed: single deficit
- Poor phonological awareness and slow naming speed: double deficit

Profile: Generalized Reading Problem

- Listening comprehension: at or below grade level
- Word identification: poor
- Word attack and spelling: poor
- Poor phonological awareness or slow naming speed: single deficit
- Poor phonological awareness and slow naming speed: double deficit
- Lower overall oral language skills

XII. SUMMARY

I pointed out early in this chapter that assessing the many aspects of developmental reading disabilities can seem daunting. As with so many areas in child language, the unsurmountable can be surmounted with a strategic plan to guide the process. Using Adams' (1990) approach considering four processors in reading helps to set the theoretical backdrop needed to strategically work through assessing developmental reading disabilities. Working from this foundation, we saw that to assess the phonological core of the reading problem we must assess the many areas that can impact a student's ability to:

use the phonological code to hold sounds and words in memory
use the phonological code in phonological awareness
use the phonological code in verbal output
use the phonological code in word retrieval

To assess the verbal naming speed core, we must assess the areas that can affect a student's:

verbal naming speed

Then, working from these five primary areas, this chapter focused on how to tease out the various language domains that must be assessed to clearly define and delimit the mulitvaried problems inherent in developmental reading disabilities. The speech–language specialist is in a key position to identify early and later literacy problems. Understanding the oral–written language continuum is the basis for planning and implementing an effective assessment for identifying potential literacy problems as well as identifying the many aspects inherent in language based reading problems.

Having completed the discussion on assessment, issues relevant for teaching/remediating, including activities for the phonological, orthographic, meaning and context processors will be presented in Chapters 5 and 6. Suggested activities and materials will be recommended in appendices for Chapters 5 and 6.

XIV. CLINICAL COMPETENCIES.

To perform the assessment of developmental reading disabilities the teacher/clinician/student will demonstrate the following competencies:

A. Select appropriate assessment tools for the phonologic, orthographic, meaning, and context processors operating in development reading disabilities.

B. Identify the performance profiles of developmental dyslexia and generalized reading problems.

C. Differentiate differences among four reading groups based on naming speed, phonological awareness, and reading comprehension.

XV. INFORMATION ON TESTS SUGGESTED IN THIS CHAPTER

Test: *Adapting 40,000 Selected Words*
Authors: Blockcolsky, V.D., Frazer, J.M., & Frazer, D.H. (1998)
Age Range: children and adults
Available Through: Academic Press
Test Description: This book is a sourcebook of words sorted by consonant sounds in the English language, arranged by the number of syllables.

Test: *Assessing Semantic Skills through Everyday Themes* (ASSET)
Authors: Barrett, M., Zachman, L., & Huisingh, R. (1988)
Age Range: 3–9 years
Available Through: LinguiSystems
Test Description: This tool assesses receptive and expressive semantics in preschool and early elementary children.

Test: *Assessment Link between Phonology and Articulation*
Author: Lowe, R.J. (1995)
Age Range: 3:0–8:11 years
Available Through: Speech & Language Resources
Test Description: This tool assesses a subject's phonetic inventory through a traditional sound-in position analysis, and deviant use of phonological processes.

Test: *Assessment of Phonological Processes—Revised* (APP-R)
Author: Hodson, B.W. (1986)
Age Range: 3–12 years
Available Through: Pro-Ed
Test Description: The APP-R identifies a student's use of phonological processes.

Test: *Bankson–Bernthal Test of Phonology*
Authors: Bankson, N.W., & Bernthal, J.E. (1990)
Age Range: 3–9 years
Publisher: Applied Symbolix, Inc.
Available Through: Pro-Ed
Test Description: This tool assesses auditory discrimination in quiet and noise.

Test: *Basic Reading Inventory*

Author: Johns, J.L. (2001)

Grades: pre-primer–8th grade

Available Through: Kendall/Hunt Publishing Company

Test Description: This tool measures word identification and reading comprehension to determine the student's reading level including 6 levels: independent reading level, instructional reading level, frustration level, strategies for word identification, strengths and weaknesses in comprehension, and listening level.

Test: *Boehm Test of Basic Concepts—Third Edition* (BOEHM-3)

Author: Boehm, A. E. (2000)

Grades: K–2

Available Through: Pro-Ed

Test Description: This tool measures 50 basic concepts most frequently occurring in K–2 grade curricula.

Test: *Boehm Test of Basic Concepts, Preschool Third Edition* (BOEHM-3 Preschool)

Author: Boehm, A. E. (2000)

Grades: Preschool

Available Through: Pro-Ed

Test Description: This tool measures basic relational concepts.

Test: *Burns–Roe Informal Reading Inventory*

Authors: Burns, & Roe, B.D. (1998)

Grade Range: K–12

Available Through: Riverside Publishing

Test Description: This tool assesses reading and offers quantitative information in the following: independent, instructional frustration reading levels, and listening comprehension level. It also offers qualitative information through a word recognition miscue analysis and a comprehension question analysis. It can be used for retelling and assessing use of context clues.

Test: *Carrow Auditory–Visual Abilities Test* (CAVAT)

Author: Carrow-Woolfolk, E. (1981)

Age Range: 4–10 years

Available Through: DLM–Teaching Resources

Test Description: This tool measures auditory and visual perceptual, motor, and memory skills in children.

Test: *Clinical Evaluation of Language Fundamentals* (CELF-3)
Authors: Semel, E., Wiig, E., & Secord, W., (1995)
Age Range: 6:0–21 years.
Available Through: Psychological Corporation
Test Description: The CELF-3 assesses word classes, word associations, rapid automatic naming of colors and shapes, and rapid alternating sequences of colored shapes.

Test: *Clinical Evaluation of Language Fundamentals—Preschool* (CELF-P)
Authors: Wiig, E., Secord, W., & Semel, E., (1992)
Age Range: 3:0–6:11 years
Available Through: Psychological Corporation
Test Description: The CELF-P assesses receptive language through linguistic concepts, sentence structure, basic concepts, linguistic concepts, sentence structure and oral directions. Expressive language is assessed through recalling sentences in context, formulating labels, word structure, recalling sentences, formulated sentences, and word structures.

Test: *Comprehensive Assessment of Spoken Language* (CASL)
Author: Publisher's Project Staff (1999)
Age Range: 3–21 years
Available Through: American Guidance Service, Inc.
Test Description: The CASL provides in-depth assessment of oral language processing systems of auditory comprehension, oral expression and word retrieval, knowledge and use of words and grammatical structures of language, and the ability to use language for special tasks requiring higher-level cognitive functions, and knowledge and use of language in communicative contexts.

Test: *Comprehensive Receptive and Expressive Vocabulary Test—2* (CREVT2)
Authors: Wallace, G., & Hammill, D.D. (2002)
Age Range: 4:0–89:11 years
Available Through: Pro-Ed
Test Description: The CREVT2 assesses receptive and expressive vocabulary at the one word level.

Test: *Comprehensive Test of Phonological Processing* (CTOPP)

Authors: Wagner, R.K., Torgesen, J.K., & Rashotte, C.A. (1999)

Age Range: 5–24 years

Available Through: Pro-Ed

Test Description: The CTOPP assesses phonological processing skills and rapid automatized naming of colors, letters, numbers, and objects.

Test: *Decoding Skills Test* (DST)

Authors: Richardson, E. & Dibenedetto, B. (1985)

Age Range: Grades 1–5

Available Through: York Press

Test Description: The DST identifies strengths and weaknesses in the following areas: basal vocabulary, phonic patterns and contextual decoding.

Test: *Detroit Tests of Learning Aptitude—4* (DTLA-4)

Author: Hammill, D.D. (1998)

Age Range: 6–17 years

Available Through: Pro-Ed

Test Description: The DTLA-4 assesses a student's language, attention and motor skills, general intelligence, and discrete abilities. Identifies strengths and weaknesses in the following areas: basal vocabulary, phonic patterns and contextual decoding.

Test: *Developmental Test of Visual–Motor Integration—4th Edition* (VMI)

Authors: Beery, K.E., & Buktencia, N.A. (1997)

Age Range: 28 weeks–17 years

Available Through: Western Psychological Services

Test Description: The VMI assesses visual–motor integration.

Test: *Developmental Test of Visual Perception, Second Edition* (DTVP:2)

Authors: Hammill, D.D., Pearson, N.A., & Voress, J.K. (1993)

Age Range: 4–9 years

Available Through: Stoelting Co.

Test Description: The DTVP:2 assesses eye-hand coordination, copying, spatial relations, position in space, figure–ground, visual closure, visual–motor speed, and form constancy.

Test: *Dynamic Assessment & Intervention: Improving Children's Narrative Abilities*

Authors: Miller, L., Gilliam, R.B., & Pena, E.D. (2001)

Age Range: 5–9 years

Available Through: Pro-Ed

Test Description: This tool identifies strengths and weaknesses in elementary aged children's narrative abilities.

Test: *Expressive One-Word Picture Vocabulary Test—2000*

Author: Gardner, M.F. (2000)

Age Range: 2–18:11 years

Available Through: Pro-Ed

Test Description: This tool assesses verbal expression of language through providing names of pictured items.

Test: *Fluharty—2*

Author: Fluharty, M.B. (2000)

Age Range: 3:0–6:11 years

Available Through: American Guidance Services, Inc.

Test Description: This tool assesses articulation, repeating sentences, following directives and answering questions, describing actions, and sequencing events.

Test: *Goldman–Fristoe–Woodcock Test of Auditory Discrimination*

Authors: Goldman, R., Fristoe, M., & Woodcock, R.W. (1990)

Age Range: 3–70+ years

Available Through: The Speech Bin

Test Description: This tool assesses auditory discrimination in quiet and noise.

Test: *Gray Oral Reading Tests—Diagnostic* (GORT-D)

Authors: Wiederholt, J.L., & Bryant, B.R. (1991)

Age Range: 5:6–12:11 years

Available Through: Pro-Ed

Test Description: The GORT-D measures growth in oral reading by measuring three cue systems believed to affect reading proficiency: meaning cues, function cues, and graphic/phonemic cues.

Test: *Gray Oral Reading Tests—Fourth Edition* (GORT-4)

Authors: Wiederholt, J.L., & Bryant, B.R. (2001)

Age Range: 6:0–18:11 years

Available Through: Pro-Ed

Test Description: The GORT-4 measures growth in oral reading providing a fluency score derived by combining the reader's performance in rate and accuracy.

Test: *Gray Silent Reading Tests* (GSRT)

Authors: Wiederholt, J.L., & Blalock, G. (2000)

Age Range: 7–25 years

Available Through: Pro-Ed

Test Description: The GSRT measures a reader's silent reading comprehension ability.

Test: *Illinois Test of Psycholinguistic Abilities—Third Edition* (ITPA-3)

Authors: Hammill, D.D., Mather, N., & Roberts, R. (2001)

Age Range: 5:0–12:11 years

Available Through: Pro-Ed

Test Description: This tool determines children's specific strengths and weaknesses among linguistic abilities.

Test: *Khan–Lewis Phonological Analysis* (KLPA)

Authors: Khan, L. & Lewis, N. (1986)

Age Range: 2:5–11 years

Available Through: Pro-Ed

Test Description: The KLPA assesses 15 common phonological processes.

Test: *Language Processing Test—Revised* (LPT-R)

Authors: Richard, G.J. & Hanner, M.A. (1995)

Age Range: 5–11 years

Available Through: LinguiSystems

Test Description: The LPT-R identifies processing abilities in the following areas: labeling, associations, similarities, multiple meanings, stating functions, categorization, differences, and attributes.

Test: *Lindamood Auditory Conceptualization Test* (LAC)

Authors: Lindamood, C. & Lindamood, P. (1971)

Age Range: All ages

Available Through: Pro-Ed

Test Description: The LAC identifies strengths and weaknesses in the following areas: speech sound discrimination and segmentation of spoken words into phonemic units.

Test: *Nelson–Denny Reading Test CD–ROM Forms G and H*

Authors: Brown, J.I., Fishco, V.V., & Hanna, G.S. (2000)

Age Range: 9–16 years, Adult

Available Through: Riverside Publishing

Test Description: This tool identifies strengths and weaknesses in vocabulary, reading comprehension, and reading rate.

Test: *Oral and Written Language Scales (OWLS): Written Expression*

Author: Carrow-Woolfolk, E. (1995)

Age Range: 5–21 years

Available Through: Pro-Ed

Test Description: The OWLS Written Expression measures use of conventions (handwriting, spelling, punctuation), the use of syntactical forms (modifiers, phrases, sentence structures) and the ability to communicate meaningfully (relevance, cohesiveness, organization).

Test: *Peabody Individual Achievement Tests—Revised* (PIAT-R/NU)

Author: Markwardt, F.C. (1997)

Age Range: 5:0–22 years

Available Through: American Guidance Service

Test Description: The PIAT provides a wide-range, screening measure of achievement in mathematics, reading, spelling, general information, and written expression.

Test: *Peabody Picture Vocabulary Test—III*

Author: Dunn, L.M. & Dunn, L.M. (1997)

Age Range: 2:6–90+ years

Available Through: American Guidance Services

Test Description: The PPVT-III measures receptive vocabulary at the one-word level.

Test: *Phonological Awareness Skills Program* (PASP)

Author: Rosner, J. (1999)

Age Range: 4–10 years

Available Through: Pro-Ed

Test Description: The PASP identifies strengths and weaknesses in the following areas: phonological awareness at the syllable and phoneme level.

Test: *Phonological Awareness Test* (PAT)

Authors: Robertson, C., & Salter, W. (1997)

Age Range: 5–9 years

Available Through: LinguiSystems

Test Description: The PAT identifies strengths and weaknesses in the following areas: rhyming, segmentation, isolation, deletion, substitution, blending, graphemes, decoding, and invented spelling.

Test: *Pre-Literacy Skills Screening* (PLSS)

Authors: Crumrine, L, & Lonegan, H. (1999)

Grade Range: Kindergarten

Available Through: Pro-Ed

Test Description: The PLSS identifies incoming kindergarten children who may be at risk for literacy problems. It examines phonological awareness, word retrieval, and letter recognition.

Test: *Pre-School Language Scale* (PLS-4)

Authors: Zimmerman, I.L., Steiner, V.G., and Pond, R.E. (1992)

Grade Range: birth through 6 years

Available Through: Psychological Corporation

Test Description: The PLS-4 evaluates receptive and expressive language skills in the areas of attention, semantics, structure, and integrative thinking skills. For children birth–2:11 years, items target interaction, attention, and vocal/gestural behaviors. For 5 and 6 year olds, items include early literacy and phonological awareness.

Test: *Qualitative Reading Inventory* (QRI)

Authors: Leslie, L., & Caldwell, J. (1990)

Grade Range: Primer–Junior high

Available Through: HarperCollins Publishers

Test Description: The QRI is an informal reading inventory that assesses reading comprehension of words lists and narrative and expository passages.

Test: *Receptive One-Word Picture Vocabulary Test—2000*
Author: Gardner, M.F. (2000)
Age Range: 2–18:11 years
Available Through: Pro-Ed
Test Description: This tool assesses single word receptive vocabulary.

Test: *Ross Information Processing Assessment—Primary* (RIPA-P)
Author: Ross-Swain, D. (1999)
Age Range: 5–12 years
Available Through: Pro-Ed
Test Description: The RIPA-P assesses immediate memory, spatial orientation, recent memory and recall of general information. Subtests suitable for 8-12 year olds include: temporal orientation, problem solving, organization, and abstract reasoning.

Test: *Slosson Oral Reading Test—Revised* (SORT-R3)
Authors: Slosson, R.L, & Nicholson, C.L. (2002)
Age Range: Preschool–adult
Available Through: Slosson Educational Publications, Inc.
Test Description: The SORT-R3 assesses word recognition skills.

Test: *Structured Photographic Expressive Language Test—II* (SPELT-II-Revised)
Authors: Dawson, J., & Stephens, J.I. (1995)
Age Range: 4:0–9:5 years
Available Through: Janelle Publications, Inc. & Psychological Corporation
Test Description: The SPELT-II assesses a child's generation of specific morphological and syntactical structures through use of color photographs.

Test: *Structured Photographic Expressive Language Test—Primary* (SPELT-P)
Authors: Werner, E.O, & Dawson Kresheck, J.D. (1983)
Age Range: 3:0–5:11 years

Available Through: Janelle Publications, Inc.

Test Description: The SPELT-P is a screening instrument to allow the examiner to identify those children who may have difficulty in their expression of early developing morphological and syntactic features.

Test: *Slosson Written Expression Test* (SWET)

Authors: Hofler, D.B., Erford, B.T., & Amoriell, W.J. (2001)

Age Range: 8–17 years

Available Through: Slosson Educational Publications, Inc.

Test Description: The SWET is a screening test for spelling, capitalization, punctuation, sentence length and type–token ratio.

Test: *Test for Examining Expressive Morphology* (TEEM)

Authors: Shipley, K.G., Stone, T.A., & Sue, M.B. (1983)

Age Range: 3–7 years

Available Through: Pro-Ed

Test Description: The TEEM assesses expressive morpheme development including present progressives, plurals, possessives, past tenses, third–person singulars, and derived adjectives.

Test: *Test of Adolescent and Adult Language: Third Edition* (TOAL-3)

Authors: Hammill, D.D., Brown, V.L., Larson, S.C., & Wiederholt, J.L. (1994)

Age Range: 12–24 years

Available Through: Pro-Ed

Test Description: The TOAL-3 assesses adolescent and adult vocabulary (semantics) across listening, speaking, reading, and writing.

Test: *Test for Auditory Comprehension of Language:* (TACL-3)—(3rd ed.)

Author: Carrow-Woolfolk, E. (1999)

Age Range: 3:0–9:11 years

Available Through: Pro-Ed

Test Description: The TACL-3 assesses strengths and weaknesses in a student's ability to understand spoken language in three subtests: Vocabulary, Grammatical Morphemes, and Elaborated Phrases and Sentences.

Test: *Test of Auditory Analysis Skills* (TAAS)

Author: Rosner, J. (1979)

Age Range: K–3

Available Through: The Speech Bin

Test Description: The TAAS assesses phonemic analysis and synthesis skills focusing on children's abilities to process sequencing of sounds and syllables in words.

Test: *Test of Auditory-Perceptual Skills—Revised* (TAPS-R)

Author: Gardner, M.F. (1996)

Age Range: 4–13 years

Available Through: Psychological and Educational Publications, Inc.

Test Description: The TAPS-R measures auditory perceptual skills of processing, word and sequential memory, interpretation of oral directions, and discrimination. The Upper Level (TAPS:UL) assess the same skills in 12–18 year olds.

Test: *Test of Adolescent/Adult Word Finding* (TAWF)

Author: German, D.J. (1990)

Age Range: 12–80 years

Available Through: Pro-Ed

Test Description: The TWF-2 assesses word finding skills through the following activities: picture naming of nouns and verbs, sentence completion naming, description naming and category naming.

Test: *Test of Auditory Reasoning and Processing Skills* (TARPS)

Author: Gardner, M.F. (1992)

Age Range: 5–14 years

Available Through: Psychological and Educational Publications, Inc.

Test Description: TARPS measures how well children understand, interpret, draw conclusions, and make inferences from auditorally presented information.

Test: *Test of Early Language Development—Third edition* (TELD-3)

Authors: Hresko, W.P., Reid, D.K., & Hammill, D.D. (1999)

Age Range: 2:0–7:11 years

Available Through: Pro-Ed

Test Description: The TELD-3 identifies strengths and weaknesses in receptive and expressive syntax and semantics.

Test: *Test of Early Reading Ability: 3rd Edition* (TERA-3)

Authors: Reid, D.K., Hresko, W.P., & Hammill, D.D. (2001)

Age Range: 3:6–8:6 years.

Available Through: Pro-Ed

Test Description: The TERA-3 identifies strengths and weaknesses in the following areas: knowledge of contextual meaning, alphabet, and conventions.

Test: *Test of Early Written Language, 2nd edition* (TEWL-2)

Authors: Hresko, W.P., Herron, S.R., & Peak, P.K. (1996)

Age Range: 4:0–10:11 years

Available Through: Pro-Ed

Test Description: The TEWL-2 identifies strengths and weaknesses in the following areas: spelling, capitalization, punctuation, sentence construction and metacognitive knowledge. The Contextual subtests include story format, cohesion, thematic maturity, ideation, and story structure.

Test: *Test of Language Development—Primary* (TOLD-P:3)

Authors: Newcomer, P.L. & Hammill, D.D. (1997)

Age Range: 4:0–8:11 years

Available Through: Pro-Ed

Test Description: The TOLD-P:3 assesses oral language in the following areas: picture vocabulary, relational and oral vocabulary, grammatic understanding, sentence imitation, grammatic completion, word discrimination, phonemic analysis, and word articulation.

Test: *Test of Language Development—Intermediate* (TOLD-I:3)

Authors: Hammill, D.D. & Newcomer, P.L. (1997)

Age Range: 8:0–12:11 years

Available Through: Pro-Ed

Test Description: The TOLD-I:3 assesses a student's understanding and meaningful use of spoken language in the following areas: generals, malapropisms, picture vocabulary, sentence combining, word ordering, and grammatic comprehension.

Test: *Test of Memory and Learning* (TOMAL)

Authors: Reynolds, C.R., & Bigler, E.D. (1994)

Age Range: 5–19 years

Available Through: Pro-Ed

Test Description: The TOMAL assesses verbal, nonverbal, composite memory and delayed recall in the following: oral language in the following areas: memory-for-stories, facial memory, word/visual memory, digits forward/backward, manual imitation, visual sequential memory, paired recall, memory-for-location, and letters forward/backward.

Test: *Test of Pragmatic Language* (TOPL)

Authors: Phelps-Teraski, D., & Phelps-Gunn, T. (1992)

Age Range: 5:0–13:11 years

Available Through: Pro-Ed

Test Description: The TOPL assesses pragmatic language abilities within six subcomponents of pragmatic language: physical setting, audience, topic, purpose (speech acts), visual–gestural cues, and abstraction.

Test: *Test of Reading Comprehension—Third Edition* (TORC-3)

Authors: Brown, V.L., Hammill, D.D., & Wiederholt, J.L. (1995)

Age Range: 7:0–17:11 years

Available Through: Pro-Ed

Test Description: The TORC-3 provides a general reading comprehension score including: general vocabulary, syntactic similarities, paragraph reading, and sentence sequencing.

Test: *Test of Visual–Motor Skills—Revised* (TVMS-R)

Authors: Gardner, M.F. (1995)

Age Range: 3–13:11 years

Available Through: Psychological and Educational Publications, Inc.

Test Description: The TVPMS-R measures eye–hand motor accuracy, motor control, motor coordination, and/or gestalt interpretation.

Test: *Test of Visual–Perceptual Skills—Revised* (TVPS-R)

Authors: Gardner, M.F. (1996)

Age Range: 4–13 years

Available Through: Psychological and Educational Publications, Inc.

Test Description: The TVPS-R measures dimensions of visual–perceptual function including visual discrimination, visual memory, visual–spatial relationships, visual form constancy, visual sequential memory, visual figure–ground, and visual closure.

Test: *Test of Visual–Perceptual Skills—Upper Limits* (TVPS-UL)
Authors: Gardner, M.F. (1997)
Age Range: 12–18 years
Available Through: Psychological and Educational Publications, Inc.
Test Description: The TVPS-R measures dimensions of visual–perceptual function including visual discrimination, visual memory, visual–spatial relationships, visual form constancy, visual sequential memory, visual figure–ground, and visual closure.

Test: *Test of Word Finding—2* (TWF-2)
Author: German, D.J. (2000)
Age Range: 4:0–12:11 years
Available Through: Pro-Ed
Test Description: The TWF-2 assesses word finding skills through the following activities: picture naming, sentence completion, picture naming of verbs, and picture naming of categories.

Test: *Test of Word Finding in Discourse* (TWFD)
Author: German, D.J. (1991)
Age Range: 6:6–12:11 years
Available Through: Pro-Ed
Test Description: The TWFD assesses word finding skills in both single word naming and narrative discourse.

Test: *Test of Word Reading Efficiency* (TOWRE)
Authors: Torgesen, J.K,, Wagner, R., & Rashotte, C.A. (1999)
Age Range: 6:0–24:11 years
Available Through: Pro-Ed
Test Description: The TOWRE assesses word–reading accuracy and fluency. The Sight Word Efficiency subtest assesses the number of real printed words that can be accurately identified within 45 seconds, and the Phonetic Decoding Efficiency subtest measures the number of pronounceable printed nonwords that can be accurately decoded within 45 seconds.

Test: *Test of Written Language—3* (TOWL-3)

Authors: Hammill, D.D., & Larsen, S.C. (1996)

Age Range: 7:6–17:11 years

Available Through: Pro-Ed

Test Description: The TOWL-3 assesses writing competence through spontaneous formats including contextual conventions, contextual language and story construction, and contrived formats including vocabulary, spelling, style, logical sentences, and sentence combining.

Test: *Test of Written Spelling—4th Edition* (TWS-4)

Authors: Larsen, S.C., Hammill, D.D., & Moats, L. (1999)

Grade Range: 1–12 years

Available Through: Pro-Ed

Test Description: The TWS-4 assesses spelling ability.

Test: *The Help Test (Elementary): A Test of Language Competence*

Author: Lazzari, A.M. (1996)

Age Range: 6–11:11 years

Available Through: LinguiSystems

Test Description: The Help Test identifies vocabulary strengths and weaknesses in the following areas: semantics, specific vocabulary, general vocabulary, and defining.

Test: *The Word Test—Elementary Revised*

Authors: Huisingh, R., Bowers, L., LoGiudice, C., Orman, J., & Barrett, M. (1990)

Age Range: 6–11:11 years

Available Through: LinguiSystems

Test Description: The Help Test identifies vocabulary strengths and weaknesses in the following areas: semantics, specific vocabulary, general vocabulary, and defining.

Test: *Token Test for Children*

Author: DiSimoni, F. (1978)

Age Range: 3–12 years

Available Through: The Speech Bin

Test Description: The Token assesses a student's ability to process and follow increasingly complex spoken directions.

Test: *Wepman Auditory Discrimination Test—Second Edition* (ADT)
Author: Reynolds, W.M. (1997)
Age Range: 4:0–8:11 years
Available Through: Western Psychological Services
Test Description: This test assesses auditory discrimination abilities.

Test: *Woodcock–Johnson III Tests of Cognitive Abilities* (WJ III)
Authors: Woodcock, R.W., McGrew, K.S., & Mather, N. (2001)
Age Range: 2–90+ years.
Available Through: Riverside Publishing Company
Test Description: The WJ III identifies strengths and weaknesses in the following areas: Comprehension–Knowledge, Long-term retrieval, Visual–spatial thinking, Auditory processing, Fluid reasoning, Processing speed, and Short-term memory.

Test: *Woodcock Language Proficiency Test—Revised* (WLPB-R)
Author: Woodcock, R.W. (1991)
Age Range: 2–90+ years.
Available Through: Riverside Publishing Company
Test Description: The WLPB-R identifies strengths and weaknesses in the following areas: letter–word identification, word attack skills (decoding nonreal words), passage comprehension, and strengths and weaknesses in reading vocabulary (reading words and supplying appropriate meanings).

Test: *Woodcock Diagnostic Reading Battery* (WDRB)
Author: Woodcock, R.W. (1997)
Age Range: 4–90+ years
Available Through: Riverside Publishing Company
Test Description: The WDRB identifies strengths and weaknesses in the following areas: letter word identification, word attack, passage comprehension, reading vocabulary, incomplete words, sound blending, oral vocabulary, listening comprehension, memory for sentences, and visual matching.

Test: *Woodcock–Johnson III* (WJIII)
Author: Woodcock, R.W., McGrew, K.S., & Mather, N. (2001)
Age Range: 2–90+ years.

Available Through: Riverside Publishing Company

Test Description: The WLPB-R identifies strengths and weaknesses in the following areas: reading, oral language, math, written language, and academic knowledge.

Test: *Word Test—R (Elementary)*

Authors: Huisingh, R., Barrett, M., Zachman, L., Blagden, C., & Orman, J. (1991)

Age Range: 7:0–11:11 years

Available Through: LinguiSystems

Test Description: The Word Test Revised identifies strengths and weaknesses in word associations, synonyms, semantic absurdities, antonyms, definitions, and multiple definitions.

Test: *Word Test—Adolescent*

Authors: Bowers, L., Huisingh, R., Barrett, M., Orman, J., & LoGiudice, C. (1989)

Age Range: 12:0–17:11 years

Available Through: LinguiSystems

Test Description: The Word Test—Adolescent identifies strengths and weaknesses in vocabulary and semantic skills in the following areas: brand names, synonyms, signs of the times, and definitions.

CHAPTER

5

Treatment of Developmental Reading Disabilities: Part I

I.   INTRODUCTION

Lyon (1997) as cited by McCardle et al. (2001) pointed out that reading problems "are not confined or defined by intelligence, race, or ethnicity," and literacy problems will cause a myriad of problems for students within and beyond the classroom. Literacy, therefore "is not just an educational issue, but a public health issue, as there are many downstream sequelae of reading problems in an individual's life" (p. 184). According to the American Speech–Language–Hearing Association (2001), speech language specialists have many roles and responsibilities in their support of literacy. "In general they must ensure that students with special needs receive intervention that builds on and encourages the reciprocal relationships between spoken and written language. Such intervention should focus on the underlying goal of improving language and communication across both spoken and written language forms" (p. 27).

Adams' (1990) model of reading processors was described in Chapter 2 and referred to again in Chapter 4 to help define and delimit the many areas to assess in language-based reading disabilities. Similarly, to impose an overall structure to the numerous components that must be considered in supporting literacy, Adams' model is revisited once again in this chapter. Recall the four broad subcomponents of reading that must work together efficiently to be successful in reading: the phonological, orthographic, meaning, and context processors. As Adams explained "the four processors work together, continuously receiving information from and returning feedback to each other . . . Within each of these processors, knowledge is represented by interconnected sets of simpler units" (p. 21). *The phonological processor* handles the auditory image of any particular word, syllable, or phoneme. The ability to form and mentally hold strong phonological representations while we process and/or verbally produce language, decode the printed form of our language, and/or encode to produce the written form of our language is critical. *The orthographic processor* involves visual information from the printed page. Orthographic processing is "the ability to form, store, and access orthographic representations" (Stanovich, West & Cunningham, 1991, p. 220.) This processor is important for the reader to store individual letters as well as sublexical word parts (-ing) and letter patterns (-at). *The meaning processor* stores familiar word meanings "as interassociated sets of more primitive meaning elements" (Adams, 1990, p. 143). Finally, *the context processor* is in charge of constructing a coherent, ongoing interpretation of the text. The suggested interventions in Chapters 5 and 6 are presented under the headings of these four processors.

As discussed in the previous two chapters, at least two core deficits underlie language-based reading problems: phonological processing and verbal naming speed. In Chapter 4 we examined how to assess the many areas that can impact upon a student's ability to:

use the phonological code to hold sounds and words in memory
use the phonological code in phonological awareness
use the phonological code in verbal output
use the phonological code in word retrieval

And to assess the verbal naming speed core, we examined how to assess the areas that can impact upon a student's:

verbal naming speed.

In Chapter 4, charts and discussions centered on the intertwining abilities that emanate from the above five areas. Numerous areas were presented, illustrating how the oral language base of a reading problem has the potential of contaminating many abilities across the oral–written language continuum. A summary of assessment areas and corresponding methods that target the phonological processor are presented in this chapter followed by research on phonological awareness training and a listing of suggested materials in Appendix 5.1. Methods that target the orthographic, meaning, and context processors are presented in Chapter 6. In both Chapters 5 and 6, I have described the steps of methods I use in my own instruction/therapy with students demonstrating developmental reading disabilities. Of course, depending upon the nature and severity of each student's problem, I select where to begin within each processor according to each student's needs. However, if, for example, I find a student who needs to "begin at the beginning," I begin with Teaching Goal #1 and work through Goal #9 under the phonological processor. As the student's phonological processing increases, I add goals included under the orthographic, meaning, and context processors. Stated differently, I never work through the processors from phonological through context. Rather, as the student's performance increases in one I add goals from the other three processors so that instruction across the processors is simultaneous as well as sequential, with each goal providing a scaffold for the next. Under many of the goals, I include selected materials and carryover activities that I have found to be particularly effective in my own sessions.

II. METHODS THAT TARGET THE PHONOLOGICAL PROCESSOR

The relationship among phonological processing, oral and written language was presented in Chapter 2. To better understand the discussion of intervention for the phonological processor, some thoughts as to how auditory processing and phonological awareness relate were presented in Chapter 4. In summary, auditory processing is a lower level ongoing activity occurring as the brain recognizes and interprets heard sounds. Phonological awareness is a complex cognitive activity involving intentional manipulation of language units. Torgesen and Mathes (2000) noted that "phonological awareness is most commonly defined as one's sensitivity to, or explicit awareness of, the phonological structure of words in one's language. In short, it involves the ability to notice, think about, or manipulate the individual sounds in words" (p. 2).

Section A below presents suggested goals and activities for the ongoing activity of auditory processing while Section B presents suggested goals and activities for the intentional acts inherent in phonological awareness. Section C presents suggested activities for increasing verbal output (vocabulary, syntax/morphology, and narrative). Important considerations about phonological awareness instruction are included in Section IV. Although some materials are suggested with the teaching goals, Appendix 5.1 lists recommended materials for use with the phonological processor. See Appendix B for a list of all goals suggested in Chapters 5 and 6.

A. Ongoing Activity of Auditory Processing.

If the student's ability to use the phonetic/phonological code to hold sounds and *words in memory is weak*, teaching goals may include any of the following, the first six of which are frequently referred to as auditory processing/perceptual skills (See Lucker & Wood, 2000).

1. **Goal 1: To increase auditory decoding through decreasing phonemic discrimination problems.**

   Suggested Activities: the student is asked to recognize and identify similarities and differences in speech sounds. 1) Ask the student to identify whether words you say begin/end with the same/different sounds. 2) Ask the student to identify whether the middle sound in monosyllabic words you say are the same/different. For a rich source of consonant–vowel and vowel–consonant syllable training targets see Sloan's (1986) program.

2. **Goal 2: To increase auditory decoding through decreasing temporal pattern recognition/use problems.**

   Suggested Activities: 1) The student is asked to differentiate between long and short sounds (/s/ versus /k/). 2); The student is asked to blend individual sounds to form simple words where the time between presentation of individual phonemes becomes increasingly shorter; 3) The student is asked to identify where one word ends and another begins in 2–3 word phrases, for example: "the rat's hat" or "the rat sat;" 4) The student is asked to identify the difference in meaning of two utterances containing the same words but varying in time between sounds responsible for changing the meaning, for example, "Look out the door" versus "Look out! The door!" (Lucker & Wood, 2000); 5) Bellis (2001) recommended prosody training to help students learn to recognize and use rhythm, stress, and intonational aspects of language. Examples included varying syllabic stress, altering prosody within sentences, altering tone of voice, reading aloud with exaggerated prosodic features. An adaptation of *Melodic Intonation Therapy* (Helm-Estabrooks, Nicholas, & Morgan, 1989) might be useful here; 6) Teach nursery rhymes stressing various words and rhythms (Mayer, 2001).

3. **Goal 3: To decrease auditory processing problems secondary to auditory figure/ground problems.**

    Suggested Activities: The student is asked to recognize a relevant auditory stimulus against a background of competing noise. 1) Tape record various background noises such as cafeteria noise or classroom noise, and play a tape while you ask the student to follow a variety of sequential directions presented orally; 2) Teach the student to identify noisy environments that are difficult for him/her and what needs to be done to alter the environment to enhance listening and understanding what is being said, for instance, moving to a quieter location, or closing the door.

4. **Goal 4: To decrease auditory processing problems secondary to auditory selective attention problems.**

    Suggested Activities: The student is asked to focus selectively on various sounds or spoken words for increased lengths of time. 1) Tape record familiar sounds such as cars, telephones, doorbells, and musical instruments occurring numerous times. Have the student listen to the tape and indicate each time one of the designated sounds is heard, or ask the student to tell how many times one of the designated sounds is heard; 2) Repeat above activity with tape recorded taps against a background of noises. The student is asked to tell how many taps are heard. Vary the rate of presentation of stimuli to accomodate difficulties in rapid processing of auditory input; 3) Ask the student to close his/her eyes for one minute. Then ask the student to tell how many environmental sounds were heard during the minute.

5. **Goal 5: To decrease auditory processing problems secondary to poor auditory memory.**

    Suggested Activities: 1) The student is asked to retain increasingly longer lists of letters, numbers, or words with the addition of strategies such as: holding up certain number of fingers to help recall the number of details the teacher says and pre-focusing questions to help student listen for and recall certain bits of information presented orally. Ask the student to listen for information such as the color or size of something you will read about, or ask the same question following your reading of the material. It is particularly helpful to ask the student to restate what he or she is to listen for prior to reading the material (Mayer, 2001). If the student is to listen for a particular number, it is helpful to have him or her print the number as soon as it is read aloud from the passage. Similarly, if the student knows sound–symbol associations, it helps to have him or her print the first letter of the word he or she is to be listening for in the passage; 2) Bellis (2001) recommended compensatory strategies to "increase motivation and self-confidence on the part of the student and to help him/her become an active, rather than passive, listener" (p. 7). Her examples included the following: a) specific training in language rules such as listening for tag words such as "first," "last," "next," "before," and "after"; causal words such as "because," and "since" adversative terms such as "but," "however," and "although"; and words that imply relationships among words such as "neither," "nor," and "or;" b) chunking information, for instance saying 48 rather than as two separate numbers 4 and 8; c) verbal rehearsal, also known as reauditorization; d) paraphrasing information: restating what was heard in somewhat different terms; e) helping the student sequence instructions; and f) dividing steps of large project into discrete steps.

6. **Goal 6: To decrease auditory processing problems through increasing binaural integration (a.k.a. auditory closure/synthesis).**

    Suggested Activities: The student is asked to take the individual pieces of messages to form a whole message. Bellis (2001) recommended the following activities to help students learn to fill in missing components of a message to arrive at a meaningful whole: 1) Missing word exercises. The student fills in missing words in familiar passages and then less familiar passages. Begin, for instance, by having the student fill in missing words to known nursery rhymes ("Mary had a little _____"); 2) Missing syllable exercise. The student fills in missing syllables: "there are 26 letters in the al-pha ___" (p. 208); 3) Missing phoneme exercises. The student fills in missing phonemes: "I like to (w)atch (t)ele(v)ision" (p. 208); 4) Phoneme training. According to Bellis, "the purpose of phoneme training is to help the child learn to develop accurate phonemic representation to improve speech-to-print skills" (p. 210). She recommended Sloan's (1986) program which asks the student to discriminate between words with minimal contrast phoneme pairs.

7. **Goal 7: To increase simple receptive language.**

    Suggested Activity: The student is asked to carry out increasingly complex commands presented through the auditory channel.

8. **Goal 8: To increase listening comprehension.**

    Suggested Activity: The student is asked to listen to increasingly complex sentences and short paragraphs and to verbally answer questions about the material.

9. **Goal 9: To increase verbal repetition.**

    Suggested Activity: The student is asked to verbally repeat increasingly complex words, sentences, and sayings such as limericks and tongue twisters. Use contrastive stress techniques, emphasizing various words in utterances to call the student's attention to them. For instance, ask the student to repeat "Hey diddle diddle, the cat and the FIDDLE" (stressing the last word.) Repeat this activity, this time stressing the word "THE" instead of "fiddle." This will call the student's attention to words in the phrase that are typically stressed, for example, "fiddle," and those that are not, for example, "the."

B. Intentional Acts Inherent in Phonological Awareness.

If the student's ability to use the phonological code in *phonological awareness is impaired*, teaching goals may include any of the following six goals.

By moving from words, to syllables, to phonemes, the child is encouraged to focus on increasingly smaller units of the speech stream, and gradually shift attention from the content (meaning) of language to the form (syntax, morphology, and sounds) of language. Activities selected for inclusion in this program have been culled from the literature. (See for example, Adams, 1990; Blachman, 1994a & b; Donnelly et al., 1992; Fox & Routh, 1984; Hatcher, 1994; O'Connor et al., 1993; Pickering, 1993a & b; Rosner, 1979; Swank, 1994; and Yopp, 1992.) Suggestions for a developmental ordering of activities appear in some of these sources; however, the complete listing of activities did not emanate from a single source. Materials for increasing phonological awareness can be found at the end of this chapter. These activities can be found in three sources tied directly to children's literature. (See Goldsworthy, 1998 and 2001; and Goldsworthy & Pieretti, 2003.)

1. **Goal 1: To increase phonological awareness at the word level: implicit teaching.**

Knowing that sentences are composed of words is the first level of language awareness in children entering school (Donnelly, Thomsen, Huber, & Schoemer, 1992). Bowey and Tunmer (1984) cited findings by Papandropoulou and Sinclair (1974) as to the emergence of word awareness. The definition of "word" given by 4- and 5-year-old children suggested that at that age, words are not viewed as having an autonomous existence. Rather, preschool- and kindergarten-aged children identified words as words because of the existence of objects or actions to which they refer. Children aged 6 1/2 to 8 years old viewed words as "bits of a story" (i.e., a sequence of words carrying meaning). Eight- to 10-year-olds were able to define "word," indicating the influence of formal instruction. Bowey and Tunmer concluded that before learning to use the label "word" correctly, a child must "become aware of the word as a unit of language, larger than phonemes and smaller than phrases, and syntactically distinct from bound morphemes . . . this insight may not be easily attained" (p. 79). The activities presented in this section were selected to provide an enjoyable, informal means by which students may become sensitive to the speech stream at the word level.

Suggested Activities:

a. Reading Aloud.

Read to students and occasionally point to specific words as you read. Encourage the student to help turn the pages, hold the book, and eventually point to some of the words as you read. Among books that call particular attention to words are those included in Table 5-1.

Table 5-1. Suggested Word-Level Books for Use in Reading Aloud to Students.

Wordless Books

Example: One Frog Too Many (Mayer & Mayer, 1975)

Encourage the student to make up and tell you a story as you print his/her words on Post-Its that you stick onto the book pages. The student sees that spoken words are recoded into print.

Books with Patterning and Predictable Language

Example: Napping House (Wood & Wood, 1984)

"There is a house, a napping house, where everyone is sleeping.

And in that house there is a bed, a cozy bed in a napping house, where everyone is sleeping." After reading this aloud two to three times to a student, encourage him/her to fill in words you omit as you read it aloud again. "There is a house, a _____ house."

Books with Pictures Inserted Along Lines of Print

Example: P.B. Bear's Birthday Party (Davis, 1994)

"Meet P.B. Bear (picture of a bear). The P. stands for Pajama, because his (picture of pjs) are his favorite clothes. (picture of a bed) time is his favorite time of day. One morning, (picture of bear) woke up early . . . ." The student is asked to "read" the pictured items as you read the text. Reinforce the student for helping you read the book.

Books with Play on Words

Example: A Chocolate Moose for Dinner (Gwynne, 1976)

"Mommy says she had a chocolate moose for dinner last night" (picture of a moose). "After dinner she toasted dad" (picture of dad in toaster). Explain the two or three different definitions of words to the student.

Also see Appendix D.

b. Singing Songs.

Singing songs that accentuate single words out of the auditory stream is helpful, for example, "Pop! goes the weasel" (Yopp & Troyer, 1992); any of the "Wee Sings," or other versions of finger plays or nursery rhymes where words stand out.

c. Identifying Missing Words.

Place a number of objects or pictures on the table. Ask the student to hide his or her eyes as you remove or replace one or more of the objects or pictures. The student is to guess what has been removed, thereby learning about word removal and replacement.

2.   **Goal 2: To increase phonological awareness at the word level: explicit teaching.**

Suggested Activities:

a. Identifying Words and Sentences.

As you read to the student ask him or her to point to words and sentences. Explain that the first word in a sentence begins with a capital letter and that sentences end with punctuation marks, "period/the dot." Show the student how words are separated on the page by the spaces between them.

b. Explaining Words and Sentences.

The student explains how we can tell when there is a word or sentence on the page and gives some information about what a word and/or a sentence is.

c. Filling in Words as Adult Reads.

Omit words as you read and allow time for the student to "read" the omitted words.

d. Counting Words Heard or Seen.

Ask the student to count the number of words he or she hears/sees as you read from a book. Provide blocks for the student to tap/count and then ask the student to tell you the number of words/blocks counted.

e. Rearranging Words to Make Sentences.

To increase the student's semantic–syntactic and memory abilities, provide increasingly longer sentences with the words out of order. Ask the student to rearrange the words so they make sense.

3. **Goal 3: To increase phonological awareness at the syllable level: implicit teaching.**

We learned in Chapter 2 that children's development of oral language transitions from storage of gestalt holophrases ("shoesnsox") to discovery of word parts and finally phonemes. Between 18 to 20 months until approximately 36 months, the child discovers some regularities about language. The holophrastic forms that were being stored earlier will now be decomposed into parts as the child learns about and applies grammatical rules. Phrases are broken into words and words into parts as the child learns about how to divide phrases into parts and meld parts back into wholes. Alegria, Pignot, and Morais (1982) concluded that first-graders, who had been reading for 4 months, were able to reverse the order of two words spoken to them, because they had developed insight into the sublexical structure of words. Explicit syllable segmentation is easier than segmenting phonemes, because consonant segments of a phonemic message are usually folded into the vowel at the acoustic level, which makes them more difficult to segment.

Suggested Activities:

a. Reading Aloud.

Read to students and occasionally point to specific words as you read. Explain that words are made up of parts, sometimes one, two, three, and so forth, and provide examples from books such as those listed in Table 5-2. Use pictures or books with compound words to provide the opportunity of hearing language sequenced orally. Compound words allow the student to attend to the story line while word parts are emphasized.

Table 5-2. Suggested Syllable-Level Books to Use in Reading Aloud to Students.

Books with Poems and Rhymes

Example: If I Had A Paka (Pomerantz, 1993)

"You take the blueberry, I'll take the dewberry. You don't want the blueberry, OK take the bayberry." Explain to the student that words have different parts, and that these parts can be changed, for instance if we substitute "blue" for "dew" in "dewberry," the new word is "blueberry."

Example: Pets in Trumpets (Most, 1991)

"Why did the musician find a dog in his trumpet?"

"Because he always finds a pet in his trum*pet*."

"What happens when a greedy gorilla eats too many bananas?"

"Greedy gor*illa* gets ill." Draw the student's attention to "hidden" syllables in words, for example, "pet" in "trumpet."

Example: Tikki Tikki Tembo (Mosel, 1968)

"Tikki Tikki Tembo No Sa Rembo Chari Bari Ruchi Pip Peri Pembo." Ask the student to repeat parts of this phrase. Ask him/her to count number of syllables, for instance, six syllables in "Tikki Tikki Tembo."

Also see Appendix D.

---

4. **Goal 4: To increase phonological awareness at the syllable level: explicit teaching.**

    Suggested Activities:

    a. **Syllable Tapping in Poems and Rhymes.**

    Nursery rhymes are used and the student is asked to tap each syllable on his or her knees or on the table. Hatcher (1994) suggested varying the speed and amount of support you give. Children might also find it easier to tap alternately with their left and right hands rather than to use one hand all the time. Ideally, by the end of this activity, children should be able to tap their leg(s) while they, or you, recite the rhyme (p. 24).

b. **Differentiating Real Compound Words from Nonreal, Compound Words.**

The student is asked to indicate when a word is "real," for example, "Is baseball a word?" Is "ballbase a word?"

c. **Differentiating Real, Noncompound Words from Nonreal, Noncompound Words.**

As in the activity previously described using noncompound words, the student is asked to identify real and nonreal words, for example, "Is quickly a word?" "Is ly-quick a word?" Nonsense words are used here and in later activities in this program to promote generalization of phonological awareness ability, not just word knowledge.

d. **Identifying the Missing Syllable.**

Ask the student to name each of two pictures shown, for example, "cow and "boy." Then, ask the student to identify which part of the word is missing when you cover one picture, for example, the cow. Fade the use of pictures when the child understands the task.

e. **Syllable Counting.**

Ask the student to count the number of syllables in words as you read words. Use blocks if the student needs tangible manipulatives to help count.

f. **Deleting a Syllable.**

The student is asked to say a word, for example, "butterfly," then is asked to say it again but to leave out a specified part of the word, for example, "don't say butter," or "don't say fly."

g. **Defining Syllables.**

The student is taught that a syllable is a part of a word and is asked to provide the same definition. It may help the student's understanding to show the pieces of a 3- to 4-piece puzzle. Like a part of a puzzle, a syllable is a part of a word.

h. Identifying the Common (Hidden) Syllable in Words.

The student is asked to tell if a particular syllable is heard in words, for example, "Is the word 'dog' in the word 'doghouse?'" "Is it in hotdog?" "Is it in housepet?"

i. Adding a Syllable.

Ask the student to add another part (prefix or suffix) to the word you say, for example, "add '-ing' to the end of 'begin.'" Increasingly complex words—"photo, photograph, photographer, photography, photographic" can facilitate phonological maturity (see Chapter 2).

j. Substituting a Syllable.

Ask the student to substitute (replace) a part of a word, for example, ask the student to say "baseball." Then, instead of "base" say "foot."

k. Reversing Syllables in Compound Words.

Ask the student to reverse or switch the parts in a compound word, for example, "Switch the two parts of 'horsefly'" (flyhorse)

l. Reversing Syllables in Noncompound, Bisyllabic Words.

As in the previous task, using noncompound, two-syllable words, ask the student to reverse or switch the parts, for example, "Switch the two parts of 'flower'" (erflow).

5. **Goal 5: To increase phonological awareness at the phoneme level: implicit teaching.**

As noted in Chapter 2, if language is developing normally the child acquires approximately 400 expressive words by 28 to 30 months, then discovers and applies morphological rules (Locke, 1997, p. 277). As the child learns to segment words into syllables, overlapping articulatory gestures lead the child to discover the phoneme, a speech sound that can stand alone. The child becomes aware of minimal pairs (words differing from each other by one sound). The discovery of phonemes leads to the child's discovery of morphological endings, such as making a word plural by adding -s or -es, or changing word tenses. Kamhi and Catts (1999) explained that grammatical morphemes are "words and inflections that convey subtle meaning and serve specific grammatical and pragmatic functions . . . (they) . . . modulate meaning" (pp. 2–3). The ASHA Guidelines (2001) proposed that "regardless of their ages, children who struggle to learn word decoding and encoding require intervention focused on explicit awareness of phonemes in words, the association of phonemes with alphabetic symbols, and the ability to segment and blend phonemes in words and manipulate them in other words" (p. 18).

Suggested Activities:

a. Reading Aloud.

As in the previous goals for phonological awareness training, use books that emphasize specific sounds. Books with alliteration and assonance are particularly relevant for this activity. See Table 5-3 for suggested books.

Table 5-3. Suggested Phoneme-Level Books for Use in Reading Aloud with Students.

Example: Double Trouble in Walla Walla (Clements, 1997)

Lulu: "I feel like a nit-wit. Homework is higgledy-piggledy." Draw the student's attention to initial phoneme changes in "nit" and "wit," and in "higgledy" and "piggledy."

"Last night it was in tip-top shape, but now it's a big mish-mash." Draw the student's attention to medial phoneme changes in "tip" and "top," and in "mish" and "mash."

Example: Pets in Trumpets (Most, 1991)

"Why were the mice invited to the picnic?"

"Because the mice brought the ice."

"Why did the witch let children hold her broomstick?"

"Because the witch had an itch." Draw the student's attention to how a word can be changed by omitting the first phoneme, for example, deleting /m/ from "mice" leaves "ice," and omitting /w/ from "witch" leaves "itch."

Books with Alliteration:

Example: Anamalia (Base, 1986)

"Diabolical dragons daintily devouring delicious delicacies."

"Eight enormous elephants expertly eating easter eggs." The emphasis here is on the repetition of initial phonemes.

Table 5-3. Suggested Phoneme-Level Books for Use in Reading Aloud with Students (continued).

Example: Listen to the Rain (Martin & Archambault, 1988)

"Listen to the rain the roaring pouring rain, leaving all outdoors a muddle, a mishy, mushy, muddy puddle." The emphasis here is on repetition of initial phonemes and the changing medial phonemes.

Example: One Odd Old Owl (Adshead, 1993)

"In the forest of Nod by a slumbering stream, there's a tall, twisting tree that grew out of a dream. Down through its branches, silently snoozing, slides a slow, sleepy Snail disturbed from her snoozing! Again, the emphasis is on repetition of initial phonemes.

Use the next three books to draw the student's attention to changing words through changing initial phonemes.

Books with Rhyme

Example: There's a Wocket in My Pocket. (Geisel, 1974)

"Did you ever have the feeling there's a wasket in your basket? Or a nureau in your bureau? Or a woset in your closet?"

Example: Cock-a-doodle-moo! (Most, 1996)

The cow tries to learn to say "cock-a-doodle-doo." She says, "Mock-a-moodle-moo" then "Rock-a-pododle-moo!" and "cock-a-doodle-moo!"

Books with Assonance

Example: Six Sick Sheep (Cole & Calmenson, 1993)

"You've no need to lite a night-light on a light night like tonight."

Also see Appendix D.

---

b. **Storytelling.**

As in previous goals to increase phonological awareness, accentuate specific phonemes.

c. **Auditory Bombardment/Sound for a Day or a Week.**

As the student is engaged in an activity, for example, drawing or putting a puzzle together, read a story that contains many instances of a certain sound, or name pictures that begin with the same phoneme (Hodson & Paden, 1991). "A sound for a day" or "A sound for a week" can be accomplished by asking the student to find pictures or objects that begin with the same sound and glueing them into an ABC book. Objects beginning with the same first sound can be found around the room and put into a "sound" bag or box (Catts, 1991a). Pickering (1994) suggested "sound boxes" where each box contains several objects beginning with the same initial sound. When the student has become familiar with objects in the boxes, the teacher mixes up the objects and the student is instructed to sort the objects by initial sounds.

6. **Goal 6: To increase phonological awareness at the phoneme level: explicit teaching.**

Results of their research led Treiman and Zukowski (1991) to conclude that children become aware of onsets, rimes, and finally single phonemes. Their data indicated that shared onsets (beginning consonants) were more difficult to identify than shared rimes (rest of word after initial consonant is removed, e.g., -at).

Suggested Activities:

a. **Blending Sounds in Monosyllabic Words Divided into Onset–Rime Beginning with Two Consonant Cluster.**

Ask the student to put sounds together to make a word, for example, "Say /sp/ /ot/ to make a word."

b. **Blending Sounds in Monosyllabic Words Divided into Onset–Rime Beginning with a Single Consonant.**

Ask the student to put sounds together to make a word, for example, "h + ot." Sublexical word parts, or phonograms, will be introduced in print in Chapter 6. It is useful, therefore, to introduce them as stimuli materials for these activities. Jenkins and Bowen (1994) suggested the teacher introduce word "families," for example, the "it" family.

Suggested Materials:

Printing short stories that students can observe while manipulating corresponding pictured cues helps them "memorize unknown words while focusing on the underlined 'it family' words to learn the significance of one-to-one correspondence between sound and symbol in reading" (p. 34). Jenkins and Bowen (1994) suggested one of Jenkins' stories:

> <u>Kit</u> the Indian and the <u>Pit</u>
>
> <u>Kit</u> dug a <u>pit</u>. <u>Kit</u> got wood for the <u>pit</u>.
>
> The wood <u>fit</u> in the <u>pit</u>. <u>Kit</u> <u>lit</u> a fire.
>
> <u>Kit</u> put meat over the <u>pit</u> to cook. <u>Kit</u>,
>
> <u>sit</u> and wait. <u>Kit</u> took the meat off with
>
> a <u>mit(t)</u>. <u>Kit</u> <u>bit</u> the meat. <u>Kit</u> said <u>it</u>
>
> was good. (p. 34)

c. Sound play–initial sound.

Tell the student you are going to play a game making up new words for pictures or objects. For example, label things in the room by making them all begin with the /b/ sound. "Chair" becomes "bair," "desk" becomes "besk."

d. Sound Play–Final Sound.

Tell the student you are going to play a game making up a new language by adding a sound to the end of words that name things in the room, for example, "desky" or "lampy" (Catts, 1991b).

e. Supplying the Rhyming Word in Known Nursery Rhymes.

Read a nursery rhyme known by the student, for example, "Humpty Dumpty." Read it again leaving out certain rhyming words and ask the student to fill in the missing word, for example, "Humpty Dumpty sat on a wall" "Humpty Dumpty had a great _____" (student supplies "fall").

f. Producing Rhyme Using Content Words.

Ball (1993) found that "the ability to provide rhymes on demand is relatively low in terms of explicitness and is easy to assess" (p. 133). Ask the student to generate a word that rhymes with a word you say, for example, "Tell me a word that rhymes with 'cat'"

g. Producing Rhyme Using Noncontent Words.

As in the previous task, use noncontent words, for example, "Tell me a word that rhymes with 'of.'"

h. Recognizing Rhyme.

Ask the student if two words rhyme, for example, "Does 'cat' rhyme with 'hat?'" "Does 'cat' rhyme with 'coat'?"

i. Sound Categorization or Identifying Rhyme Oddity.

Ball (1993) explained that "categorizing words by rhyme requires the child to group words together that contain the same rhyme" (p. 24). Bradley and Bryant (1983, 1985) referred to this as an "oddity task." Ball (1993) provided the following example:

Children are presented with four pictures of objects, three of which rhyme and one that is the "odd one out." (With younger children, it is suggested that two rhyming pictures and one nonrhyming picture be used.) After naming each of the pictures, children must select the card that does not belong with the others because it does not rhyme (p. 24).

j. Matching Rhyme.

Ask the student to choose one of three words that rhyme with a stimulus word (e.g., "Which word rhymes with coat? 'boat,' 'cat,' 'dog'?") Ball (1993) found that a rhyme judgment task "taxes more memory than either the production or categorization tasks described above." Ball found the use of printed letters to represent common sounds in the words helps when children experience difficulty with this activity. "The addition of letters adds a concrete, visual component to the task and may facilitate an understanding of the commonalities between the spoken words and their orthographic representations" (p. 24).

k. Sound Matching.

Ask the student to identify which of two to four words begin with a particular sound, for example, "Which words begin with the /s/ sound: sink, soup, soap, cat)." Do this with pictures, if needed, and then repeat the activity without pictures.

l. **Generating Words Beginning with a Particular Sound.**

Ask the student to tell you one to four word(s) that start(s) with a certain phoneme, for example, "the /k/ sound."

m. **Blending Three Continuous Sounds to Form a Monosyllabic Word.**

Ask the student to put three sounds together to make a word, and then to tell you what the word is. For example, ask the student to "say sssss-aaaa—mmmmm. What's the word?" Choose words beginning with continuant sounds, for example, /m/, /n/, /s/, /f/, /sh/, /th/, /r/, /h/, /l/, and /w/.

n. **Blending Three Noncontinuous Sounds to Form a Monosyllabic Word.**

Ask the student to put sounds together to make a word, and then to tell you what the word is. For example, ask the student to "say c-a-t. What's the word?" Choose words beginning with noncontinuant sounds, for example, /p/, /b/, /t/, /d/, k/, and /g/.

Yopp and Troyer (1992) suggested a motivating, blending game "What am I thinking of?" The teacher names a category (e.g., animals). "The teacher then gives a clue—then separate sounds in the word," for example, "/k/-/ow/" articulating each of the sounds separately. The students are asked to blend the sounds together to discover the animal the teacher has in mind (p. 700).

o. **Supplying the Initial Sound.**

Ask the student to tell you what sound is missing in the beginning of one of the words you say, for example, "Can, -an. What sound do you hear in 'can' that is missing in '-an'?"

p. **Supplying the Final Sound.**

Ask the student to tell you what sound is missing at the end of one of the words you say, for example, "Can, Ca- What sound do you hear at the end of 'can' that is missing in 'ca-'?"

q. Judging the Initial Consonant Same.

Ask the student to identify which of three to four words begins with the same sound heard in the beginning of a stimulus word. For example, "Which word begins with the same first sound you hear in 'cat?': 'boat,' 'hat,' 'cow'?"

r. Judging the Final Consonant Same.

Ask the student to identify which of three to four words ends with the same sound heard in the end of a stimulus word. For example, "Which word ends with the same sound you hear at the end of cat? 'cow,' 'hat,' 'dog'?"

s. Identifying Initial (Continuant) Sound.

Ask the student to identify what sound is heard at the beginning of one to four stimulus word(s). For example, "What is the first sound you hear in 'mom,' 'me,' 'moo,' 'mine'?" (Choose words beginning with continuant sounds—/m/, /n/, /s/, /r/, /f/, /h/, /l/, /v/, /w/, and /z/.)

t. Identifying the Initial (Stop) Sound.

Ask the student to identify what sound is heard at the beginning of one to four stimulus word(s). For example, "What is the first sound you hear in these words, 'put,' 'pet,' 'pat,' 'pot'?" (Choose words beginning with stop sounds—/p/, /b/, /t/, /d/, /k/, and /g/.)

u. Identifying the Initial Consonant Different

(also referred to as a phonological oddity task). Ask the student to identify which one of three to four words begins with a different sound. For example, "Which word has a different beginning sound? 'bat,' 'horse,' 'ball,' 'banana'?"

v. Identifying the Final Consonant Different.

Ask the student to identify which one of three to four words ends with a different sound. For example, "Which word has a different ending sound? 'cat,' 'coat,' 'dog,' 'sit'?"

w. Substituting the Initial Sound.

Ask the student to change the first sound in a word. For example, "Say cat. Now say it with a /s/ instead of /k/ in the beginning."

x. Substituting the Final Sound.

Ask the student to change the last sound in a word, for example, "Say cat. Now say it with an /n/ instead of /t/ at the end."

y. Matching the Initial Sound-to-Word Using Real, Content Words.

Ask the student to tell you if a word begins with a particular sound. Suggest either the correct or incorrect answer. For example, "Does cat begin with /k/?" or "Does cat begin with /t/?"

z. Matching the Initial Sound-to-Word Using Nonreal or Noncontent Words.

Ask the student to tell you if a word begins with a particular sound. Suggest either the correct or incorrect answer. For example, "Does gat begin with /g/?" or " Does gat begin with /m/?"

aa. Matching the Final Sound-to-Word Using Real, Content Words.

Ask the student to tell you if a word ends with a particular sound suggesting either the correct or incorrect answer, for example, "Does cat end with /t/?" or "Does cat end with /g/?"

bb. Matching the Final Sound-to-Word Using Nonreal or Noncontent Words.

Ask the student to tell you if a word ends with a particular sound. Suggest either the correct or incorrect answer. For example, "Does gat end with /t/?" or "Does gat end with /b/?"

cc. **Segmenting the Initial Sound in Real, Content Words.**

Ask the student to identify the first sound in a word. For example, "What's the first sound in cat?" Segmenting the first or last sound (C:VC or CV:C) is easier for students than segmenting the word into three separate sounds C:V:C

dd. **Segmenting the Initial Sound in Nonreal or Noncontent Words.**

Ask the student to identify the first sound in a word, for example, "What's the first sound in gat?"

ee. **Segmenting the Final Sound in Real Content Words.**

Ask the student to identify the last sound in a word, for example, "What's the last sound in cat?"

ff. **Segmenting the Final Sound in Nonreal or Noncontent Words.**

Ask the student to identify the last sound in a word. For example, "What's the last sound in gat?"

gg. **Segmenting the Middle Sound in Real, Content Words.**

Ask the student to identify the middle sound in a word. For example, "What's the middle sound in cat?"

hh. **Segmenting the Middle Sound in Nonreal or Noncontent Words.**

Ask the student to identify the middle sound in a word. For example, "What's the middle sound in gat?"

ii. **Counting and Segmenting All Sounds in Real, Content Words.**

Ask the student to identify all sounds in a word. Begin with three-sound monosyllabic words. For example, "How many sounds do you hear in the word 'cat'?" or "What three sounds do you hear in the word cat?"

jj. Counting and Segmenting All Sounds in Nonreal or Noncontent Words.

Ask the student to identify all sounds in a word. Begin with three-sound monosyllabic words. For example, "What three sounds do you hear in the word zog?"

kk. Deleting the Initial Sound.

Ask the student to omit the first sound of a word. For example, "Say cat. Say it again but don't say /k/."

ll. Deleting the Final Sound.

Ask the student to omit the last sound of a word. For example, "Say cat. Say it again but don't say /t/."

mm. Deleting Sounds within Words.

Ask the student to omit a sound in a word. For example, "Say slip. Say it again but don't say /l/."

nn. Substituting Sounds in Words.

Ask the student to substitute a sound in a word. For example, "Say slip. Say it again but instead of /l/ say /k/."

oo. Saying Words Backward or Sound Reversing.

Ask the student to say words backwards. For example: "if we say 'tall' backward, the word is 'lot.'"

pp. Switching First Sounds in Words.

Ask the student to switch the first sounds in two words. For example: "If we switch the first sounds in 'feet sank' the new words are 'seet fank.'"

qq. Learning a "Secret Language," for example, "Pig Latin."

Ask the student to put the first consonant of a word at the end and add a long /a/ sound, for example, "lamp" becomes "amplay."

All the activities suggested above have been used successfully with students in my clinical practice. Although an attempt has been made to order the activities in a developmental hierarchy, some students may have more or less difficulty with specific activities, depending on their experience with oral and written language. Therefore, the order of activities should be flexible. I move to the next activity when the student demonstrates competence with a preceding activity. Similarly, if a particular task is too difficult for a student, I provide more experience with a previous activity and/or move to the next activity.

C. Activities for Increasing Verbal Output.

If the student's ability to use the phonological code in *verbal output is weak*, teaching goals may include any of the following:

1. Goal 1: To increase oral vocabulary.

See Sections A and B above, and use traditional language therapy goals for increasing vocabulary.

2. Goal 2: To increase syntax/morphology.

See Sections A and B above, and use traditional language therapy goals for increasing syntax/morphology.

3. Goal 3: To increase oral narrative skills.

See Sections A and B above, and use traditional language therapy goals for increasing narrative skills.

Suggested Activity:

a. Storytelling.

Sequencing stories that use pictures or books provides the opportunity of hearing language sequenced orally. Asking students to tell what they think happens next in the story helps to keep them actively involved in the storytelling as well as providing them with experiences for learning to predict. *Never Ending Stories* (Discovery Toys, 1993) is an excellent game for increasing story telling abilities. Cards drawn from envelopes including people, places, events, help structure the developing oral narrative. I use children's books across all my language therapy. A source I find particularly helpful is Gebers' (1995) *Books Are for Talking, Too!* This sourcebook provides numerous suggestions as to what kind of language constructions and concepts can be found in various books. Students usually begin to fill in words and phrases you omit after hearing the story read to the them two-to-three times. Some examples of language constructions modeled in various books include: *Arthur's Nose* (Brown, 1976): possessive nouns, personal pronouns, possessive pronouns, and reflexive pronouns; *Drummer Hoff* (Emberley, 1967): rhyming, regular and irregular past tense, storytelling, and auditory memory; *King Bidgood's in the Bathtub* (Wood, 1985): expectation/prediction, storytelling; *The Snowy Day* (Keats, 1962): personal pronouns, present progressive tense, past tense, relating personal experiences, and storytelling; *Harry and the Terrible Whatzit* (Gackenbach, 1984): prepositions, regular and irregular past tense, adjectives, and drawing inferences; and *Hiccup* (Mayer, 1976): personal pronouns, expectation/prediction, storytelling, discussion, and drawing inferences.

4.   **Goal 4: To increase ability to say complex words.**

See Sections A and B above.

Suggested Activity:

a.   **Increase rate of saying increasingly complex words.**

Use sources such as *40,000 Selected Words* (Blockcolsky, Frazer, & Frazer, 1987), or workbooks for apraxia of speech for rich sources of increasingly complex words. Ask the student to read or repeat after you verbally produce the words. Verbally stress one or another of the syllables and/or tap as you say each syllable asking the student to do the same. Then ask the student to say/read the same words as quickly as possible. Time the student's verbal production and encourage him/her to increase the rate of production without sacrificing accuracy of responses.

5.   **Goal 5: To decrease use of phonological processes/deviations.**

See Sections A and B above and use traditional language therapy goals for decreasing phonological processes/deviations.

D. Activities to Increase Word Retrieval.

If the student's ability to use the phonological code *in word retrieval is weak*, teaching goals may include any of the following:

1. Goal 1: To increase word finding abilities.

2. Goal 2: To increase word finding abilities in discourse.

Suggested Activities:

a. Teaching about phonological and perceptual components of words.

Wing (1990) found that 6-year-old language-impaired students benefitted more from a treatment approach focusing on phonological and perceptual components of the retrieval process than a more traditional approach that focused on semantic associations and organization of the semantic store. Pictures representing age-appropriate vocabulary were cut from a picture dictionary and mounted on cards. Training stimuli included two- to five-syllable words and monosyllabic words that contained three to six phonemes. Other materials included rhyming objects and rhyme cards. Two groups of activities were included:

i. *Phonological segmentation activities* were included to increase metalinguistic awareness of phonological structure and the ability to retrieve all phonological segments of a word when only a portion of the representation was initially retrieved (e.g., the initial sound or a syllable). The students named one picture at a time, segmented the name as they touched a series of small squares on a paper grid, and then counted the number of squares they had touched. They also matched objects and pictures whose names rhymed, and they supplied rhyming words for words presented auditorally.

ii. *Imagery activities* were used to increase the ability to process visual and auditory perceptual information and integrate this with related, stored information and, thereby, facilitate efficient retrieval of verbal labels in the form of auditory images. The pictures used for segmentation activities were presented again, and students were asked to close their eyes and "see the picture in your mind and hear my voice saying the name of it in your mind" (p. 154). With the pictures facing down, the students were asked to name the pictures. To encourage visual and auditory image retention, the students were asked to identify a black and white copy of the pictures in an array of six pictures. Names of pictured objects were given to the students if they had difficulty retrieving them.

To practice holding several words in immediate memory, the students played two games. One involved showing the students three of the pictured objects. One student walked to a door and back rehearsing the words silently and named them for the rest of the students on returning to the group. Second, a guessing game was played in which several of the pictures were displayed on the table. While one student looked away, another student touched one of the pictures visible to the other students. The first student then looked at the pictures and tried to guess which one had been touched by using clues given by the group including initial sound or number of syllables in the word.

McGregor (1994) reported on the efficacy of using phonological information in treating word-finding problems in two boys with mild to moderate expressive language delays with age-appropriate receptive language abilities and phonological skills. Testing results for the boys indicated "their inconsistent naming provided evidence that they knew the words to some extent but could not always find them accurately" (p. 1383). Age-appropriate scores on the *Goldman–Fristoe–Woodcock Auditory Skills Test Battery* (Goldman, Fristoe, & Woodcock, 1974) provided evidence of normal short-term memory for novel single words by both subjects. McGregor interpreted the finding that neither boy could repeat any of the three-syllable stimuli on the test correctly to indicate "phonological encoding deficits that become increasingly apparent as phonological complexity increases" (p. 1384).

Using black and white line drawings, two sets of stimuli included eight target words (e.g., chef), eight semantically related words (e.g., maid), and eight phonologically similar words with the same initial sound and the same number of syllables as the target (e.g., shelf). Both semantically and phonologically related stimulus words were included because generalization would most likely occur because of the "presumed organization of the lexicon wherein semantically and phonologically related items are linked" (p. 1384).

Two approaches were incorporated in the training sessions. To elaborate on their storage of phonological output information, the subjects were trained to produce the first sound in the name of the pictured item and then determined the number of syllables in the stimulus words, which were either one- or three-syllables long. Two cards were given to the subjects to aid in counting syllable number(s). One card had the number 1 with one sticker and the second card had the number 3 with three stickers. The visual aids helped the subjects in tapping out and saying how many syllables were in target words. "After a few sessions, each child could orally segment the word into syllables with the aid of the cards and thereby identify the number of syllables with high levels of accuracy" (p.1385).

The purpose of the second aspect of training was to give the subjects practice retrieving trained items, and when unable to do so, to practice the use of cueing. Each subject named the pictured item and was instructed to "think about the first sound in the word or how long the word is if you have trouble remembering" (p. 1385). The number of syllables or first sound of the word was provided if the subject experienced difficulty. McGregor noted that with the cues the two boys "could always find the target word" (p. 1385).

A generalization effect was noted following treatment. The few phonological substitution errors "i.e., a word that is similar in segments and/or word shape to the target, such as rouge for rose" (p. 1381) made by the subjects during pretreatment were not made during posttreatment probing. McGregor interpreted this to mean "the phonological-based treatment may have had the general effect of reducing phonological errors on trained words and words that were semantically and phonologically related to those words" (p. 1391). McGregor concluded:

> The fact that phonological information did serve to reduce semantic errors in word finding provides support for a model of lexical storage and access where phonological and semantic information are represented in independent but

linked components and where semantic representations activate phonological output stores (p. 1391).

b. Retrieval strategies.

Three categories of word finding problems suggested by German (2001a) were described in Chapter 3.

i) The speaker who produces primarily lemma-related errors (slip of the tongue errors) fails to retrieve the target word lemma (meaning and syntax) to match the concept elicited by the stimulus. This speaker tends to be a fast, inaccurate word retriever and German recommended teaching this student to: 1) Pause reflectively: the student is taught to "screen and disregard competing lemmas to reduce their fast inaccurate responses" (p. 14); 2) Use semantic associate cue: the student is taught to link/associate "an intermediate word that frequently co-occurs with the target word in other contexts (color blue linked to jeans [blue jeans])" (p. 14); 3) Use 2 different attribute strategies: *Imagery cueing*: the student is taught to picture the target word referent to self cue retrieval; and *Gesture cueing*: the student is taught to motorically gesture the action associated with the target word.

ii) The speaker who produces primarily word-form-related errors (tip of the tongue errors) fails to retrieve the target word's syllabic and/or phonological form to match the concept elicited by the stimulus. This speaker tends to be a slow, accurate word retriever and German recommended teaching this student to use: 1) Phonemic associate cueing: the student is taught to "associate an intermediate word that is phonemically linked to the target word to aid future retrieval of that target word's form" for instance "daffy for daffodil" (p. 15); 2) Two semantic alternate strategies: *synonym substituting*: the student is taught to substitute acceptable word substitions while talking; and *category substituting*: the student is taught to use a category name for the word not retrieved; 3) Two attribute cueing strategies: *phonemic cueing*: the student is taught to think of the target word's first sound, vowel nucleus or syllable to self cue the word's retrieval; and *graphemic cueing*: the student is taught to spell the target word to cue the word's retrieval.

iii. The speaker who produces primarily word–form–segment-related errors (twist of the tongue errors) retrieves part of the target word's syllables or sounds and phonemic prompting does not help. This speaker tends to be a slow, inaccurate word retriever and German recommended teaching this student to use: 1) Segmenting plus rehearsal: the student is taught to segment target words into syllables and to focus on the phonological structure of target words (see Section B above). The student is taught to rehearse this strategy with words alone, then in phrases, sentences, and then in discourse; 2) Rhythm plus rehearsal: the student identifies target word and is taught to clap or make rhythmic taps while verbally producing each of the word's syllables.

E. Activities to Improve Reading.

If the student's ability to use the phonological code in *reading is weak*, teaching goals may include any of the following.

1. **Goal 1: To increase auditory processing and phonological awareness abilities**

   See Sections A and B above.

2. **Goal 2: To increase word attack skills** (see Chapter 6).

F. Summary of goals included under this processor.

If the student's ability to use the phonetic/phonological code to *hold sounds and words in memory is weak*, teaching goals may include any of the following, the first six of which are frequently referred to as auditory processing/perceptual skills.

1. **Goal 1: To increase auditory decoding through decreasing phonemic discrimination problems.**

2. **Goal 2: To increase auditory decoding through decreasing temporal pattern recognition/use problems.**

3. **Goal 3: To decrease auditory processing problems secondary to auditory figure/ground problems.**

4. Goal 4: To decrease auditory processing problems secondary to auditory selective attention problems.

5. Goal 5: To decrease auditory processing problems secondary to poor auditory memory.

6. Goal 6: To decrease auditory processing problems through increasing binaural integration (a.k.a. auditory closure/synthesis).

7. Goal 7: To increase simple receptive language.

8. Goal 8: To increase listening comprehension.

9. Goal 9: To increase verbal repetition.

If the student's ability to use the phonological code in *phonological awareness* is impaired, teaching goals may include any of the following six goals.

1. Goal 1: To increase phonological awareness at the word level: implicit teaching.

2. Goal 2: To increase phonological awareness at the word level: explicit teaching.

3. Goal 3: To increase phonological awareness at the syllable level: implicit teaching.

4. Goal 4: To increase phonological awareness at the syllable level: explicit teaching.

5. Goal 5: To increase phonological awareness at the phoneme level: implicit teaching.

6. Goal 6: To increase phonological awareness at the phoneme level: explicit teaching.

If the student's ability to use the phonological code in *verbal output is weak*, teaching goals may include any of the following:

1. Goal 1: To increase oral vocabulary.

2. Goal 2: To increase syntax/morphology.

3. Goal 3: To increase oral narrative skills.

4. Goal 4: To increase ability to say complex words.

5. Goal 5: To decrease use of phonological processes/deviations.

If the student's ability to use the phonological code in *word retrieval is weak*, teaching goals may include any of the following:

1. Goal 1: To increase isolated word finding abilities

2. Goal 2: To increase word finding abilities in discourse

If the student's ability to use the phonological code in *reading is weak*, teaching goals may include:

1. Goal 1: To increase auditory processing and phonological awareness abilities (see #1 and #2 above).

2. Goal 2: To increase word attack skills (see Chapter 6).

III. RATIONALE FOR INCLUSION OF PHONOLOGICAL AWARENESS

The importance of phonological processing to reading acquisition was emphasized in Chapter 3 through discussion of the many trajectories related to this processing. Intervention research over the course of two decades "has affirmed the importance of phonological awareness and its relation to reading acquisition" (Smith et al., 1995). Griffith and Olson (1992) proposed that phonological awareness has emerged as a better predictor of reading ability than more global measures such as Intelligence Quotient or general language proficiency. Ellis (1997) declared that phonological awareness has the potential of unraveling the mysteries of reading for countless thousands of individuals (pp. 13–15).

A. Does phonological awareness instruction work?

Studies in the United States and abroad have demonstrated that systematic instruction in phonological awareness for kindergarten and first-grade students has a positive impact on initial reading and spelling acquisition, particularly when the instruction includes teaching students to make connections between sound segments of words and the letters that represent the words and sound segments. See, for example, Bradley and Bryant, (1983, 1985), Ball and Blachman (1988, 1991), and Lundberg (1988), Blachman (1994a & b), Torgesen et al. (1994), Harbers (1999), and Gillon (2000).

O'Connor, Jenkins, Leicester, and Slocum (1993) found significant improvement in special education preschoolers following training in three categories of phonological awareness tasks: rhyming, blending, and segmenting. Finding little or no generalization within a category (from one type of blending task to another type of blending task) or between categories (from blending to segmenting), O'Connor et al. concluded that phonological awareness skills "may be more isolated and specific than the global term phonological awareness implies" (p. 544). In their study, Foorman et al. (1997) found that phonological awareness activities in kindergarten can lead to "significant gains in phonological processing skills relative to children in the same curriculum who do not receive this training" (p. 4). Research by Scanlon and Vellutino (1997) revealed that children at-risk for reading problems, who were reading at above-average levels in first grade, usually came from kindergarten classes with more phoneme awareness instruction and invented spelling. Vellutino and Scanlon (1991) studied 297 second and third graders, and 171 sixth and seventh graders. While phonologically based skills were found to be the most important determinants of word identification in both groups, this was especially true during the beginning stages of reading. The Vellutino group concluded "the research quite strongly endorses the practice of incorporating activities that foster the development of both alphabetic coding and phoneme awareness as part of the instructional program" (p. 439). Van Kleeck (1994) explained that the importance of phonological awareness in achieving insight into the alphabetic principle "seems to provide unequivocal support for a phonics approach to early reading instruction" (p. 79). Finally, Smith et al. (1995) reviewed twenty eight sources including 13 primary studies and 15 secondary sources on phonological awareness training, and concluded that "since phonological awareness has been established as one of the prerequisites for reading acquisition, phonological awareness instruction is obligatory, not optional" (p. 2).

B. Instruction by whom and for how long?

The connection between phonological awareness and reading acquisition has become clear, and training in these skills provides the perfect meeting place for parents, teachers, speech–language specialists, and other educators, for example, resource specialists, reading teachers, and tutors. Hatcher (1994) observed that an important implication of the relationship between phonological awareness and reading "particularly for teachers and speech therapists, is that training in phonological skills might help prevent children experiencing undue difficulty in learning to read" (p. 1). The instruction can be done on an individual basis or in a group setting. Ball (1997) found that when teachers incorporate sound-based activities through books providing play with rhyme, alliteration, and invented spellings, "they seize (the) opportunity to heighten for some children the connections between sound and print" (p. 23).

The speech–language specialist works most directly with young children with developmental language problems. Because of their backgrounds in linguistics, phonetics, language acquisition, and childhood language disorders, speech–language specialists represent a natural bridge to training of other educators and adults as well as implementing phonological awareness training to students on their caseloads and/or work collaboratively in classroom environments. The addition of phonological awareness testing to this specialist's battery is entirely appropriate because of the oral–written language continuum and because early oral language problems so frequently evolve into later reading, writing, spelling problems. The speech–language specialist is in a critical position to train parents and other professionals about phonological awareness. It would seem the natural linkage for the speech–language specialist to implement phonological awareness training, and the resource specialist to follow up with explicit phonics instruction. In his position as director of the National Institute of Child Health and Human Development (NICHD), Lyon (1997) considered speech–language specialists as "gems" in the shift toward integrating phonological awareness training into reading. Lyon noted that the nature of speech-language specialists' curriculum and clinical training prepares them to integrate practice with theory. They "know how to interpret the data, know the importance of phonological awareness, . . . (and) need to explicitly and daily translate what they know about language and reading to teachers" (p. 5). The ASHA Guidelines (2001) pointed to many strengths speech–language specialists bring to phonological awareness instruction including the following:

> Knowledge of phonology also helps SLPs tailor lessons for success. They know how to reduce stimulus complexity in sound–segmentation activities for example, by mixing continuant and stop sounds to maximize discriminability. They also understand how place and man-

ner of articulation, coupled with voicing, affect sound production and how sounds are affected by their position in words and surrounding contexts (pp. 7–8).

Intervention studies report positive results with phonological awareness training incorporated into the listening–oral language curriculum. Activities are variously implemented in the classroom and outside the class in small group instruction. Blake-Davies (1994) found increased decoding abilities in elementary school-age boys after 2 hours twice weekly of individualized phonological awareness training over 6 consecutive weeks by a speech–language specialist. Yopp and Troyer (1992) reported measurable gains in phonemic awareness skills after training by teachers in one activity 15 to 20 minutes daily over 2 weeks. Foorman et al. (1997) reported significant gains in phonological processing skills in children who received 15 to 20 minutes of daily phonological awareness training relative to other children who did not receive this training. Ball (1997) compared performance on phoneme awareness, reading phonetically regular words, and sophistication of developmental spellings in three groups of kindergarten children. The group who received phonological awareness training showed significant gains compared with children in the other two control groups: one with children who participated in language activities and letter–sound instruction, and one with children who received no intervention. The phonological awareness training occurred outside the classroom for 20 minutes four times each week. Pieretti (2001) reported increased reading scores and faster naming speed in double-deficit readers enrolled in a program including approximately 10 minutes of phonological awareness instruction once weekly for eight weeks. Sawyer (1994) reported that college-aged students with sixth grade reading abilities and phonological awareness problems benefitted from sixteen 10-minute sessions twice weekly for 8 weeks. Students commented "Why didn't someone show me this before;" "Now reading and spelling make sense;" "I feel so much more in control;" and "This is helping me in my writing class too."

Because a number of programs reported gains in phonological awareness after 15 to 20 minute sessions, Blachman (1991, 1994) recommended inclusion of these activities in the classroom to foster literacy acquisition. Lyon (1995b) emphasized that "instruction must be intense, of sufficient duration, and informed by a knowledge of linguistic development and its relationship to the development and structure of written language."

IV. VARIABLES THAT INFLUENCE THE EFFECTIVENESS OF EARLY READING AND PHONOLOGICAL AWARENESS INSTRUCTION

The ability to read does not emerge spontaneously, but rather through regular and active engagement with print. For a child who is well prepared to learn to read, the beginning of formal reading instruction should not be an abrupt step, but a further step on a journey already well underway. While preschool knowledge about written language is typically developed at home, schools can play an important role. Print awareness, letter familiarity, and phonemic awareness can all be developed through classroom instruction in preschool, kindergarten, and first grade.

A. **The following activities were recommended for use prior to formal reading instruction by Adams (1990) and summarized by Stahl et al. (1990):**

1. The single most important activity for building the knowledge and skills eventually required for reading appears to be reading aloud to children regularly and interactively.

2. Language experience activities and the use of big books are excellent means of establishing print awareness (although they are less useful as primary vehicles for reading instruction itself).

3. Some children have difficulty conceiving of spoken language as consisting of individual words. The concept of "word" can be developed easily, though, through exposure to written text or through direct instruction. Children should also be helped to appreciate the relationship between the lengths of spoken and written words.

4. Activities designed to develop young children's awareness of words, syllables, and phonemes significantly increase their later success in learning to read and write. The impact of phonemic training on reading acquisition is especially strong when phonemes are taught together with the letters by which they are represented (pp. 124–125).

B. **In her conclusions about effective techniques for teaching children who are beginning to read, including phonics instruction, Adams (1990) observed the following:**

1. Approaches in which systematic code instruction is included along with the reading of meaningful connected text result in superior reading achievement overall, for both low-readiness and better prepared students.

2. Programs for all children, good and poor readers, should strive to maintain an appropriate balance between phonics activities and the reading and appreciation of informative and engaging texts.

3. Classroom encouragement of invented spellings is a promising approach toward the development of phonemic awareness and knowledge of spelling patterns.

4. Because most phonemes cannot be pronounced without a vowel, many programs avoid or limit the use of isolated phonemes in their instruction. This practice often leads to potentially confusing instruction. The advantages of asking students to articulate phonemes in isolation outweigh the disadvantages.

5. Although rules and generalizations cannot substitute for direct practice with the words to which they pertain, they may be useful for either directing students' attention to a particular spelling pattern, or providing strategies for coping with difficult decoding patterns (Stahl et al., 1990, pp. 125–126).

C. Included among Lyon's (1997) findings as to variables that influence the effectiveness of phonological awareness training were the following:

1. While phonological awareness training is a necessary component for the development of early reading skill, it is not sufficient.

2. Children who display deficits in phonological awareness and rapid naming ability appear to be the most difficult to remediate.

3. Such children require instructional formats that provide substantial intensity, consistency, and long duration.

4. Teachers must be trained in depth about the structure of spoken and written language. A complete understanding of the components of phonological processing and how the components relate to word recognition and decoding skills is critical.

5.   Classroom settings that promote the ability to instruct children in an explicit manner with maximum intensity and duration are required.

D. **In their review of twenty-eight studies of phonological awareness instruction, Smith et al. (1995) found that the following five curriculum designs should be considered instructional priorities during phonological awareness instruction.**

1.   Use Conspicuous Strategies:

the explicit teaching about words, syllables, and sounds. Phonological awareness needs to be obvious and salient because phonemes are elusive and because children pay attention to meaning, not sounds. The individual who is instructing students needs to model specific sounds and "how they feel" in the mouth, for instance, talks about how "sat" and "at" are different because "I didn't say /s/, the sound that is made by putting my teeth together and letting air out the front of my mouth like a 'snake sound.'" Students should then produce specific sounds and then touch or move concrete representations of a sound while verbally producing them, for example "/s/ /-at/". The concrete representations can be blank tiles or tiles with letters printed on them. I like using plastic chips or wooden blocks, or I ask the student to draw lines or dashes to represent words, syllables or sounds.

2.   Mediated Scaffolding:

what the teacher/speech language–specialist does to facilitate the task. The sources reviewed identified four dimensions that can be adjusted in terms of range of difficulty:

a. Word length: simple words contain 1–3 phonemes: (-a, -at, sat); difficult words contain 3+ phonemes (class, swing, pumpkin).

b. Size of phonological unit: simple units are compounds words, syllables, onset–rimes (carwash, kitt-y, S-am); difficult units include individual phonemes (for example: /m/, /n/ /s/).

  c. Position of phonemes in words: phonemes in the initial and then final position in words are easier, while phonemes in medial position of words are more difficult.

  d. Phonological properties of phonemes and clusters: continuant sounds (for example "Say 'mmmmman'") is easier than consonant clusters (for example ("What's the beginning sound in 'school'?" and later developing phonemes such as /r/ and /l/.

  Materials can be scaffolded through use of puppets, stories, pictures, tiles, and alphabet tiles. Teacher scaffolding comes through modeling how phonemes are produced, and how they sound and feel in the mouth, and through verbally stressing target phonemes students are to identify and manipulate.

3. **Strategic Integration:**

  when previously learned phonological skills are paired with letters in the following sequence:

  a. Begin instruction in phonological awareness using simple units and focus on initial sounds.

  b. When these are mastered, introduce corresponding graphemes (printed letters).

  c. Increase complexity of phonological units.

  d. Begin to have students decode words as you continue to work on phonological awareness with them.

4. **Primed Background Knowledge:**

  relevant learned strategies with sounds that will facilitate new learning. For example, detecting individual phonemes is relevant to segmenting phonemes, therefore review sound detection ("what is the first sound in 'cat'?") prior to introducing phoneme segmentation ("what are the 3 sounds in 'cat'?")

5. **Judicious Review:**

  progressing from easy to more difficult features. This must include guided practice ranging from teacher modeling to verbal prompt to use of particular strategies. Finally, the studies reviewed recommended that daily review is important to developing phonological awareness.

V. SUMMARY

The focus of this chapter has been on relevant issues for teaching/remediating the phonological processor. Chapter 6 will focus on activities for teaching/remediating the orthographic, meaning and context processors.

VI. CLINICAL COMPETENCIES.

To remediate developmental reading problems the teacher/clinician/student will demonstrate the following competencies:

A. Determine goals to teach/remediate the phonological processor.

B. Develop curriculum-relevant goals to foster literacy acquisition.

C. Collaborate with other professionals to support literacy.

APPENDIX 5.1. SUGGESTED MATERIALS TO STRENGTHEN PHONOLOGICAL PROCESSOR

A Sound Start: Phonemic Awareness Lessons for Reading Success
Authors: McCormick, C.E., Throneburg, R.N., & Smitley, J.M. (2002)
Publishing Co.: The Guilford Press
Contents:
1) Activities promoting phonemic awareness for whole class and small groups.
2) Activities promoting phonemic awareness for students needing additional, more intensive instruction.
3) Activities promoting phonemic awareness through focusing on auditory, visual, and motoric properties of English consonant phonemes.

Alphabet Sounds Box

Author: none (1994)

Publishing Co.: Lakeshore Learning Materials

Contents:

1) A large wooden box with 26 boxes, each for a different letter of the alphabet.

2) Small objects to place in the boxes according to initial sound/letter.

3) Picture cards and plastic upper and lower-case letters.

Auditory Discrimination and Memory Intermediate/Advanced

Author: Pickering, Joyce S. (1993)

Publishing Co.: The June Shelton School & Evaluation Center

Contents: Six sections of activities for Auditory Discrimination and Memory for various vowel and consonant sounds.

Barnaby's Burrow: An Auditory Processing Game

Author: Truman, B. (2000)

Publishing Co.: LinguiSystems

Contents: Activities involving Barnaby the rabbit and rhyming, segmenting, sound substitution, sound blending.

Barnaby's Burrow: An Auditory Processing Game

Author: Truman, B. (2000)

Publishing Co.: LinguiSystems

Contents: Activities involving Barnaby the rabbit and rhyming, segmenting, sound substitution, sound blending.

Blend It, End It!

Author: Keopke, H. (2000)

Publishing Co.: LinguiSystems

Contents:

1) Activities for phonological awareness skills, phonics and spelling skills.

2) Players flip disks to determine whether target will be a word beginning (blend) or ending. Players write words incorporating target. Includes 36 initial word blends including: bl-, cr-, fr-, pl-, spl-, st-, ak-, th-, tw- and 108 word endings including: -ark, -ace, -all, -eak, -ear, -ice, -ill, -old, -uff.

Books Are for Talking Too!

Author: Gebers, J.L. (1995)

Publishing Co.: Pro-Ed

Contents:

1) Materials for helping preschool through Grade 12 students transition from oral language to literacy.

2) Listings of books appropriate for preschool and kindergarten, grades 1-5, and grades 6-12.

3) An index that helps you easily find books to achieve specific language goals.

Earobics

Author: Cognitive Concepts Inc. (1998)

Publishing Co.: Cognitive Concepts

Contents:

1) Software to increase phonological awareness and auditory processing skills critical for reading and writing success.

2) Step 1 includes six interactive games and 309 levels

3) Step 2 includes five interactive games and 593 levels for building auditory and listening skills, such as: sound-symbol correspondence; phoneme identification and sequencing; auditory, syllable, and phoneme segmentation; and rhyming.

(HELP-4) Handbook of Exercises for Language Processing

Authors: Lazzari, A.M. & Peters, P.M. (1989)

Publishing Co.: LinguiSystems

Contents:

1) Phonological awareness activities at the word level including counting words and rearranging words in sentences.

2) Phonological awareness activities at the syllable level including adding, segmenting, and identifying syllables.

3) Phonological awareness activities at the sound level including rhyming, blending, sound identification, and segmentation.

Handbook of Exercises for Language Processing: for Auditory Processing

Authors: Lazzari, A.M. & Peters, P.M. (1994)

Publishing Co.: LinguiSystems

Contents:

1) Activities for recognizing and identifying initial and medial sounds in words.

2) Activities for recognizing blends and digraphs.

3) Activities for recognizing vowels and dipthongs.

4) Activities for discriminating sounds in words in sentences.

5) Activities for phonemes substitution in words in sentences.

Helping Children Overcome Learning Difficulties

Author: Rosner, J. (1993)

Publishing Co.: Walker and Company

Contents:

1) Activities for phonological awareness at the syllable level including identification and deletion.

2) Activities for phonological awareness at the phoneme level including identification and deletion, and substitution.

Ladders to Literacy: A Kindergarten Activity Book

Authors: O'Connor, R. E., Notari-Syverson, A., & Vadasy, P. F. (1998)

Publishing Co.: Brookes Publishing Co.

Contents:

1) Activities for print awareness such as shared storybook reading, making books, photography, sorting objects, transition to reading words, and integrating spelling and reading.

2) Activities for phonological awareness such as rhythmic activities, listening to songs, clapping syllables, rhyming, isolating sounds, blending, and segmenting.

3) Activities for oral language such as show and tell, book review/story grammar, special words, and brainstorming.

Ladders to Literacy: A Preschool Activity Book

Authors: Notari-Syverson, A., O'Connor, R. E., & Vadasy, P. F. (1998)

Publishing Co.: Brookes Publishing Co.

Contents:

1) Activities for print/book awareness such as shared storybook reading, following recipes, recording constructions, my first journal, and museum exhibit.

2) Activities for metalinguistic awareness such as rhythmic activities, listening to songs, nursery rhymes, rhyming games, playing with sounds in words, blending, play with miniature toys, and pretend play.

3) Activities for oral language such as show and tell, talking about books, book buddy, special words, let's say it another way, interviews, movie reviews, brainstorming, and showtime.

Language!

Author: Greene, J.F. (2000)

Publishing Co.: Sopris West

Contents: Sounds and Letters for Readers and Spellers establishes phoneme awareness in emerging readers and spellers including phoneme isolation, segmentation and counting, blending, rhyming, deletion, substitution, reversal, and pig Latin.

LocoTour Software

Authors: Scarry-Larkin, M., & Price, E. (1999)

Available through: Dimensions Speech, Language and Learning Services, North

Contents: Software for enhancing literacy–phoneme awareness.

1) Activities showing video/photos demonstrating mouth movements of sounds.

2) Activities to reinforce sound/symbol relationships.

3) Activities to reinforce sound and syllable awareness.

More than Words: Activities for Phonological Awareness and Comprehension

Authors: Donnelly, K., Thomsen, S., Huber, L., & Schoemer, D. (1992)

Publishing Co.: Communication Skill Builders

Contents:

1) Activities for phonological awareness including sentences to words (content and noncontent words), words to syllables (1–4 syllable words), rhyming, sound blending, and words to sounds.

2) Activities for reading comprehension including before, during and after reading.

More Story Making: Using Predicatable Literature to Develop Communication

Authors: Peura-Jones, R.E., & DeBoer, C.J. (2000)

Publishing Co.: Thinking Publications

Contents:

1) Activities that allow you to simultaneously develop phonological awareness skills and speech and language development.

Once Upon a Sound: Literature-Based Phonological Activities
Authors: Smith-Kiewel, L. & Claeys, T.M. (1998)
Publishing Co.: Thinking Publications
Contents: Activities that allow you to simultaneously develop literacy, phonological awareness, and phonology using children's classic stories.

Phonemic Awareness Fun Deck
Author: Webber, S.G. (1998)
Publishing Co.: Super Duper
Contents: 19 sets (3 cards each) of colorfully illustrated rhyming words.

Phonological Awareness in Words and Sentences (PAWS)
Authors: Academic Communication Associates (2000)
Publishing Co.: Academic Communication Associates
Contents:
1) Activities for strengthening awareness of sound patterns in words, sentences, and short stories.
2) Skills include identifying sounds in words, vowel changes, syllables within words, and rhyming words within sentences; finding words that start or end with the same sound; forming compound words; comparing syllable patterns within words; changing sounds to create new words; and combining consonants to create blends.
3) Activities include consonants, vowels, dipthongs, and blends in words and sentences.

Phonological Awareness Skills Program (PASP)
Author: Rosner, J. (1999)
Publishing Co: Pro-Ed
Contents: Activities for phonological awareness at the syllable and phoneme level.

Phonemic Awareness in Young Children: A Classroom Curriculum
Authors: Donnelly, K. Thomsen, S., Huber, L., & Schoemer, D. (1998)
Publishing Co.: Communication Skill Builders
Contents:
1) An asessment test for detecting rhymes, counting syllables, matching initial sounds, counting phonemes, comparing word lengths, and representing phonemes with letters.

2) Listening activities including listening to sounds and listening to sequences of sounds.

3) Activities for rhyming including poetry, songs, jingles; rhyme stories; word rhyming, and action rhyming.

Phonological Awareness Shuffle
Author: Flynn, M. (1998)
Publishing Co.: LinguiSystems
Contents: Activities for consonant blend rhyming.

Phonological Awareness Training for Reading
Authors: Torgesen, J. & Bryant, B. (1994)
Publishing Co.: Pro-Ed
Contents: Activities for phonemes including segmentation, blending, and rhyming.

"Say and Do" Phonemic Awareness Stories and Activities
Authors: Super Duper Publications, illustrated by Rishforth, P. (1998)
Publishing Co.: Pro-Ed
Contents:
1) Activities for rhyme including recognition, completion, and production.
2) Activities for phoneme identification.

Sound Effects
Author: Spector, C.C. (1999)
Publishing Co.: Thinking Publications
Contents:
1) Activities for strengthening the distinction between how words sound and how they are spelled.
2) Activities to enhance student's divergent thinking skills, mental associations, and vocabulary.
3) Activities to facilitate discussions about humor based on phoneme changes.

Sound Search: Reauditorization Sentences
Author: Flynn, M.L. (1999)
Publishing Co.: LinguiSystems

Contents:

1) Activities for expanding phonological processing through listening to and reauditorizing words and sentences.

2) Activities for identifying orthographic patterns and identify short and long vowel sounds.

Sound Wizard: Strategy-Building Games for Phonological Awareness
Author: Lencher, O. (2001)
Publishing Co.: Thinking Publications
Contents: 18 strategy-based card games to help children learn and practice: rhyme recognition and production; syllable segmentation, deletion, and blending; sound identification and matching; sound blending; sound–symbol correspondence; and sound manipulation.

Sounds Abound: Listening, Rhyming, and Reading
Authors: Catts, H. & Vartiainen, T. (1993)
Publishing Co.: LinguiSystems
Contents:

1) Activities for rhyme including rhyme judgment, production, and play.

2) Activities for word beginnings and endings including sound judgment, production, and play.

3) Activities for segmenting and blending syllables and phonemes.

Sounds and Letters for Readers and Spellers
Author: Greene, J. (1997)
Publishing Co.: Sopris West
Contents: Phoneme awareness drills including isolation, segmentation, counting, blending, rhyming, and substitution.

Sounds Good to Me: Phonological Awareness
Author: Bryant, J.E. (1998)
Publishing Co.: Thinking Publications
Contents:

1) Activities to enhance phonological awareness, as well as speech, language, and early literacy skills.

2) Over 100 poems that emphasize sound words such as "buzz," "swish," "slurp," and "clickety-clack."

Sourcebook of Phonological Awareness Activities: Children's Classic Literature
Author: Goldsworthy, C. (1998)

Publishing Co.: Singular Publishing Group, Inc.

Contents:

1) Activities integrating children's classic literature for phonological awareness at the word level including segmentation, blending, isolation, and deletion.

2) Activities integrating children's classic literature for phonological awareness at the syllable level including segmentation, blending, isolation, and deletion.

3) Activities integrating children's classic literature for phonological awareness at the phoneme level including segmentation, blending, isolation, and deletion.

Sourcebook of Phonological Awareness Activities: Children's Core Literature
Author: Goldsworthy, C. (2001)

Publishing Co.: Singular Publishing Group, Inc.

Contents:

1) Activities integrating children's core literature for phonological awareness at the word level including segmentation, blending, isolation, and deletion.

2) Activities integrating children's core literature for phonological awareness at the syllable level including segmentation, blending, isolation, and deletion.

3) Activities integrating children's core literature for phonological awareness at the phoneme level including segmentation, blending, isolation, and deletion.

Sourcebook of Phonological Awareness Activities: Children's Core Literature Grades 3–5
Authors: Goldsworthy, C. & Pieretti, R. (2003)

Publishing Co.: Thomson Delmar Learning

Contents:

1) Activities integrating children's core literature for phonological awareness at the word level including segmentation, blending, isolation, and deletion.

2) Activities integrating children's core literature for phonological awareness at the syllable level including segmentation, blending, isolation, and deletion.

4) Activities integrating children's core literature for phonological awareness at the phoneme level including segmentation, blending, isolation, and deletion.

Strong Rhythms and Rhymes: Language and Literacy Development through Sentence Combining
Authors: Strong, C.J. & Strong, W. (1999)

Publishing Co.: Thinking Publications

Contents: Chants to be used to increase phonological awareness and syntax skills.

Take Home: Phonological Awareness

Authors: Robertson, C. & Salter, W. (1998)

Publishing Co.: LinguiSystems

Contents: Take home activities for generalization of phonological awareness training including phoneme isolation, segmentation, blending, rhyming, deletion, substitution, reversal, and pig Latin.

The Green Readiness Book: Auditory and General Readiness Activities for Reading and Arithmetic

Author: Rosner, J. (1986)

Publishing Co.: Walker and Company

Contents: Activities including rhythm and tempo, copying and classifying sounds, identifying syllables in multisyllabic words, auditory discrimination, reordering sounds, sound identification, omission and substitution.

The Lindamood Phoneme Sequencing Program for Reading, Spelling, and Speech (3rd Edition) (LIPS-3)

Authors: Lindamood, P. & Lindamood, P. (1998)

Publishing Co.: Pro-Ed

Contents: Activities to develop phoneme-sequencing ability through materials including mouth drawings and manipulatives.

The Literacy Link: A Multisensory Approach to Sound–Symbol Connections

Author: Northrup, P.S. (2002)

Publishing Co.: Thinking Publications

Contents: Activities to increase rhyming; initial consonant identification; knowledge of word families; phoneme blending and segmentation; articulatory features of each sound; and phoneme–grapheme correspondence.

Tongue Twisters

Contents: Activities for alliteration (first letter in word sounds the same). Available through local book stores, libraries, and teachers supply stores.

The Phonological Awareness Companion

Author: The Wellington County Board of Education (1995)

Publishing Co.: LinguiSystems

Contents: Activities for phonological awareness including word counting, syllable segmentation and blending, and phoneme substitution and rhyming.

The Phonological Awareness Kit

Authors: Robertson, C. & Salter, W. (1995)

Publishing Co.: LinguiSystems

Contents:

1) Activities for phonological awareness at the word level including segmentation, blending, isolation, and deletion.

2) Activities for phonological awareness at the syllable level including segmentation, blending, isolation, and deletion.

3) Activities for phonological awareness at the phoneme level including segmentation, blending, isolation, and deletion.

The Phonological Awareness Kit-Intermediate

Authors: Robertson, C. & Salter, W. (1997)

Publishing Co.: LinguiSystems

Contents:

1) Activities for phonological awareness at the syllable level including segmentation, blending, isolation, and deletion.

2) Activities for phonological awareness at the phoneme level including segmentation, blending, isolation, and deletion.

The Phonological Awareness Skills Program

Author: Rosner, J. (1999)

Publishing Co.: Pro-Ed

Contents: Activities for syllable deletion, sound omission and deletion, and sound substitution.

The Sounds Abound Program

Authors: Lenchner, O. & Podhajski, B. (1998)

Publishing Co.: LinguiSystems

Contents:

1) Activities for rhyme including recognition, completion, and production.

2) Activities for syllable segmentation and deletion.

3) Activities for phoneme recognition, segmentation, deletion, substitution, and blending.

Word Scramble: A Phonological Awareness and Word-Building Game

Author: Johnson, P.F. (1998)

Publishing Co.: LinguiSystems

Contents:

1) Activities for phonological awareness skills, listening skills, decoding skills, word flexibility, articulation skills, and thinking skills.

2) Players create words through matching letter tiles to gameboard.

Word Scramble 2: A Word-Building Game

Author: Johnson, P.F. (2000)

Publishing Co.: LinguiSystems

Contents:

1) Activities for students who have a good grasp of basic CVC words, vowel sounds, and consonant blends. Word Scramble 2 helps students build root words, prefixes and suffixes.

2) Players read and write words, define words, use words in sentences, and ask questions using the target words.

Working Out with Phonological Awareness

Authors: Schreiber, L.R., Sterling-Orth, A., Thurs, S.A., and McKinley, N.L. (2000)

Publishing Co.: Thinking Publications

Contents: Activities spanning six phonological awareness skill areas: segmenting syllables, rhyming, blending syllables and sounds, segmenting sounds, manipulating sounds, and working with clusters.

> To support literacy beyond the phonological processor, we must move beyond the sound level and help our students transition into print. Chapter 6 presents teaching goals and activities and suggested materials for use in targeting the orthographic, meaning and context processors.

CHAPTER

6

Treatment of Developmental Reading Disabilities: Part 2

OUTLINE

Appendix 6.2. Suggested materials to strengthen the meaning processor

Appendix 6.3. Suggested materials to strengthen the context processor

I. INTRODUCTION

"Regardless of their ages, children who struggle to learn word decoding and encoding require intervention focused on explicit awareness of phonemes in words, the association of phonemes with alphabetic symbols, and the ability to segment and blend phonemes in words and manipulate them in other ways" (ASHA Guidelines, 2001, p. 18). Phonological awareness training has the greatest impact on reading when combined with explicit instruction of the alphabetic principle and its application to decoding and spelling words (Ball & Blachman, 1991; Bradley & Bryant, 1985; Torgesen, 1998). To that end, and in keeping with the format of this book, Adams' (1990) model of reading processors will be used once again in this chapter as it has been in Chapters 2, 4 and 5. Accordingly, four processors work together for successful reading: the phonological, orthographic, meaning, and context processors (see Chapter 2 for an explanation of this model.)

The importance of looking at verbal naming speed was emphasized in Chapter 3. Wolf (2001) summarized three reasons many researchers have looked beyond the phonological-core deficit as the sole contributor to developmental reading disabilities. These are: 1) The growing need to explain the "heterogeneity of reading disabilities and the complexity of reading breakdown—especially in the area of fluency" (p. xii); 2) Increased awareness of the "multiple, underlying sources that can contribute to or impede fluency development" (p. xiii); 3) The growing body of research demonstrating children's reading problems may be related to phonological processing problems, or naming speed problems, or both (p. xiii).

A discussion of assessment areas and corresponding tests for the four processors was presented in Chapter 4. Suggested goals, activities, and materials to strengthen the phonological processor were presented in Chapter 5. Goals and activities that target the orthographic, meaning and context processors are presented in this chapter. Recall that the *orthographic processor* involves visual information from the printed page. This processor is important for the reader to store individual letters as well as sublexical word parts (-ing) and letter patterns (-at). The *meaning processor* stores familiar word meanings, and the *context processor* is in charge of constructing a coherent, ongoing interpretation of the text.

In both Chapters 5 and 6, I have described the steps of methods I use in my own instruction/therapy with students demonstrating developmental reading disabilities. Of course, depending upon the nature and severity of each student's problem, I decide where to begin within each processor according to each student's needs. However, for example, I find a student who needs to "begin at the beginning," I would begin with Teaching Goal #1 and work through Goal #9 under the phonological processor. As the student's phonological processing increases, I add goals included under the orthographic, meaning, and context processors. Stated differently, I never work through the processors from phonological through context. Focusing all our attention on one processor to the exclusion of the others only helps the student become more proficient with goals for that processor. For example, emphasizing only goals targeting the phonological processors results in a student becoming more proficient at auditory processing, phonological awareness, and word attack skills. This student is likely to become a good decoder with poor reading comprehension. It is far more beneficial to monitor the student's progress, and as his/her performance increases in the use of one processor, add goals from the other three processors so that instruction across the processors is simultaneous as well as sequential, with each goal providing a scaffold for the next. Under many of the goals, I include selected materials and activities I have found to be particularly effective in my own sessions.

II. METHODS THAT TARGET THE ORTHOGRAPHIC PROCESSOR

As students with developmental reading disabilities become more proficient with the phonological aspects of language through the goals and activities in Chapter 5, transition into print is made smoother through use of techniques and materials that coincide with the language-based treatment goals and activities presented under the next sections.

A. Activities to Strengthen the Orthographic Processor.

If the student's ability to use the *orthographic processor is weak*, teaching goals may include any of the following.

1.   **Goal 1: To increase phonological awareness skills at the phoneme level using print.**

Suggested Activities:

a. **Introduce graphemes.**

When the student is at the phoneme level in explicit phonological awareness instruction, introduce some of the corresponding graphemes (letters), for instance, the graphemes: -a -t -m. Be sure the student recognizes and can verbally name the graphemes as well as verbally produce the sounds that correspond with the graphemes. Then combine graphemes into word families, such as "-at" and "-am" families (also known as rimes or phonograms.) Ask the student to name each word family, or ask "What is the word part?" Now work through the following activities to strenghthen the automaticity of naming onset–rimes. According to The Literacy Volunteer Connection (2001) onsets and rimes (phonograms) are "an economical use of students' attention and capacity for learning" with 37 rimes needed to generate 500 words frequently used by children in grades 1 to 3. "When teaching the use of phonograms, we get a lot of bang for the buck!" (p. 1). And Adams (1990) explained that exercises with phonograms fulfill the desirable goal of reinforcing the integrity of frequent spelling patterns even as they are part of different words (p. 132).

b. **Substituting the medial sound in words using plastic letters or print.**

Ask the student to change the middle sound of a word to make a new word. For example, "Change 'pat' to 'pet.'" Ask the student to manipulate the corresponding plastic letters or to print the letters of the word. The student changes the middle sound verbally as he/she replaces [a] with [e] and moves the plastic letters or prints the letters.

c. **Connecting sound segments and letters through Elkonin boxes.**

Blachman (1994) summarized the steps in Elkonin's (1973) phoneme segmentation activities.

i. The student is given a picture of a person or object, whose name is in the student's vocabulary. Early training should include words beginning with fricatives—/f/, /s/, /v/—or nasals—/m/ and /n/, because these sounds are produced easily in isolation.

ii. "Boxes" are drawn below the picture, and the number of boxes corresponds to the number of phonemes in the pictured word. For example, three boxes are placed below a picture of a man or a ship.

iii. The student is given colored chips ("tokens") all in one color. The student slowly says the name of the picture and places a chip in each of the corresponding boxes under the picture. After the student understands this activity, different colored chips are given to him or her to place in the boxes under the picture. Consonants are now represented by one color, and vowels are represented by another color.

iv. After the student can manipulate the tokens to represent vowels and consonants, letters are printed on the chips, and the student continues the activity. The tokens are eventually replaced with letter tiles.

In their *"Say-it-and-move it"* procedure, Ball and Blachman (1988) asked the student to represent two to three sound items with tiles that are stored above the picture on a card (see Figure 6-1). The student is taught to pronounce each sound as he or she moves each tile down to a line below the pictured item. The blended sounds are repeated and represent the name of the pictured item.

d. Introduce carryover games.

I have found a number of games that are useful for young children crossing the bridge from phonological to orthographic processors. In Game One, *Bug Bites*, of *Alphabug Soup* (Learning Resources, undated), letter disks are turned letter-side-up in a pool on the game board. Students are asked to name words that begin with the letters they select, and then they put the letters into a "soup pot." In Game Two, *All-You-Can-Eat Bug Buffet*, "bug disks" are turned letter-side-up next to vowel circles and in a "spell-off," students write as many words as possible using the letters they have selected.

In the three-dimensional game, *UpWords* (1988), students spell words with stackable letter tiles on a gameboard to score points. Words are built by placing letters across or down on the board as well as by stacking letters on top of letters already on the board to form different words.

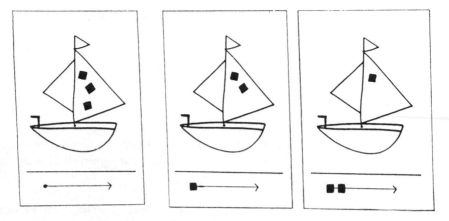

Say-it-and-move-it instructional sequence. Step 1: Children store all tiles/ disks on the picture. Step 2: After repeating the stimulus item, children slide one tile/disk below the line as they pronounce slowly the first pho- neme. Step 3: The second phoneme is pronounced slowly as children move the second tile/disk below the line. The original blended item is then repeated.

Figure 6–1. Say It and Move It. (From "Phonome Training: Effect on Reading Readiness" by E. W. Ball and B. A. Blachman, 1988, *Annals of Dyslexia, 38*, p. 221. Copyright 1988 Orton Dyslexia Society, Inc. Reprinted with permission.)

Boggle Jr. (1998) offers two formats helpful for students at this point in the instructional program. *Match It–Spell It* introduces simple letter matching. Picture/word cards are placed in a game tray. The student sees a picture, for instance of a pig, with the word "pig" printed below the picture. You tell the student that the printed word says "pig," and ask the student to find the corresponding letter cubes to place in the slot in the tray directly below the letters in the word, thereby engaging in simple letter matching. The second game, *Cover It*, encourages the student to find letters and spell words from memory. This time, the word under the picture is covered. The student glances at the word briefly, covers the word, and now finds corresponding cubes to spell the word from memory.

2. **Goal 2: To increase visual discrimination abilities to facilitate use of the orthographic processor.**

Suggested Activity:

a. Visual discrimination activities.

I like introducing *Think-It-Through Tiles*: Beginning Reading Visual Discrimination booklets (Discovery Toys, 2000) at this point. By working their way through four booklets, students develop increasingly precise visual discrimination abilities necessary for use of the orthographic processor. They begin with deciding which letter-like objects are identical and progress to matching words. As they make decisions about which items match in a booklet, they place tiles into a plastic case. When they complete a page, they close the case, flip it over, open it, and see if the pattern formed by their answers matches the one in the booklet. This is highly motivating, and I have not worked with a student yet who did not ask for "the blue case" during this part of my instructional program.

3. **Goal 3: To increase rapid naming of sublexical units (word families/word parts/ or onset–rimes (phonograms) to increase word identification and fluency in reading, and to increase spelling of words.**

Suggested Activities:

a. Introduce Making Words Lessons.

Cunningham and Cunningham (1992) proposed that "Making Words" lessons facilitate decoding and spelling abilities. Steps in planning and teaching a Making Words lesson are presented in Table 6–1. Steps in an initial Making Words lesson are summarized below. See Table 6–2 for more specific suggestions.

Begin with two letters, "i" and "n," to form the word "in."
Add a letter to make the three-letter word "pin."
Change letters, one at a time, to show how words can be made. Turn "pin" into "pig," and "pig" into "rig" (a big truck), and "rig" into "rip."
Add a letter to "rip" to form a four-letter word "rips."
Change a letter, for example, "rips" into "nips" (a young puppy nips at your feet), "nips" to "spin," and "spin" to "snip."
Letters are added up to a total of six to form "spring."

Table 6-1. Steps in Planning and Teaching a Making Words Lesson.

Planning Steps

1. Decide what the final word in the lesson will be. In choosing this word, consider its number of vowels, child interest, curriculum tie-ins you can make, and letter-sound patterns you can draw children's attention to through the word sorting at the end.

2. Make a list of shorter words that can be made from the letters of the final word.

3. From all the words you listed, pick 12–15 words that include: (a) words that you can sort for the patterns(s) you want to emphasize; (b) little words and big words so that the lesson is a multilevel lesson; (c) words that can be made with the same letters in different places (e.g., barn, bran) so children are reminded that when spelling words, the order of the letters is crucial; (d) a proper name or two to remind them where we use capital letters; and (e) words that most of the students have in their listening vocabularies.

4. Write all the words on index cards and order them from shortest to longest.

5. Once you have the two-letter, three-letter, etc., words together, order them further so that you can emphasize letter patterns and how changing the position of the letters or changing or adding just one letter results in a dfferent word.

6. Store the cards in an envelope. Write on the envelope the words in order and the patterns you will sort for at the end.

Steps in Teaching

1. Place the large letter cards in a pocket chart or along the chalk ledge.

2. Have designated children give one letter to each child. (Let the passer keep the reclosable bag containing that lettter and have the same child collect that letter when the lesson is over.)

3. Hold up and name the letters on the large letter cards, and have the children hold up their matching small letter cards.

4. Write the numeral 2 (or 3, if there are no two-letter words in this lesson) on the board. Tell them to take two letters and make the first word. Use the word in a sentence after you say it.

5. Have a child who has the first word made correctly make the same word with the large letter cards. Encourage anyone who did not make the word correctly at first to fix the word when they see it made correctly.

6. Continue having them make words, erasing and changing the number on the board to indicate the number of letters needed. Use the words in simple sentences to make sure the children understand their meanings. Remember to cue them as to whether they are just changing one letter, changing letters around, or taking all their letters out to make a word from scratch. Cue them when the word you want them to make is a proper name, and send a child who has started that name with a capital letter to make the word with the big letters.

Table 6-1. Steps in Planning and Teaching a Making Words Lesson (continued).

7. Before telling them the last word, ask "Has anyone figured out what word we can make with all our letters?" If so, congratulate them and have one of them make it with the big letters. If not, say something like, "I love it when I can stump you. Use all your letters and make _____."

8. Once all the words have been made, take the index cards on which you have written the words, and place them one at a time (in the same order children made them) along the chalk ledge or in the pocket chart. Have children say and spell the words with you as you do this. Use these words for sorting and pointing out patterns. Pick a word and point out a particular spelling pattern, and ask children to find the others with that same pattern. Line these words up so that the pattern is visible.

9. To get maximum transfer to reading and writing, have the children use the patterns they have sorted to spell a few new words that you say.

Note: Some teachers have chosen to do steps 1–7 on one day and steps 8 and 9 on the following day.

Source: Reprinted with permission from "Making Words: Enhancing the Invented Spelling-Decoding Connection" by P.M. Cunningham and J.W. Cunningham, 1992, pp. 106–115. *The Reading Teacher, 46.*

Table 6-2. Sample Making Words Lesson.

These lessons go from very simple (5–6 letters with only 1 vowel) to moderate (6–8 letters with 2 vowels) to complex (at least 9 letters, unlimited vowels). List the letters with all the vowel letters first and then all the consonant letters in alphabetical order so as not to give any clues to the big word that will end the lesson. Words separated by a / indicate places in the lesson where the same letters can be rearranged to form a different word.

Lessons using only one vowel:

Letter cards:	u k n r s t
Words to make:	us nut rut run sun sunk runs ruts/rust tusk stun stunk trunk trunks
Sort for:	rhymes s pairs (run runs; rut ruts; trunk trunks)
Letter cards:	o p r s s t
Words to make:	or top/pot rot port stop/spot sort sorts stops/spots sport sports
Sort for:	or o s pairs
Letter cards:	e d n p s s
Words to make:	Ed Ned/end/den pen pens dens/send sped spend spends
Sort for:	rhymes names s pairs

Table 6–2. Sample Making Words Lesson (continued).

Lessons using only one vowel:

Letter cards:	a h l p s s
Words to make:	Al pal/lap Sal sap has/ash sash lash pass pals/laps/slap
	slaps slash splash
Sort for:	rhymes names s pairs

Letter cards:	a c c h r s t
Words to make:	art/tar car cat cart cars/scar star scat cash rash trash
	crash chart scratch
Sort for:	a ar rhymes

Letter cards:	i c k r s t
Words to make:	is kit sit sir stir sick Rick tick skit skirt stick trick
	tricks
Sort for:	i ir sk rhymes

Lessons with two vowels, 6–8 letters:

Letter cards:	e u d h a n r t
Words to make:	red Ted Ned/den/end her hut herd turn hunt hurt under hunted
	turned thunder
Sort for:	u ur e er ed pairs

Letter cards:	e u l r s t t
Words to make:	us use/Sue let set true rule test rest rust trust result
	turtle turtles
Sort for:	e u ue rhymes

Letter cards:	a e c h p r t
Words to make:	at art car cat hat chat cart heat heap cheap cheat/teach
	peach preach chapter
Sort for:	c h ch a ar rhymes

Letter cards:	a o c r r s t t
Words to make:	at rat rot cot cat/act coat cast cost coast toast roast actor
	carrot carrots tractors
Sort for:	a o oa rhymes act actor

Letter cards:	a e l n p s t
Words to make:	pat pet pen pan pal pale/peal pets/pest pane plan plane plant
	plate/pleat planets
Sort for:	a e ea a-e p pl rhymes

Letter cards:	a u y d h r s t
Words to make:	say day dry try shy stay tray rust dust duty dusty rusty
	stray sturdy Thursday
Sort for:	ay y-try rusty tr st

Table 6–2. Sample Making Words Lesson (continued).

Letter cards:	a u b b h s t t
Words to make:	us bus/sub tub/but bat/tab hut hat that bath stab tubs/stub bathtubs
Sort for:	a u th rhymes
Letter cards:	e i d f n r s
Words to make:	Ed red rid end fin fine fire ride side send dine diner rides fires friends
Sort for:	e i i-e s pairs rhymes
Letter cards:	a e h n p r t
Words to make:	an at hat pat pan pen pet net ate/eat heat neat path parent panther
Sort for:	a e ea rhymes
Letter cards:	e i k n s t t
Words to make:	it in ink kit sit net/ten tin tint tent skit skin/sink stink kittens
Sort for:	i e sk rhymes
Letter cards:	a e g m n s t
Words to make:	man men met mat Nat net/ten tan mean/mane mate/meat neat stem steam magnets
Sort for:	a e ea a-e rhymes
Letter cards:	e e n p r s t
Words to make:	see ten teen tree step/pest rest rent sent steep stern enter serpent/present
Sort for	e ee er rhymes
Letter cards:	a e g n r s t
Words to make:	ant age sag rag rage star stag stage great/grate grant agent range strange
Sort for:	st gr g-rag rage rhymes
	Lessons for big words:
Letters on strips:	a a a e i b c h i l p t
Words to make:	itch able cable table batch patch pitch petal label chapel capital capable alphabet alphabetical
Sort for:	el le al itch atch
Letters on strips:	a a e e u h k q r s t
Words to make:	use heat rake take shake quake quart earth reuse square quaker retake reheat/heater karate request earthquake
Sort for:	qu re ake-take rake quake shake retake earthquakes
Letters on strips:	a e e i o g n n r t
Words to make:	got gene genie giant tiger great/grate orange nation ration ignore enrage entire engine ignorant nitrogen tangerine generation
Sort for:	en tion g g (got gene)

Table 6–2. Sample Making Words Lesson (continued).

Letters on strips:	e i u m n n r s s t t
Words to make:	sun set tie use rest rise trust untie unrest misuse sunset
	sunrise sunnier sunniest mistrust instruments
Sort for:	un mis er est sun sunnier sunniest sunset sunrise

Letters on strips:	e o o y c c l m r s t
Words to make:	room cost sore/rose rosy loot lose loser motor storm roomy
	cycle cycler stormy sorely costly looter motorcycles
Sort for:	ly y (rose rosy; room roomy) er

Letters on strips:	a e e e u m p r r t t
Words to make:	treat trump temper tamper repeat mature mutter trumpet
	pretreat repeater tamperer mutterer trumpeter premature
	temperature
Sort for:	pre ture er

Letters on strips:	e e o o c d k p r w
Words to make:	row cow pow owe owed word work wood cook coop cord cork
	droop power powder cowpoke woodpecker
Sort for:	oo(wood coop) ow(cow owe) or(work cork)

Source: Reprinted with permission from "Making Words: Enhancing the Invented Spelling-Decoding Connection" by P. M. Cunningham and J. W. Cunningham, 1992, pp. 106–115. *The Reading Teacher, 46.*

b. Introduce Modified RAVE-O onset–rime activities.

In an attempt to design a therapy program consistent with the ASHA guidelines, a study was conducted as part of a Master's Thesis at California State University, Sacramento (Pieretti, 2001). This study built on a program that is part of ongoing research at the Center for Reading and Language Research at Tufts University in Medford, Massachusetts. Wolf, Miller, and Donnelly (2000) described Retrieval, Automaticity, Vocabulary Elaboration and Orthography (RAVE-O) as "a program that directly addresses the need for automaticity in phonological, orthographic, and semantic systems and the connections between these systems" (Wolf, 1999, p. 19). RAVE-O is currently being used in regular education classrooms in Medford, Massachusetts. Wolf et al. (2000) summarized RAVE-O's three primary goals which are "conceptually and practically interwoven with no one goal predominating" (p. 377). See Table 6-3.

Table 6-3. Three Primary Goals of the RAVE-O Program.

1. RAVE-O's primary goal is the "development of fluency in reading outcome behaviors including word identification, word attack, and comprehension" (p. 377).

2. RAVE-O emphasizes the "interconnectedness of lexical and sublexical processes" to facilitate reading fluency (p. 377). To that end, RAVE-O activities are aimed at increasing automaticity in the following underlying component skills, and as such, are included in this chapter under the orthographic processor. These include:

   • "vision-related processes such as left-to-right scanning, letter recognition, and, in particular, orthographic pattern recognition.

   • "auditory processes that include faster initial and final phoneme and rime identification" (p. 377).

3. RAVE-O's third goal focuses on metalinguistic strategies wherein students are taught "magic tricks" to increase their control over the reading process.

Because RAVE-O "is grounded in the belief that word recognition is facilitated by semantic knowledge," core words are selected to use in the sublexical onset-rime activities and again as words to study in multiple meaning activities, to be discussed under the meaning processor in this chapter. Likewise, lexical retrieval strategies are included in the RAVE-O program and will be discussed in this chapter under the meaning processor.

Pieretti's study was a modification of the RAVE-O program in an attempt to fit the scope and caseload demands of speech–language specialists. Specifically, Pieretti questioned the feasibility of speech–language specialists' inclusion of these activities for students with language-based reading disabilities in an attempt to support literacy. Furthermore, this study set out to measure the impact a modified RAVE-O program would have on language-reading disabled students as compared with more traditional top-down language therapy. (See Chapter 3 for a discussion single and double-deficit language–reading problems.) Six participants, aged 8 years 7 months to 10 years, 11 months were identified as having double-deficit language–reading problems. Three students were placed in a modified RAVE-O treatment program. The activities included were bottom-up approaches including systematic phonological awareness instruction, onset–rime word family activities, multiple meanings word study, word-webbing, and journal writing. The activities were tied directly to the phonological awareness activities completed, so that core words used in phonological awareness instruction were the same words used in the other activities named. Because automaticity is central to RAVE-O, a timed element was added to increase automaticity of reading rime patterns in the card sorting activity. The three participants in the Traditional Language Therapy group received a more traditional top-down language therapy approach working on vocabulary expansion, synonyms and antonyms, listening comprehension, oral vocabulary, and verbal analogies. All participants were seen for 45-minute sessions for a total of eight individual sessions.

Results of the study revealed important trends. The modified RAVE-O group increased more than two times the composite standard score point increases of the Traditional Language Therapy Group on the Phonological Awareness Composite, the Alternate Phonological Awareness Composite and the Phonological Memory Composite of the *Comprehensive Test of Phonological Processing* (CTOPP). The modified RAVE-O group demonstrated an increase of seven points on the CTOPP Rapid Naming Composite, while the Traditional Language Therapy group revealed no improvement in this ability. The modified RAVE-O group demonstrated a marked improvement in Word Attack skills on the *Woodcock Language Proficiency Battery—Revised* (WLPB-R), whereas the Traditional group actually demonstrated a decrease in word attack skills. The modified RAVE-O group also revealed more than three times the standard score point increase of the Traditional Language Therapy group on Passage Comprehension on the WLPB-R. Finally, the modified RAVE-O group demonstrated significantly higher standard score points on four of five WLPB-R oral language subtests. Pieretti and Goldsworthy (2001) concluded that while this study's findings "have the potential of being the basis of a much larger research project," they strongly suggest that speech–language specialists "can target oral language goals while simultaneously supporting literacy in a combination that provides maximum benefit to students across oral–written language" (p. 9).

4. **Goal 4: To increase word attack, word identification, and spelling abilities through exposure to increasingly complex print.**

    Suggested Activities:

    a. **Show the student how to sound out words:**

In a summary of 30 years of research by the National Institute of Child Health and Human Development (NICHD), Grossen (1997) concluded that to teach students the process of sounding out, it is important "to move sequentially from left to right through spellings as they 'sound out,' or say the sound for each spelling" (p. 10). It is helpful for you to model how to sound out words pointing to letters from left to right as you read.

b. Introduce decodable text in reading.

Furthermore, the NICHD report recommended using connected, decodable text for children to practice the sound–spelling relationships. "Decodable text is composed of words that use the sound–spelling correspondences that children have learned to that point and a limited number of sight words that have been systematically taught" (p. 10). The NICHD compared two different texts to illustrate the effectiveness of decodable text in providing students "the opportunity to practice their new knowledge of sound–letter relationships in the context of connected reading" (p. 10). The first example from a meaning-based program with an unintegrated phonic component was: "The dog is up." Because the students had learned the sound–letter relationships [d], [m], [s], [r], and [t], they were able to read only this much of the sentence by applying what they had learned in the phonic component: "___ d__ __ __." In the second example, the sounds the students learned thus far were: [a], [s], [m], [b], [t], [ee], [f], [g], and [l]. In the example: "Sam sees a big fist," the students were able to read the following by using the sound–spelling relationships they had learned: "Sam sees a big fist" (p. 10). In other words, the sentence in the second example is 100% decodable.

There are a number of excellent decodable texts, and included among my favorites are the *J & J Language Readers* (Greene & Woods, 2000) with the corresponding *Language! Curriculum* (Greene, 2000). The *J & J Language Readers* offer a comprehensive series of 54 books containing 108 stories incorporating vocabulary, oral language expansion, written expression, spelling, comprehension, and higher level thinking skills with readability extending from primer through sixth grade. The materials support a systematic, cumulative language approach for students with special language–learning needs. Rather than presenting sound–symbol relationships randomly, as is the case with most phonics programs, the *J & J* series presents the alphabetic code of English orthography in a sequential, cumulative format. The systematic phonology and vocabulary presented in this program supports phonology programs such as Project Read, Orton–Gillingham, Slingerland, Distar, and Alphabetic Phonics. The word families included in the beginning units coincide with work already covered under Goal 3 in this section. For instance, Unit 1 introduces "-am" and "-at;" Unit 2 introduces "-al;" Unit 3 introduces "-an" and "-ad;" and Unit 4 introduces "-ig," "-ac," and "in."

I have found the *J & J* materials to be an excellent place to begin with students demonstrating the reading problems described in this book. The systematic presentation of phonology and vocabulary helps students learn the alphabetic principle without struggling with difficult vocabulary. Students benefit from this plus the comprehension and higher order thinking skills built into the material.

c. Introduce carryover activities.

After a student masters approximately three word families, I ask them to print words we have made while manipulating plastic tiles or seen in our decodable texts. This activity, which involves printing on lined paper or on an erasable white board, becomes part of all sessions. I keep an array of colored pencils, pens, crayons, and the latest "fad" in writing utensils (currently sparkly gel pens) in my office. I also introduce a computer program I believe offers significant carryover work, *Ultimate Phonics Reading Program Words and Sentences* (Spencer Learning, 2000). In this program, the student can read words and sentences, and then click on the printed word list or sentence list on the screen to hear a speaker produce correct answers. We discuss whether or not the student's reading matched what we heard the speaker say. Each of the 262 lessons contains a word list and a sentence list. For example, Lesson 2 Word List contains the following: at, am, an, ad, Al, sad, Sal, sap, sat, Sam, sag, rat, ram, rag, ran, rap, can, cap, cat, cab, hat, ham, had, Hal. Lesson 2 Sentence List contains the following: Sad Sam sat. Sam had a rag. Can a rag sag? Hal had a cap. Sal had a can. A rat ran at a ham. A cat ran at a rat. A cat can rap a rat. Coincidentally, there is nice overlap of stimulus items in the *J & J* readers and the *Ultimate Phonics Reading Program*.

An educational computer program I find useful at this point is *Treasure Mountain* (The Learning Company, 1997). The game part of the program is to collect clues to win points. The educational value lies in reading and solving the puzzles to gain clues. For instance: "I use my eyes to look around. I use my ears to _____ a sound." Word choices: hear, smell, see. Another example is: "vest vote vine vat. These words all start with v. Do you see one more v word? Please pick it out for me." Word choices: very, fine, west.

d. Introduce the Wilson Reading System

(Wilson, 1996). This program, which can be used with elementary-aged students through adults, is based on Orton–Gillingham (see International Dyslexia Association) philosophy and on current reading research. Students learn about the reliability of the printed English language as they work from sounds to syllables, words to sentences, and from stories to books. The Wilson promotional material describes what students do in this multisensory program: "Students learn by hearing sounds; manipulating color-coded sound, syllable and word cards; performing finger-tapping exercises; writing down spoken words and sentences; reading aloud, repeating what they have read in their own words, and hearing others read it as well. Skills and knowledge are reinforced verbally, aurally, tactually, and visually—and learned well" (p. 4). Organized around six syllable types found in English, the *Wilson Reading System* sounds are taught only in relationship to the syllable type under study. All materials are phonetically controlled with word lists, sentences and paragraphs incorporating only word structure elements taught in or up to the corresponding lesson.

e. Increase phonological maturity.

We learned in Chapter 2 that practice with oral language leads native English speakers to assimilate rules and develop an implicit knowledge of how to pronounce the different forms words take when prefixes and suffixes are added. Recall how the first vowel in the words "telegraph," "Canada," and "contract" sound different from each other because of their placement in the stressed syllable. When suffixes are added, the stress shifts to the next syllable to the right as in "telegraphy," "Canadian," and "contractual." The native speaker's lexicon contains one rule to mediate both instances, that is, "pronounce all vowels as 'uh' when in unstressed syllables." As a result of being phonologically mature, the speaker has internalized the rule neutralizing unstressed vowels, and the phonologic rule will be used automatically when attempting to recover the phonetic aspect (i.e., the pronunciation of printed words).

Phonological maturity, then, allows the reader to relate phonological and phonetic representations of the language. Without this maturity, the reader's decoding, fluency, and comprehension are jeopardized. The phonologically immature reader will "get stuck" with one or two pronunciations of words, and will experience difficulty pronouncing printed words correctly. It is as if this reader cannot shift the syllabic emphasis easily. One of my students, for instance, attempted to read the word "abdomen." Time after time he said "abdohnmen" or "abedomen,"emphasizing the middle syllable, and finally said: "Okay, I know what the word is I just can't pronounce it. I heard this word before in the doctor's office," indicating he knew the word but could not translate from print.

Increasing a student's phonological maturity can come through explicitly teaching them how to divide words into syllables and to shift the vocal emphasis from first to middle to last syllables. Lists of multisyllabic words or words with the same root word and different affixes (for instance: photo, photographer, photography, photograph) are helpful in increasing students' phonological maturity. Sources containing increasingly longer and complex utterances are also useful with this activity. The following list, for example, is included as stimulus items in Exercise 10 in the *Audio Workbook for the Verbally Apraxic Adult* (Richards & Fallon, 1988).

Exercise 10. The student can read the following words and phrases.

moment	momentary	momentarily	I'll be with you momentarily.
public	publicly	publicity	She received much publicity.
purpose	purposely	purposefully	She performed purposefully.
time	timeless	timelessness	The house had a sense of timelessness.
boast	boastful	boastfully	He said it boastfully.
peace	peaceful	peacefully	She behaved peacefully.

Reading across different genres such as narrative, expository, poetry, and humor can provide valuable sources of materials to facilitate phonological maturity. Usually, this is a student who has imprecise lexical entries and has become passive in figuring out if the speaker said "inpendix, appendix, or dependix," and has not had the courage to ask for clarification of meaning. Working on roots and affixes will be important to consider (see later discussion in this chapter on context processor, IV.A, GOAL 2.)

B. Summary of goals included under this processor

If the student's ability to use the *orthographic processor is weak*, teaching goals may include any of the following:

1. **Goal 1: To increase phonological awareness skills at the phoneme level using print.**

2. **Goal 2: To increase visual discrimination abilities to facilitate use of the orthographic processor.**

3. **Goal 3: To increase rapid naming of sublexical units, that is, word families/word parts/ phonograms/onset–rimes, to increase word identification and fluency in reading, and to increase spelling of words.**

4. **Goal 4: To increase word attack, word identification, and spelling abilities through exposure to increasingly complex print.**

III. METHODS THAT TARGET THE MEANING PROCESSOR

Students with developmental reading disabilities frequently display problems in reading comprehension because: 1) their underlying language processing problem interferes with their developing vocabulary. While writing this book, I was reminded once again about how frequently our students mix up words and word meanings. 7-year-old Talia, for example, told her mother "I think my teacher is dyslexic." Her mother asked "Why do you think that?" Talia replied "Because she's so thin" (meaning anorexic). And 8-year-old Michael told his mother we were working on "verbal allergies" (meaning analogies); 2) they expend too much energy decoding and losing sight of the meaning; 3) the length of time it takes to decode a passage taxes short-term memory; 4) they may not be focused on the task; 5) they may not be motivated to read; 6) they may be practicing "learned helplessness" where the student has learned to rely on others to explain the passage; and 7) the Matthew Effect, described earlier in this book, wherein low decoding skills lead to diminished vocabulary growth.

Tattershall (1999) listed the following reasons why reading comprehension is difficult for students with language difficulties. Materials contain unfamiliar topics; they are abstract; information presented is dry and impersonal; contain quick topic changes; are overloaded with new concepts or vocabulary; contain complicated sentences; contain unusual format; contain very short and few examples; require reading between the lines; contain unclear referents; and are poorly written.

Beyond helping students in areas discussed earlier in this chapter, the speech–language specialist can provide knowledge about language comprehension, assessment tools, remediation techniques, and materials to enhance vocabulary and syntactic aspects needed to comprehend written language. As speech–language specialists become increasingly involved in supporting literacy, whether on a consultation/collaborative basis in classrooms or in individual sessions, the reading comprehension problems students with developmental reading disabilities demonstrate must be addressed. A myriad of texts and materials are available for use in remediating higher level text comprehension problems (see, for example, Catts & Kamhi, 1999; Kameenui & Simmons, 1990; and Maria, 1990). Knowledge and experience in training metalinguistic skills allows speech–language specialists to contribute significantly in improving active strategy use to enhance reading comprehension.

Explaining that strategic reading involves two components of metacognition—awareness and self-control, Paris (1991) defined comprehension strategies as "actions that readers take before, during, and after reading to elaborate and reflect on the meaning they construct while reading" (p. 33). The ASHA Guidelines (2001) maintained that "good readers and writers are those who are strategic, that is, they know why they are reading/writing a particular text and have strategies they can bring to bear on these tasks" (p. 16). Activities for fostering active strategy use are grouped below as three goals: increasing reading comprehension *before*, *during*, and *after* reading.

A. Activities to Strengthen the Meaning Processor.

If the student's ability to use the *meaning processor is weak*, teaching goals may include any of the following:

1. **Goal 1: To increase reading comprehension: teaching active strategies before reading.**

It is important to teach active strategies before reading. Because conventional reading tests do not measure the reader's use of active strategies to enhance understanding of the author's intended meaning, the examiner may wish to select alternatives such as constructing informal measures from those presented by Paris (1991).

Suggested Activities:

a. **Introduce Think-Along Passages (TAPs).**

Paris suggested developing TAPs for narrative and expository passages for various grade levels (see Appendix A: Paris). TAPs take approximately 20 minutes to administer and yield qualitative and quantitative information. Paris suggested that TAPs also can be used as cognitive modeling exercises for students to observe how teachers think as they read.

Paris explained that the cloze procedure (filling in missing words) assists in assessing strategy use, because "the ability to fill-in missing words requires . . . many strategies (including) inferencing, rereading, and looking ahead in the text for clues to the meaning" (p. 38). Good performance on cloze tasks correlates with fluent reading and high metacognitive ability. Additional advantages of cloze tasks include: 1) A variety of formats, including blank spaces for missing words; word choices can be listed in "word banks" on the page; and multiple alternatives can be printed above the blanks; 2) Single or multiple words can be omitted; 3) The task can be transformed into a writing task by asking the student to write the missing words; 4) Activities can be presented individually or in groups; 5) Cloze activities can be used for instructional purposes through modeling successful thinking and discussing possible choices. Both of these activities foster active strategy use for use in comprehending text (pp. 38–39).

Paris also suggested that comprehension monitoring can be assessed through an error detection task where the text has been altered to contain anomalies, for example, easily pronounceable nonsense words; scrambled word order in clauses; contradictions; change in pronominal references; and/or change in syntactic agreement within text. Finally, Paris suggested using reading miscue analyses to assess a student's active strategy use. Miscue analyses provide a qualitative as well as a quantitative analysis of a student's reading through recording the student's use of repetitions, substitutions, omissions, semantic and syntactic entries, and miscues while reading a passage.

b. Introduce Project Read (Greene & Enfield, 1991).

According to Greene (1993) the "first widely employed method shown to be successful in teaching dyslexics to read, write, and spell" was the Orton–Gillingham method (p. 542). Modifications of the Orton method that have "produced excellent results with dyslexics in diverse settings include: Alpha to Omega; Alphabetic Phonics; Project Read; and Slingerland" (p. 542). The specific techniques used in Project Read can be learned through workshops on various aspects of the method including Phonology, Comprehension, and Written Expression (Javens, personal communication, 1993).

Project Read is a system of learning that is used as a strategy by the student. Utilizing a visual, auditory, tactile approach, Project Read is a systematic, structured, developmental approach based on the links of the language. Because the system moves from cognitive to evaluative, from concrete to abstract, and from part to whole rather than the reverse, it is particularly useful for "parts to the whole, noninductive, visual–kinesthetic learners" (Javens, 1993). Guided practice and generalization are built into all components of the program.

Geared toward students enrolled in the first through sixth grades, Project Read includes three components: phonology, reading comprehension, and written expression.

i. *The phonology component* is intended primarily for students in Grades 1 to 3, but it can be used with older students who experience written language problems. Students gain experience with sound–symbol relationships; learn to break apart words into sounds; and learn five patterns of syllabication through the use of hand signs, tapping words out, finger spelling, and practice with the materials. Because transfer is the goal of this method, the exercises and teaching in Project Read are highly redundant.

ii. *The comprehension component* is especially useful with students in Grades 4 to 12. Report forms for nonfiction and story forms for fiction, biographical, and autobiographical text are used to help students acquire and organize information.

iii. *The written expression component* focuses on the syntactic structures of the English language. Initially, a student's description of an object or event is written down by the teacher. As the student's description expands, the teacher expands what is printed on sentence strips. Symbols are used to help students learn what part of speech goes into which slot in the sentence. Finally, brainstorming, clustering, and editing are added into the written expression component of the program.

c. Introduce Schema Activation.

Good readers engage in top-down processing and activate knowledge they have of the world—the schemata. Students with developmental reading disabilities may not have had experience with the event described in print or may not realize that reading involves an interaction between decoding and activation of the reader's schema. The following suggestions may foster this activation.

Introduce the passage or book. Clay (1991) proposed that helping children learn to read new books independently requires a rich introduction to the story rather than reading the entire story to them. Because the introduction creates the scaffold, Clay offered the following nine suggestions to help formulate introductions. These should be implemented as conversations between the adult and student(s).

i. *Maintain interactive ease.* The adult talks with the students about the story and alerts them to the new features that will be covered. A student's remarks are repeated or expanded, and the interaction facilitates and models acceptable discussion which may call up memories, facilitate understanding, add new information, and/or diminish ambiguity.

ii. *Increase accessibility.* Information from many sources is pulled together and shared by the adult who anticipates what words and/or concepts may present confusion.

iii. *Prompt active reconstruction of the author's text* through linking to personal knowledge. Ask the student: "Have you ever done that?" "What do you expect will happen?"; pausing for the student to complete the sentence and/or to anticipate what will occur next; and reflecting by asking the student "How did you know that?"

iv. *Accept partially correct responses.* Commend some or all of a student's responses.

v. *Tighten the criteria of acceptability.* After reinforcing the student's partially correct answer, draw attention to neglected information by asking: "Did you notice that . . . ?"

vi. *Probing to find out what the student knows.* Ask questions, for example, "Show me the_____" "Have you seen a _____?" "Do you remember in another book_____?"

vii. *Present new knowledge.* Using a particular phrase, explain some part of the story; contrast a feature of the story with some aspect you know the student has encountered in another book; or help the student to discriminate between similar items, for example, adult desk and school desk.

viii. *Ask the student to work with new knowledge.* After telling the student about an item or action, you may ask him or her to elaborate or to find pictures of it in the book.

ix. *Provide a model.* Anticipating what might be difficult in the text, the teacher may provide a word, or sentence or intonation to help the student get ready for the story.

d. Teach vocabulary.

I have listed this teaching method under "before" strategies. Some educators, Ehern (1999) for instance, do not think that preteaching vocabulary is very useful. If vocabulary is not introduced prior to reading a passage, I suggest moving this to a "during" reading strategy.

The ASHA Guidelines (2001) emphasized the importance of assessing and teaching various aspects of oral language to facilitate comprehension and production of higher order language and metalinguistic skills including the following six: 1) Figurative–language forms: sophisticated nonliteral language uses such as idioms, metaphors, proverbs, humor, poetic language; 2) Literate lexicon: rarer and more abstract vocabulary that occurs in scholarly contexts; 3) Synonyms and antonyms: word equivalents and word opposites; 4) Inferential comprehension and reasoning: the integration of meaning within text, analogies, and verbal problem solving; 5) Syntactic complexity: clause density and linguistic cohesion; 6) Polysemous vocabulary: words that have multiple meanings (p. 13).

Pieretti's (2001) study was described under the orthographic processor. To increase students' comprehension of higher level vocabulary, **multiple meanings** of core words were taught each week. The core words were selected from children's literature, and were the same words used in the phonological awareness activities described under the orthographic processor section of this chapter. To increase the students' use of the meaning processor, thereby increasing reading comprehension, students **wrote word webs and corresponding definitions**. Word webs were used to describe and define the multiple meanings of words. For instance, the word "harp" from Jack in the Beanstalk was presented with two meanings: "a musical instrument," and "to complain." Word webs were used to encourage students to ask wh-questions for one or more meanings of each core word. They copied the web into their journals with questions such as:

Why would you use it?

When would you use it?

Who would use this?

What do you do with it?

Where would you find it?

Finally, **writing worksheets** with various word definitions were given to the students to monitor their understanding of the multiple meaning words. They were asked to read the sentences and fill in the blanks based upon context.

2. **Goal 2: To increase reading comprehension: teaching active strategies during reading.**

Suggested Activities:

a. **Introduce advance organizers.**

The teacher determines what vocabulary or concepts may be new or confusing for the student and incorporates these into an introductory paragraph or page to preview with students prior to the student reading a passage.

b. **Introduce cued texts** (Leverett & Diefendorf, 1992).

Visual cues are used to relate nouns with their pronoun referents. The first instance of a key noun is identified by printing the first letter of the name or word in a circle above it. Corresponding pronoun referents are identified by printing the first letter of the name or noun above them without the circle. I have adapted this by asking a student to read a passage and read the person or thing's name each time it is referred to in print as "he," "she," "it," "they," and so forth.

c. **Introduce structured overviews** (Leverett & Diefendorf, 1992).

The teacher identifies key vocabulary words and concepts presented in the text. These are organized into a flow chart or branching diagram, and the terms and concepts that the student knows are listed in appropriate positions within the structure.

d. **Introduce semantic webs** (Leverett & Diefendorf, 1992).

This demonstrates key concepts in stories or textbook chapters visually. Four components are used: a key question that states the purpose of the passage; web strands that answer the key question; strand supports that include details, facts, or other information to clarify or validate a strand; and the strand ties that show relationships among strands.

e. **Introduce contrast charts** (Yopp & Yopp, 1996).

Students are taught to "list the pros and cons of an issue, the advantages and disadvantages of a course of action, or the two sides of an argument as they are described in the selection" (p. 66). The example presented by the Yopps was based on Waber's (1972) book *Ira Sleeps Over*. Included under "Reasons Why Ira Should Take His Teddy Bear" in the Contrast Chart: "He's never slept without it," "They're going to tell scary stories," and "His friend's house is very dark." Included under "Reasons Why Ira Should Not Take His Teddy Bear" on the chart included: "His friend will laugh at him;" "He'll think Ira is a baby," and "His friend will laugh at the bear's name" (p. 66).

f. **Teach how to Make Plot Organizers** (Yopp & Yopp, 1996).

Using a visual display of events that occurred in a story, the Yopps teach us two forms. Using Numeroff's (1985) *If You Give a Mouse a Cookie*, you teach the student to list the events in a **circular plot organizer** by starting with the cookie in the story, with an arrow pointing to milk, and as you move to the right of the circle, the words in the story sequence are written, each time followed by an arrow indicating that this is what happened next in the story: straw, napkin, mirror, scissors, broom, wash floors, nap, box, story, pictures, paper and crayons, pen, refrigerator, and finally milk (p. 78).

Their second example involves a **cumulative story plot organizer**. Using Heilbroner's (1962) *This Is the House Where Jack Lives*, the story elements are depicted in a diagram that begins with one box in a stair-step pattern with the stairs positioned in ascending order left to right. In this case, the word "house" is in the first box, which will be printed in the bottom box for all the entries. The next columns, moving from left to right, add a box to each column, listing words to remind students of the story elements, in this case, the consequences of flooding caused by an overflowing bathtub. The second column contains the words "house" on the bottom, and "dog" on top. The third column has the word "house" on the bottom, the word "dog" in the middle, and the word "boy" on top. The twelfth and final column contains the following words in boxes from bottom to top: house, dog, boy, pail, man, mop, girl, cat, cook, lady, water, Jack (p. 79).

g. Increase reading fluency: speed and prosody.

When students continue to labor with decoding, they become "glued to the print," and, if reading aloud, they adopt a habitual, slow, monotonous, reading rate and vocal quality. Smith (1994) maintained that reading comprehension suffers when reading rate is slower than 200 words per minute "because a lesser rate would imply that words were being read as isolated units rather than as meaningful sentences" (p. 80). Meyer and Felton (1999) defined fluency as "the ability to read connected text rapidly, smoothly, effortlessly, and automatically with little conscious attention to the mechanics of reading, such as decoding" (p. 284). Three theoretical reasons for nonfluent reading include: slow recognition of individual words, lack of sensitivity to prosodic and rhythmic cues, and failure to make higher order orthographic and semantic connections (Meyer & Felton, 1999).

i.   *Use Tape Recordings.* Tape record the student's first reading of a passage, then replay it and discuss, for example, how to use inflections to indicate questions, surprise, disappointment, and so on. Rereading and retaping the student's reading can assist the student in developing a fluent and flexible reading rate. Having a student hear you read or listening to an enjoyable tape such as Cherdiet's (1993) "The Magic Fish Rap" allows him or her to hear the effects of speed and intonation.

ii. *Chunking (phrase reading)* was suggested by Henk, Helfeldt, and Platt (1986) as an important intermediate step in improving a student's reading fluency. The teacher selects somewhat familiar reading passages and divides the phrase groups into chunks by drawing slash marks in the text (or a copy of it) to indicate chunks of print. The same phrases can be printed on flashcards for drill. As the student becomes more fluent in reading the chunks of words, the slashes are erased, or more words are included within the chunks. This activity is also achieved through having the student read various poems several times.

Reading short plays is another enjoyable activity for increasing rate and fluency. Plays included in *Plays for Reading Aloud: The Book of Three* (Fischer & Hansen, 1989), for instance, are: *The Three Billy Goats Gruff, The*

Three Little Pigs, Goldilocks and the Three Bears, The Little Red Hen, The Three Spinners, and *Stone Cheese*. Words and phrases are typed in bold print drawing students' attention to the need to phrase or emphasize those words and phrases.

Another delightful source is Vozar's (1993) *Hungry Wolf! A Nursery Rap*. I demonstrate how to group the words and to use vocal intonation while reading, and then the students imitate. A sample from one of the stories, "The Hungry Wolf" follows:

> This here's the tale of a wolf that was hungry—
> Had a swollen stomach all hollow and spongy.
> Went to the barnyard lookin' for eats,
> And spied three pigs all juicy and sweet
> So he jumps the fence to grab and surprise 'em,
> But they see him and flee him with a speed that belies
> 'em. (pp. 1–2).

iii. *Choral repeated reading*. Bos and Vaughn (1988) described a modified version of two techniques—neurological impress and repeated readings. This method is recommended for students who have a sight vocabulary of at least 25 words. It includes the following steps: 1) Select a book of interest to the student that is one to two levels above his or her current instructional reading level and has frequent word repetitions. Books with patterning and predictability are recommended. The student's word recognition should be 75 to 85% correct; 2) The teacher reads several sentences or a paragraph at the beginning of the book and runs his or her finger smoothly along underneath the words as the student observes. Then, the teacher makes predictions with the student as to what they think will happen in the story; 3) The teacher and the student reread the same passage in unison while the teacher moves his or her finger along underneath the words. This step can be repeated until the student is comfortable with the passage; 4) The student now reads the same passage aloud independently; 5) The teacher and the student discuss how the passage relates to their original predictions; 6) Repeat the steps throughout the book; 7) Print on a card those words with which the student consistently demonstrated difficulty. Discuss the meaning of these words, locate the words in the text, and reread those sentences; 8) Have the student graph his or her progress.

iv. *Prosodic features of language.* Hook and Jones (2002) suggested that fluency training needs to include training to connect the "prosody of spoken language to the prosodic features of text that are signaled through punctuation" (p. 6). Structured exercises using short, three-word printed sentences can be used to illustrate variation in prosody. In the sentence, "He is happy," prosodic features can be emphasized through underlining one of the words, altering which word receives the underline and the emphasis. For example, "<u>He</u> is happy" "He <u>is</u> happy" "He is <u>happy</u>" provides the student practice in how to emphasize various words during reading, and thus, ultimately, to increase comprehension of the passage read. Students are to read the sentences until they are fluent. The authors recommend using this strategy with increasingly longer phrases and emphasizing the various meanings. For instance: "<u>Get out</u> of bed. Get out of <u>bed</u>. Get out of bed <u>now</u>." (p. 6). Further fluency practice comes with common phrases occurring frequently in text. Prepositional phrases provide excellent examples of syntactic structures for increasing prosodic features while reading, for instance "on the _____. in the _____, over the _____" (p. 6). Finally the authors suggest the printed phrases can be paired with oral intonational patterns including a variety of rate, intensity, and pitch. Students learn to infer the author's intended meaning as the sentences are read to them with prosodic variations. For instance, stressing a concept usually is accomplished when speakers slow their rate of speech and increase their volume. This is typically indicated in printed text with an exclamation point. "Practicing oral variations and then mapping the prosodic features onto the text will assist students in making the connection when reading" (p. 6).

h. Teach students to ask questions.

Students with impaired language abilities often do not realize that they need to ask questions to facilitate their listening or reading comprehension. Frequently, when they do realize they need clarification, they do not ask specific questions to help them understand what they read; for example, they may ask a "who" question when they need an answer to a "where" question.

I especially like to explain that "good readers ask questions when they do not understand something they have just read." I then model what to say, for instance: "What does this word mean?" I then fade the cues. For example, I might say: "What good question do you have for me? You can begin with 'what does this word _____'?" The next time I say: "What good question do you have for me? You can begin with 'what does this _____ _____'?" I pay particular attention to pronoun/referent relationships as most of the students I work with do not know to whom or what the pronouns refer. We practice questions such as "I don't know who 'he' refers to in this sentence."

Pritchard (2001) suggested teaching students to ask three different types of questions:

i. *Literal questions:* found directly in the text. "You can read the lines and find the answer" (p. 35).

ii. *Interpretive questions:* ask for information not directly in the text. "There are clues to the answer and you have to put them together and decide what message the author meant to send. You need to read between the lines" (p. 35).

iii. *Application questions:* ask you to "use the information you read and add it to knowledge you already have" (p. 35). This allows you to formulate new opinions and ideas. "You have to read beyond the lines" (p. 35).

i. Introduce KWL Plus.

Pritchard (2001) also advises using this well-known reading–thinking strategy that "activates and builds on the student's prior knowledge and natural curiosity to learn" (p. 20). The student identifies what is known about a subject, and makes notes about this under the K (known) column of the page. The student lists what he/she wants to know under the W (what I want to know) column, and after reading, the student lists what is learned under the L (what I learned) column. After filling out the KWL chart, students then fill out a

Concept Map with the topic in the center circle, main ideas written on spokes emanating from the circle, and smaller spokes and circles drawn off the main spokes indicating ideas related to the main ideas.

j. **Teach think aloud strategies.**

If students have learned how to ask questions about text, either through teacher modeling or specific formats described above, they are more likely to ask themselves or others pertinent questions about the passage they are reading to enhance their comprehension of the material. Baumann, Jones, and Seifert-Kessell (1993) found increased comprehension skills in fourth graders who had been taught the following think-aloud strategies.

i.   *Asking questions while reading*, for example, "Why did she go to the creek when her mother told her not to?"

ii. *Retelling:* The student retells what he or she has just read.

iii. *Offering hypotheses*, for example, "She'll probably go down there again and play when the water's down and not so high."

k. **Teach students about their learning strengths and weaknesses.**

An important component of training students with specific learning disabilities at The Churchill School in St. Louis, Missouri is to help demystify personal mysteries. Students are encouraged to discuss their learning strengths and weaknesses with teachers and other students. Teachers read a story about a student with learning problems to encourage students to discuss their feelings about the story and their own problems. According to Evers, Gilligan, and Wernig (1994) students develop a demystification portfolio—"a flight manual"—divided into the following sections.

i.   *General information:* includes inspirational poems and information on services available such as audiotapes available through Recordings for the Blind and Dyslexic.

ii. *About me:* includes statements made by the students as to their perceived strengths and limitations.

    iii. *Effective techniques* found to assist the student include descriptions of computers, tape recordings, and study guides.

    iv. *Famous people* with learning disabilities: includes articles on such persons.

    v. *Stages:* describes stages of acceptance of learning problems including denial, anger, depression, and acceptance with action.

    vi. *Book reviews* includes a reference list of books written to help students with learning problems. Levine's (1993) *All Kinds of Minds*, for instance, describes five students with varying language-learning problems. Concrete suggestions are offered for students with the following problems: attention deficits, reading disorders, memory problems, language disorders, social skills problems and/or motor skills problems.

    vii. *Vocabulary words* the student is studying.

l. Teach self-monitoring strategies.

Many studies have reported increased reading comprehension when students employ metacognitive strategies to monitor their reading. I like to train students to ask four questions: "Can I put this in my own words?" "Can I retell the story?" What don't I understand?" and "Can I guess what will happen next?" If the student needs help with "putting it in his or her own words," learning how to paraphrase may help. Summarizing work at the Kansas University Institute of Research in Learning Disabilities, Bos and Vaughn (1988) listed three steps the student needs to follow in learning a paraphrasing strategy.

    i. *Read a paragraph silently.* As you read, be sure to think about what the words mean.

    ii. *Ask yourself, "What were the main ideas and details* of this paragraph?" After reading the paragraph, ask yourself, "What were the main ideas and details?" This question helps you to think about what you just read. To help you, you may need to look quickly back over the paragraph and find the main idea and the details that are related to the main idea.

iii. *Put the main idea and details in your own words.* When you put the information into your own words, it helps you remember the information. Try to give at least two details related to the main idea (p. 140). If the student has difficulty retelling the story, he or she may benefit from being taught story retelling strategies. Bos and Vaughn summarized what points are typically included in the retelling of narratives. "In general, narrative texts can be organized into components such as the setting, the problems statement, the goals, event sequences or episodes, and the ending" (p. 141). The following story retelling strategy, SPOT the Story—suggested by Bos—was presented in Bos and Vaughn (1988).

Setting—Who, What, When, Where

Problem—What is the problem to be solved?

Order of Action—What happened to solve the problem? (correct/logical order)

Tail End—What happened in the end? (p. 143)

m. Teach the student how to predict.

If the student is unable to guess what will happen next in the story, he or she may benefit from learning how to predict what will happen next. I encourage students to check what they have already read to help them guess what will happen. I also encourage them to "peek" ahead to help them make predictions.

i. *Narrative text prediction.* Maria (1990) suggested using an inferential strategy technique because "this strategy encourages children to compare something from their own lives to something that might happen in the story" (p. 105). Maria summarized the three steps needed in this strategy. When introducing the strategy, the teacher should: a) explain why the group will use it in reading; b) then ask the children to imagine that they are going to read a text about a particular topic and ask them what they would think about before reading (p. 105).

The second step involves a discussion of three central concepts from the story. The teacher asks two questions about each concept: a) "How can you relate something you thought or did in a particular situation that is similar to the one we read about?"; b) "What do you predict about what a character will think or do in a similar situation" (p. 106).

The third step involves students answering inferential questions about the story and relating them to the predictions they made about the story and their own experiences. Maria explained "teachers who use the inferential strategy as a pre-reading technique should be sure that their during-reading and post-reading discussions focus on confirming or refuting the children's predictions and include some discussion of the process of connecting the children's ideas and the ideas presented in the text" (p. 108).

ii. *Expository test prediction.* Maria suggested that teachers will frequently need "to help children build schemata about the topics and structures" when reading expository texts (p. 167). "Schemata can be built by activating and building prior knowledge about the content and by guiding children to attend to text cues like headings and structural cue words" (p. 167).

n. Teach self-help strategies.

For example, outlining chapters, underlining, highlighting with fluorescent markers, or writing notes in margins of text are additional ways a reader can monitor reading comprehension during reading. Because so many of the students I work with are strong visual learners with artistic talents, I like to teach them how to take **picture notes.** We discuss how to select the most important ideas in a paragraph or page of text, and draw simple stick figures and block designs with a few printed words to help in recall of details.

3. **Goal 3: To increase reading comprehension: teaching active strategies after reading.**

Suggested Activities:

a. Extension of strategy use.

The joy of observing a student's reading comprehension increase through active strategy use can quickly fade when one asks how the strategies are working for the student outside the session and the student responds: "Use them outside here? Are you kidding? I only think of them in here!" Close monitoring of reading comprehension and rewards for active strategy use, rather than the conventional reinforcement for decoding and answering worksheet questions, can facilitate generalization and transfer of strategy use. Having students chart their own progress in using strategies outside the classroom, learning center, or therapy room, as well as securing support from friends and family, can foster greater independence in active strategy use.

b. The reading to writing connection.

Although it is not the purpose of this chapter to present in-depth materials for increasing written language expression, a final goal is added to emphasize the importance of bridging the oral–written language continuum through writing as part of a language-based treatment approach.

Especially helpful for readers who have gained some fluency and flexibility in reading is the notion of collaborative or shared writing, where a teacher or another student shares in the process of writing composition. Described by Mather and Lachowicz (1992), shared writing is an interactive process "making it possible for teachers to integrate oral language with written output and model the types of thinking they use when composing" (p. 27). An example provided by the authors included the instructional sequence used with a fifth grade boy with learning disabilities. After the teacher and student discussed possible topics, the student chose the topic and wrote the title, "The Pencil That Did My Homework," at the top of the lined page. After the student wrote the first sentence in the composition, the teacher read it and said "I am going to add a sentence that describes what your magic pencil looks like" (p. 28). Mather and Lachowicz explained that the teacher and student took turns contributing sentences and discussing their additions until they agreed that the story was complete.

Occasionally, they stopped and read the entire story before adding a sentence. Finally, they share–read the story when it was completed (p. 28). I have had a great deal of success training parents to help in the carryover of this assignment. Shared writing between my student and parents in composition books, journals, and running diaries, facilitates carryover of the written language goals, for instance, using descriptive words, and writing more complex plots.

Because shared writing incorporates principles of the writing process approach, "basic skills such as spelling, punctuation, and capitalization are not emphasized in the first draft" (p. 28). The authors recommended that the teacher spell the student's incorrectly spelled word correctly in the next sentence written by the teacher. Variations in shared writing may include alternating single words, sentences, or paragraphs. On revising and editing the story "the student recopies the entire story to share with others" (p. 28).

c. Restatement training.

After reading a passage, the student should be encouraged to jot down main ideas and questions he or she now has as the result of reading. Jenkins, Heliotis, Stein, and Haynes (1987) evaluated the effectiveness of restatement training on reading comprehension in 32 third through sixth grade students with learning disabilities. Scripted lessons from primary level SRA Reading level were retyped with lined spaces inserted after each paragraph.

During the first training phase, students were instructed to read each paragraph then name the most important person and major event that occurred. According to Jenkins et al. (1987), "Two questions guided students in formulating restatements: (1) Who? and (2) What's happening?" (p. 55). In the second training phase, students were encouraged to jot restatements of what just happened in the passage using three or four words. During the third training phase, narrative passages without spaces were used. Students were instructed to write their restatements on separate papers. The researchers noted the most encouraging results came during transfer tests. When asked to read silently, but not instructed to use the restatement technique, subjects in the experimental group and some in the control group made notes about each paragraph and "demonstrated higher comprehension." Further, the effects were noticed during the remote transfer test when students did not have writing materials, suggesting "they adopted a covert form of the restatement procedure" (p. 58).

d. Transform traditional stories.

Sipe (1993) suggested transforming traditional stories. For example, sixth-grade students were encouraged to revisit and re-experience favorite childhood stories and transform them into new stories by constructing a parallel story or extending the original story. Transformations differ from story retellings, which require one to be faithful to the original story, because transformations range farther afield. An adaptation of Sipe's list of ways students can transform stories follows.

i.   Change the style from old-fashioned to modern language.

ii.   Change or add to the details in the plot.

iii. Change a few of the main events in the plot.

iv.   Keep a few of the main events, but change most of the plot.

v.   Change the setting (time and place). This usually requires more changes in the characters and details.

vi.   Change the point of view.

vii. Change the characters in the story by changing their occupation, gender, or reversing their roles.

viii. Write a sequel to the original story.

ix.   Keep the words of the original story, but change the illustrations.

e. Read to students. Have students read to you.

Adults have read stories aloud to children for centuries. I concur with Trelease's (1984) notion that reading aloud to our students enhances their development of all literacy skills: reading, writing, speaking and listening. According to

Trelease: "Reading aloud is a commercial for reading," and he asks us to consider this: Just because most Americans have heard about McDonald's restaurants, it doesn't stop McDonald's from advertising. "Each year it spends more money on ads to remind people how good its products taste. Don't cut your reading advertising budget as children grow older." I usually try to read 2 to 3 pages of a book, article, or directions for making something to the student at the end of our session. I also ask that the student read 2 to 3 pages of a book to me that is not included in our regular language–reading work. Text that is at a much easier reading level than where the student currently performs is selected. I frequently audiotape record the student's reading and replay it for him/her to reinforce "how much better" the student is reading.

B. Summary of goals included under this processor

If the student's ability to use the *meaning processor is weak*, teaching goals may include any of the following:

1. **Goal 1: To increase reading comprehension: teaching active strategies <u>before</u> reading.**

2. **Goal 2: To increase reading comprehension: teaching active strategies <u>during</u> reading.**

3. **Goal 3: To increase reading comprehension: teaching active strategies <u>after</u> reading.**

IV. METHODS THAT TARGET THE CONTEXT PROCESSOR

When students with developmental reading disabilities struggle with decoding print, they typically become "glued to print" and consequently become rigid in their ability to interact with it. They laboriously sound out words and soon learn that reading is all about making the sounds the letters make. How many readers I have worked with sound out a word such as /a......n........d/, then say "and" and do not seem to understand that this is a word they use numerous times throughout their day. In beginning reading, these readers over-rely on context. You can observe them looking furtively at print and then eyes dart to any picture on the page that may help them out this time. When the pictures become fewer, these students infrequently think to use printed context to facilitate their decoding and comprehension. A student explained to me: "Why on earth would I try reading back and forward to try to help me understand? It's hard enough just to read!" Strategic readers, on the other hand, seem to intuitively know to look at the last sentence or forward in the sentence they are reading to help them understand what they are reading. Once again, students with developmental reading disabilities will need to be explicitly taught how to use the context processor.

The ASHA Guidelines (2001) supported the teaching of metacognitive strategies that support literate language:

> Intervention aimed at developing literate language should involve integrated, authentic school experiences that the student has previously identified as problematic (e.g., listening to a lecture and taking notes, writing a report, arguing a position on a controversial topic). In such contexts higher level language skill are frequently taught along with strategic language behaviors. Examples include:
>
> • Awareness of derived words taught as a word–identification strategy.
>
> • Sensitivity to high- and low-frequency words taught as a writing–revision strategy.
>
> • Main ideas taught as a writing–planning strategy.
>
> • Narrative text structure taught as a writing–planning strategy.
>
> • Complex sentence structure taught as strategies for generating and revising written texts (p. 19).

A. Activities to Strengthen the Context Processor.

If the student's ability to use the *context processor in reading is weak*, teaching goals may include any of the following.

1. Goal 1: To increase strategic use of context cues.

Adams (1990) recommended readers can be taught to analyze available contextual clues for a more precise and useful concept of a particular word. "At best, readers will thoughtfully search for and interpret cues that precede the word more remotely . . . they will additionally look for clues or definitions that might follow it" (p. 146).

Suggested Activities:

a. Introduce Reading Milestones.

In its third edition, *Reading Milestones* (2001) offers six sets of language controlled readers and workbooks. Each reading level consists of ten readers and corresponding workbooks, and a spelling book is part of the total program. This reading program is especially effective for students with hearing impairments and language delays, learning disabilities and students learning English as a second language. The readers include the following vocabulary controls: number of new words per story; number of syllables per word; multiple meaning words; idiomatic and colloquial language; figurative language; word structures (contractions, compound words, prefixes, and suffixes); inflectional endings (third-person singular, plural, past tense, possessives, and present progressive).

The comprehension skills include: understanding main ideas; locating details; sequencing; recognizing cause and effect; making interpretations (judgments and generalizations); drawing conclusions; inferring word meaning through context; and making predictions and inferences. The workbooks include literal reading skills, inferential reading skills, evaluative and critical reading skills, and study skills.

b. Responding to Cloze materials.

Use published or teacher devised Cloze materials in which the student must select one of two or three possible choices to "fit" into a blank within the sentence. If the difficulty with automatic contextual facilitation is caused by impulsive guessing, cloze procedures are helpful. Photocopy a page from high interest reading material and block out words representing various parts of speech (e.g., nouns, verbs, adjectives, prepositions, etc.). Have the student read the passage and guess what word should come next based on information provided prior to the blocked out word. A number of published materials are available, for example, *Cloze Stories for Beginning Readers* (Swinburne & Bank, 1987). In Book Two, short reading passages are presented with words missing. Four choices per blank are printed in the margin for the student to select. The following sample is from "Kitty Adopts Sonya."

Sonya was very happy because she could	1. kitten
have a pet. For her birthday, she could	bird
have a pet of her own.	fish
She thought about it for weeks. Did she	puppy
want a puppy, a kitten, a bird, or	
a _____? What should her pet be? (p. 4).	
1	

Remedia Publications' *Cloze Reading* (no date) presents a number of short stories with words in a box at the top of the page. The reader selects words from the box and writes them on the blanks throughout the story. One example follows:

POPCORN

is	of	gets
not	popcorn	steam

"Most people like to eat popcorn. It _____ fun to see it pop. It makes a lot _____ noise. What makes it pop and jump? Inside every kernel of _____ there is a small drop of water. When the kernel gets hot, this water _____ hot, too. The water turns into steam. The _____ makes the kernel pop. Just think. Popcorn is _____ really cooked" (p. 1).

c. Introduce the penciling technique.

A very successful technique to help students use contextual cues in reading was devised by Anasara as reported by Tuley (1998). Anasara asked students to use a pencil while reading to help them to focus, increase eye–brain coordination, eliminate reversals, transpositions, insertions, and omissions, and other inaccuracies. "She also believed that penciling helps students recognize syllables and affixes, identify key words and phrases, and improve reading comprehension" (p. 15). Five sequential stages of the penciling technique are outlined by Tuley as follows:

Trace the initial letter of each word: *"After the battle, the emperor, Asoka. . . ."*

Draw a line under the first letter of each word: " <u>A</u>fter <u>t</u>he <u>b</u>attle, <u>t</u>he <u>e</u>mperor, <u>A</u>soka. . ."

Draw a line under phrases and circle signal words ("words that anticipate meaning such as 'but, although, since, before, after' (p. 16). <u>After the battle</u>,ʌ <u>the emperor</u>, <u>Asoka</u>,ʌ <u>walked among</u>,ʌ " circle the word "after" if the student has difficulty recognizing signal words.

Underline as you read: "<u>After the battle, the emperor, Asoka</u>". . .

Syllabicate words and circle special elements such as affixes: "<u>After the battle, the em</u>ʌper∧or, A∧so∧ka, <u>walked among</u>,ʌ <u>the dead and dying</u>" . . . (circle "le" in "battle" and "ing" in "dying" (pp. 16-17).

d. **Direct Definition Context Clues.**

Students with developmental reading disabilities learn quite early in their reading experience to shrug their shoulders and say "I don't know what this means." Teaching them that clues come right from the words on the page is powerful. I found several helpful websites in my quest to teach more about context clues. One site: *www.manatee.k12.fl.us* suggested making a large stop sign saying "STOP—don't touch that dictionary. The meaning of the word you don't know is right here in what you are reading!" The following frequently used words in print were then defined and used in examples to teach students to focus on these words:

IS/ARE: "<u>Kit E. Kat</u> **is** <u>the son of Katy Kat</u>. <u>The Kat family members</u> **are** <u>furry cats who wear sunglasses</u>.

The context clue word *IS* ties "Kit E. Kat" to the "son of Katy Kat."

The context clue word *ARE* ties "Kat family members" to "furry cats who wear sunglasses."

Other examples:

IS/ARE CALLED: "<u>Animals that have backbones</u> **are called** <u>vertebrates</u>." "<u>An animal that is warm-blooded, has feathers, and lays eggs</u> **is called** <u>a bird</u>."

IS/ARE KNOWN AS: "<u>A shape made of three straight lines</u> **is known as** <u>a triangle</u>." "<u>Triangles that are the same shape and size</u> **are known as** <u>congruent triangles</u>."

In the context clues: "Is/are called" and "is/are known as," the meaning of the words follows the clue words.

MEANS: "<u>Make-believe</u> **means** <u>made-up</u>."

SUCH AS: "<u>I like to eat green vegetables</u> **such as** <u>broccoli and green beans</u>."

WAS/WERE: "<u>A mammoth</u> **was** <u>an elephant that lived during the Ice Ages</u>." "<u>The Ice Ages</u> **were** <u>times when much of the Earth was covered with snow</u>."

,OR ——,: "<u>Glaciers</u>, **or** <u>slowly moving rivers of ice</u>, formed over many parts of the Earth."

The following suggestions for using definition, example, and contrast context clues, were found on the following website: *http://www.ii.metu.edu.tr/nli/courses/fle126/lectures/con-textclues.html*

i. *Definition Clues:* when the writer defines a word immediately after it is used in a sentence. A definition or a synonym may be used. The words "means," "refers to," "can be defined as," "is" may be used. For example "Corona refers to the outermost part of the sun's atmosphere" (p. 2).

ii. *Example Clues:* when the writer uses examples to explain or clarify a word. For example: "*Toxic* materials, such as arsenic, asbestos, pesticides, and lead, can cause bodily damage" (p. 3).

iii. *Contrast Clues:* when the reader guesses the meaning of a word or phrase having the opposite meaning. For exam-

ple: "One of the dinner guests succumbed to the tempta-
tion to have a second piece of cake, but the others resisted" (p. 3) (contrast "succumbed" and "resisted").

e. Read back. Read forward.

Teach the student that when he/she does not understand what
the sentence is about to return to the previous sentence(s) to
read what led up to the current sentence. Likewise, teach the
student to read the next sentence(s) to facilitate understanding of the passage. I think it is important to use the words "use
contextual cues to help you solve the mystery."

2. **Goal 2: To increase understanding and recognition of morphological aspects of words: roots, prefixes and suffixes, that is, to
increase structural analysis.**

Suggested Activities:

Maria (1990) suggested that when structural analysis is combined with context, it provides a way of "connecting unfamiliar
to familiar words and learning new meanings independently.
Structural analysis instruction should not involve memorization
of lists of roots or affixes, but should consist of teaching students
to use their knowledge of word parts in known words to help get
some sense of the meanings of unknown words" (pp. 128–129).
Bebko et al. (2001) explained that "once the foundation for word
recognition is laid, students must learn to read larger words with
fluency and to determine word meaning from context" (p. 1).
Derivational morphology, in which students are taught how to
combine roots with affixes "to change parts of speech and meanings of words, . . . is far more efficient than analyzing words as
syllables" (p. 2). Many materials are available for achieving this
goal. Three are mentioned here.

In the *Tutor* series by Henry and Redding (1990), students learn
syllable patterns and prefixes and suffixes through structured,
sequential, multisensory lessons based on the Orton–Gillingham
approach. Henry and Redding explained:

> Each lesson integrates decoding and spelling. Because children with
> specific language learning disabilities often possess deficits in visual
> memory for words, memorization of an adequate sight vocabulary
> becomes impossible. Thus, by consistently utilizing auditory and
> kinesthetic modalities along with the visual pathway in a structured,

sequential, multisensory presentation, these children can learn to read and spell (Tutor 2, p. i).

Toomey's (1989) *Morph-Aid* is a good resource for teaching students how affixes and morphemes change word meanings. Toomey described the contents of *Morph-Aid* as follows:

> Thirty-three pages are devoted to specific prefixes and suffixes. Each of these pages offers the particular prefix or suffix (or contrasting pair or group) defined, utilized as derivatives, and then used in context. These pages might be used as a means of presenting or teaching the target affix or morpheme and are, therefore, referred to as Presentation Pages. On the page opposite each of the Presentation Pages is a Writing Worksheet which is meant to strengthen the presentation and discussion using written exercises. Here, the student reviews definitions, divides derivatives into roots and affixes, composes and writes original sentences, and answers questions found on the Presentation page (p. ix).

Language! (Bebko, Alexander, & Doucet, 2001) was written for seventh and eighth-graders with language learning problems. The vocabulary "was chosen for its relevance and is based on general middle-school vocabulary as well as on science and social studies words typical to those grade levels" (p. 4). Word lists included in *Language!* contain numerous contemporary everyday words as well as some words that are "more archaic or esoteric" (p. 5). I especially like the emphasis on "word families" as I use that at an earlier point in my instruction (see the discussion of onset–rime word families under the orthographic processor section of this chapter). Students are taught how to combine prefixes and suffixes with root words in units such as these:

Unit 26: roots: duc/duce/duct, ver/vert/verse
          prefixes: em, en
          suffixes: ish, ist

Unit 33: roots: spirare, found (fundere)
          prefixes: astra/astro, auto/aut, bene
          suffixes: age, ance, ancy, ence, ency, ice

B. Activities to Strengthen Writing.

If the student's ability to use the *context processor in writing* is weak, teaching goals may include any of the following.

1. **Goal 1: To increase written language formulation.**

    I find that students begin to increase their use of contextual cues in print as they move into writing their own stories. This reminds me of the reciprocity in oral-written language. At times we target various language goals as determined by assessment tools and student classroom needs only to find that another language area increased as the result of our work. In the area of written language I find my students needing tremendous amounts of structure. There are many excellent writing programs available. I'll describe a few of my favorites starting with where I begin with young children then move through more complex writing.

    Suggested Activities:

    a. **Introduce wordless books.**

       Using an assortment of wordless books I ask the student to tell the story. I write their words on Post-it papers and stick these onto the books' pages. Students literally see their words printed on papers, learn that printed words represent their spoken words, and develop oral narrative abilities.

    b. **Introduce sequencing ideas.**

       I select books that have a simple sequence of events in them, for instance, Numeroff's (1998) *If You Give a Pig a Pancake.* In the story, a girl gives a pig a pancake, and the pig wants syrup to go with the pancake. The syrup makes the pig get sticky so she needs to take a bath. As with all of Numeroff's creative stories, the events in the story continue and then conclude with the story's initial event. In this case, the pig gets sticky when hanging wallpaper. This reminds her of syrup, and after she gets the syrup, she will want a pancake. After reading the story to a student, we discuss the sequence of events and, depending on the student's ability, copy/print words to form our own written stories.

    c. **Introduce Project Read** (see the discussion in this chapter on meaning processor, section A, Goal 1b.)

    d. **Use materials that emphasize contextual cue use.**

Many materials exist that call attention to contextual cues. One I like with older students is *Bring the Classics to Life* (Edcon, various dates). In this series, a number of classic literature stories are written at lower readability levels. Each story contains a preparation section in which the student learns about the story's key words, special words and people. There is a picture and a short paragraph. The student reads the paragraph and responds to a preview question, for instance "You learned from your preview that Aunt Polly called loudly because _____." After reading the story, the student responds to a comprehension check and a vocabulary check.

e. **Introduce more complex structure of writing.**

Sturomski (1999) explained that "it is no secret that many students find learning a difficult and painful process" (p. 2). From their earliest school experiences, students with language–learning disabilities become passive learners and we must teach them about their learning strengths and weaknesses and how to be strategic learners. Sturomski proposed that our students "need to become strategic learners, not just haphazardly using whatever learning strategies or techniques they have developed on their own, but becoming consciously aware of what strategies might be useful in a given learning situation and capable of using those strategies effectively" (p. 3). Sturomski supported the following example of a strategy intervention for writing known as DEFENDS (Ellis, 1994). DEFENDS is the acronym for an approach to help "secondary students write a composition in which they must take a position and defend it (p. 5)." Each letter stands for a strategic step, as follows:

> D ecide on audience, goals, and position
> E stimate main ideas and details
> F igure best order of main ideas and details
> E xpress the position in the opening
> N ote each main idea and supporting points
> D rive home the message in the last sentence
> S earch for errors and correct (p. 5)

While there are many available materials to help increase a student's writing complexity, I particularly like *Narrative Toolbox* (Hutson-Nechkash, 2001) because students are taught about story structure under the following topics.

i.   *Story grammar octopus:* teaches the student labels for 8 grammar elements; setting, first event, response, goal, plan, attempt, outcome, and ending.

ii. *Story train:* groups story components (character, place, time, response, goal, plan, attempt, outcome, and ending) into 3 categories: setting, problem, and solution.

Many excellent computer programs are available to facilitate our students' written language formulation. I'll briefly describe two that I especially like to use with my students. *Writing Blaster* (Davidson & Associates, Inc., 1998) includes many topics and projects. Four of my favorites include:

i.   *Poetry:* contains many forms of poetry, for instance, color poem, couplet poem, name poem, Haiku poem, and limericks. The student is taught about the poem form, given examples, and can then create his/her own.

ii. *Reading and Writing:* contains many topics to increase a student's spelling, writing, and punctuation abilities. The topics I find helpful include: Words that Rhyme, Make a Sentence, Sequence, Spelling Jungle, What Am I?, and Writing is a Blast.

iii. *Storybooks:* includes a number of titles such as "My Bear Story." On the first page of the story, one or two sentences are provided to act as story starters for students such as "One day my teddy bear came to life. This is what we did that day."

iv. *Story Starters:* includes many beginning sentences for students to use to begin their stories such as the following: Title: "An animal I'd be;" First sentence: "If you could be any animal, what would you be? Why?" Title: "My Space Journey;" First sentence: "My space journey was exciting because."

In all the above examples, I work with the student in printing/writing his/her responses on paper and then help the student type the formulated written product using Writing Blaster.

Storybook Weaver Deluxe (The Learning Company, 1998) includes two excellent categories to facilitate our work with written language formulation. Story Starters, for instance, includes a number of interesting starters such as: Title: "Repairmen in Space;" Starter: "We were working on the broken satellite when a spaceship with two little green men approached us. They looked like they were smiling at us. I was wondering if they could help repair the satellite and was about to ask when . . ." In *Create-A-Story*, students fill in the Title, Author, Comment, and write their stories. A creative feature in *Story Weaver Deluxe* allows students to select backgrounds for their stories and 1,800 objects to apply to their stories. I use *Create-A-Story* in two ways. For novice or reluctant writers, I ask them to select their background and objects and then type some words, phrases, or sentences about what they selected. I ask my more experienced writers to create their stories first and then use this computer program to input the story and to finally apply background and objects. I encourage using writing as a process, encouraging writers to "just get your good thoughts down. Spelling doesn't matter right now." I draw a big square on a sheet of paper and label it the WORD BANK. I will write any word in the box the student needs to continue writing his/her story. I teach the student to edit and rewrite the story and the publishing comes with the computer program.

2.   **Goal 2: To increase syllabication and spelling abilities.**

Suggested Activity:

a. **Increase syllabication and spelling.**

There are many programs available to use in this activity. One of my favorites, *The Brody Method* (Brody, 1991) offers a structured, sequential approach to use with students who need to learn about patterns in print. Instruction in decoding, comprehension, spelling, and writing are integrated through extensive multisensory practice that leads students from one-syllable word reading to longer words in challenging text. Students begin dividing unfamiliar words into parts by using several strategies that do not depend on prior word recognition or dictionary use. Six common consonant/vowel patterns are introduced to help students identify vowel sounds and pronunciations of word parts.

Another excellent source is *Phonographix* (McGuinness & McGuinness, 1998).Under the "Teaching the Advanced Code" section of *Phonographix*, the following goals are discussed with corresponding lesson plans and practice sheets: 1) Ability to understand that sometimes two or more letters represent a sound; 2) Ability to understand that most sounds can be represented in more than one way; 3) Ability to understand that there is overlap in the code, that some components of the code can represent more than one sound.

The final sections of this program deal with multisyllable analysis.

3.   **Goal 3: To increase capitalization and punctuation.**

Any number of products are available through teacher supply stores and educational publishing companies to help students with this goal (See Appendix 6.3 for materials to use with context processor). Examples include: *100% Punctuation* (LoGiudice, M. & LoGiudice, C., 1998), *100% Punctuation LITE* (LinguiSystems staff, 2000) and two sources available through Remedia: *Punctuation* and *Capitalization*. A computer software program I use with this goal is *Writing Blaster* (Davidson & Associates, Inc., 1998): *I Can Practice Capitalization* and *I Can Practice Punctuation*.

4.   **Goal 4: To increase proofreading.**

Suggested Activity:

a. **Grade each other's papers.**

Using the student's written creation, I have found that being reinforced for finding errors on someone else's paper increases the likelihood that a student will proofread, find and correct his/her own errors. I have also found that progress on this goal is measured sooner when proofreading is limited to one item, such as proofreading for capitalization errors, then proofreading for another item such as use of question marks. Before proofreading for a third item, I ask that students proofread for both capitalization and use of questions marks. If they are successful proofreading for the first two items, I then add a third one. Students must be proficient with these three before I add proofing for a fourth item.

C. Summary of goals included under this processor

If the student's ability to use the *context processor is weak in reading*, teaching goals may include any of the following:

1. Goal 1: To increase strategic use of context cues in reading.

2. Goal 2: To increase understanding and recognition of morphological aspects of words: roots, prefixes, and suffixes, i.e., to increase structural analysis.

If the student's ability to use the *context processor in writing is weak*, teaching goals may include any of the following:

1. Goal 1: To increase written language formulation.

2. Goal 2: To increase syllabication and spelling abilities.

3. Goal 3: To increase capitalization and punctuation.

4. Goal 4: To increase proofreading.

V. SUMMARY

The purpose of this chapter has been to outline goals, methods and suggested materials to use when working to increase use of the orthographic, meaning, and context processors. The reader is reminded to review Chapter 5 for goals, methods, and suggested materials to use when working to increase use of the phonologic processor. The final chapter of this book considers some additional, relevant issues: what is good instruction, curriculum based IEP goals to support literacy, ideas about collaboration, and future directions.

VI. CLINICAL COMPETENCIES.

To remediate developmental reading problems the teacher/clinician/student will demonstrate the following competencies:

A. Determine goals to teach/remediate the orthographic processor.

B. Determine goals to teach/remediate the meaning processor.

C. Determine goals to teach/remediate the context processor.

D. Develop curriculum-relevant goals to foster literacy acquisition.

E. Collaborate with other professionals to support literacy.

APPENDIX 6.1. SUGGESTED MATERIALS TO STRENGTHEN THE ORTHOGRAHIC PROCESSOR

Alpha-Bug Soup

Publishing Co.: Learning Resources (undated)

Contents: Educational games to encourage students to spell, read and write words formed by letter disks.

Audio Workbook for the Verbally Apraxic Adult

Authors: Richards, K.B., & Fallon, M.O. (1988)

Publishing Co.: Communication Skill Builders

Contents: Materials ranging from words to complex sentences to use for increasing a student's ability to read or repeat increasingly complex utterances.

Beginning Basic Skills: Size Comparisons

Publishing Co.: Remedia Publications (undated)

Contents: Activities for early printing using tracing, writing, and coloring activities.

Fun Phonics Manipulatives

Author: Hancock, M., Pate, S., and VanHaelst, J. (1997)

Publishing Co.: Scholastic Professional Books

Contents:

1) Making and using phonetic pull-throughs to make letter–sound associations through rhyming activities.

2) Making and using pull-through interactive mini-books tie words to related meanings.

Golden Step Ahead Flash Cards

Publishing Co.: Western Publishing Company (not dated)

Contents: Good example of onset–rime flash cards for blending words. Available through teacher supply stores.

Jr. Boggle

Author: none listed (1998)

Publishing Co.: Parker Brothers

Contents:

1) Activities for object and word recognition, letter recognition and letter matching, and spelling.

2) Activities for sorting and grouping.

3) Activities for concentration and memory.

Language!

Author: Greene, J.F. (2000)

Publishing Co.: Sopris West

Contents: *J & J Readers* Level establish a solid base of phonologically regular words.

Making Big Words

Authors: Cunningham, P., & Hall, D.P. (1994)

Publishing Co.: Good Apple

Contents:

1) Activities for combining letters, onsets and rimes to make new words.

2) Activities for sorting words by letter patterns, prefixes, suffixes, and big word parts.

Making More Big Words

Authors: Cunningham, P. & Hall, D.P. (1997)

Publishing Co.: Good Apple, A division of Simon & Schuster

Contents:

1) Activities that encourage hands-on exploration of words, letter-sound relationships, and letter patterns.

2) Activities using preselected letters to make 15 to 20 words, beginning with short words and continuing with longer words.

3) Activities for sorting words by prefixes, suffixes, rimes, homophones, and other patterns.

Phonological Awareness Shuffle
Author: Flynn, M. (1998)
Publishing Co.: LinguiSystems
Contents: Activities for consonant blend rhyming with print.

Phonological Awareness Training for Reading
Author: Torgesen, J. & Bryant, B. (1994)
Publishing Co.: Pro-Ed
Contents: Activities for phoneme grapheme correspondence.

Phonics : Games & Learning Acitivites (Primary)
Author: Turly, S. (1999)
Publishing Co.: Teacher Created Material, Inc.
Contents:

1) Rhyme Wheels: onset and rime wheel that can be used for making word with pictures.

2) Roll a Word: onset and rime dice that can be used for making words.

3) Wheel of Words: onset and rime wheel that can be used for making words.

Plastic or Magnetic Letters
Contents: Good for orthographic representation of phonemes. Available through teacher supply stores.

Reading Milestones
Author: Quigley, S.P, McAnally, P.L., Rose, S. & King, C.M. (2001)
Publishing Co.: Pro-Ed
Contents: Activities for increasing orthographic abilities through word completion.

Sounds Abound: Listening, Rhyming, and Reading
Author: Catts, H. & Vartiainen, T. (1993)

Publishing Co.: LinguiSystems

Contents: Activities for putting sounds together with letters.

Sounds and Letters for Readers and Spellers

Author: Greene, J. (2000)

Publishing Co.: Sopris West

Contents: Reading, spelling, and vocabulary activities corresponding with the *Language!* Program.

Sounds Search Bingo

Author: Flynn, M. (1999)

Publishing Co.: LinguiSystems

Contents: Activities to link phonemes to graphemes.

Storybook Weaver

Publishing Co.: The Learning Company, Inc.

Contents: Educational computer program for use with developing writing skills.

Take Home: Phonological Awareness

Author: Robertson, C. & Salter, W. (1998)

Publishing Co.: LinguiSystems

Contents: Take-home activities for generalization of phoneme–grapheme correspondence.

The Phonological Awareness Kit

Author: Robertson, C. & Salter, W. (1995)

Publishing Co.: LinguiSystems

Contents: Activities for phoneme-grapheme correspondence.

The Phonological Awareness Kit–Intermediate

Author: Robertson, C. & Salter, W. (1997)

Publishing Co.: LinguiSystems

Contents: Phonetically structured activities for grapheme identification and use.

The Sounds Abound Program

Author: Lenchner, O & Podhajski, B. (1998)

Publishing Co.: LinguiSystems

Contents: Activities for phoneme-grapheme correspondence.

Think It Through: Beginning Reading. Booklets 1–3

Publishing Co.: Discovery Toys, Inc. (1979)

Contents:

1) Activities using booklets and tiles for recognition of orthographic forms from abstract patterns to words.

2) Activities using pictures, letters, and words to strengthen word structure in print.

Treating Auditory Processing Difficulties in Children

Author: Sloan, C.

Publishing Co.: Singular Publishing Group Press (1995)

Contents:

1) Activities for auditory discrimination of phonemes primarily of consonant discrimination skills including minimal contrasting pairs in consonant–vowel and vowel–consonant syllables and words of increasing complexity.

2) Activities for speech-to-print skills.

Ultimate Phonics Reading Program Words and Sentences

Author: Spencer Learning

Publishing Co.: Spencer Learning (2000)

Contents: 262 lessons comprising the following:

1) Idea or Pattern page describing the theme of the lesson.

2) Word List: lists of all the words introduced in the lesson.

3) Word Page: the words on the Word List are presented one at a time.

4) Sentence Page: lists sentences made up of words from the current and prior lessons.

UpWords

Author: Milton Bradley company

Publishing Co.: Milton Bradley Company (1997)

Contents: A 3-dimensional game to encourage formation of words by stacking letters on a gameboard.

Wilson Reading System
Author: Wilson, B.A. (1996)
Publishing Co.: Wilson Language Training
Contents:

1) Activities for teaching students the basics: sounds, sound blends and fundamental syllabication rules to establish a solid foundation.
2) Activities for higher steps covering sound options, spelling rules, morphological principles and other advanced concepts.

Word Scramble
Author: Johnson, P.F. (1998)
Publishing Co.: LinguiSystems
Contents:

1) Activities for phonological awareness skills, listening skills, decoding skills, word flexibility, articulation skills, and thinking skills.
2) Players create words through matching letter tiles to gameboard.

Word Scramble 2
Author: Johnson, P.F. (2000)
Publishing Co.: LinguiSystems
Contents:

1) Activities for root words, prefixes and suffixes.
2) Players create multisyllabic words through matching word part tiles to gameboard.

Words Their Way
Author: Bear, D.R, Invernizzi, M., Templeton, S., and Johnston, F. (1996)
Publishing Co.: Prentice Hall, Inc.
Contents: Activities for rhyming, making words, sorting word families.

APPENDIX 6.2. SUGGESTED MATERIALS TO STRENGTHEN THE MEANING PROCESSOR

100% Vocabulary Primary and 100% Vocabulary Intermediate (formerly BESST)
Authors: Rothstein,V., & (Zacker) Termansen, R. (1997)
Publishing Co.: LinguiSystems

Contents:

1) The Primary version contains exercises to help younger students begin to understand complex word relationships.

2) The Intermediate version contains exercises to help older students learn vocabulary through activities for: classification, comparison, synonyms, antonyms, absurdities, exclusion, definitions, and analogies.

Achieve Revised Red Book

Author: Huisingh, R., Bowers, L., Barrett, M., Johnson, P., LoGiuidice, C., Orman, J., Truman, B., Whiskeyman, L., & The LinguiSystems Staff. (1997)

Publishing Co.: LinguiSystems

Contents: Activities to teach vocabulary in a systematic way. Activities are centered around home and family themes.

Big Book of Blends and Digraphs

Author: Toomey, M.M. and Christy-Pallo, S. (1994)

Publishing Co.: SuperDuper School Company

Contents: Activities for vocabulary development through matching words with pictures and sentence completion.

Blooming Language Arts

Author: Zachman, L., Huisiingh, R., Barret, M. and the Staff of LinguiSystems (1988)

Publishing Co.: LinguiSystems

Contents: Activities for vocabulary expansion through thought provoking activities at the knowledge, comprehension, application, analysis, synthesis, and evaluation levels.

Could You Swim a Fast Lap Dressed Like This?

Author: Fox, C.S. and Slater, B.B. (1997).

Publishing Co.: Fox-Slater Multisensory Resources, Inc.

Contents: Materials to strengthen vocabulary through activities using a controlled reading vocabulary.

Figurative Language: A Comprehensive Program

Author: Gorman-Gard, K.A.

Publishing Co.: Thinking Publications (1992)

Contents: Materials to strengthen vocabulary through activities using a controlled reading vocabulary.

Fun Phonics Manipulatives

Author: Hancock, M., Pate, S., and VanHaelst, J. (1997)

Publishing Co.: Scholastic Professional Books

Contents:

1) Making and using pull-through predictable books to tie rhyming words to related meanings.

2) Making and using rhyming blend flip books for use in onset and rime activities that tie the words to their meanings.

Handbook of Exercises for Language Processing: For Auditory Processing

Author: Lazzari, A.M. & Peters, P.M. (1994)

Publishing Co.: LinguiSystems

Contents: Activities for vocabulary expansion through word classes, directions, details, information, questions, and sequencing.

(HELP-4) Handbook of Exercises for Language Processing

Author: Lazzari, A.M. & Peters, P.M. (1989)

Publishing Co.: LinguiSystems

Contents: Activities for building vocabulary through combining pictures and symbols.

Language!

Author: Greene, J.F. (2000)

Publishing Co.: Sopris West.

Contents: *J & J Readers* ties previously established solid base of phonologically regular words to their meanings.

Language Processing: Remediation

Author: Richard, G.J., & Hanner, M.A. (1987)

Publishing Co.: LinguiSystems

Contents: Activities to expand vocabulary through labeling, function, association, categorization, similarities, differences, multiple meanings, and attributes.

Phonics : Games & Learning Activities (Primary)
Author: Turly, S. (1999)
Publishing Co.: Teacher Created Material, Inc.
Contents: Rhyme Wheels: onset and rime wheel that can be used for making word with pictures.

Reading Milestones
Author: Quigley, S.P, McAnally, P.L., Rose, S. & King, C.M. (2001)
Publishing Co.: Pro-Ed.
Contents: Activities for increasing vocabulary through picture and word matching and sentence completion.

Take Home: Phonological Awareness
Author: Robertson, C. & Salter, W. (1998)
Publishing Co.: LinguiSystems
Contents: Take home activities for generalization of phoneme–grapheme correspondence.

Think It Through: Beginning Reading Booklet 4
Publishing Co.: Discovery Toys, Inc. (1979)
Contents: Activities for vocabulary development through matching words with pictures.

Think It Through: Phonics Fun Booklets 3–4
Publishing Co.: Discovery Toys, Inc. (1979)
Contents:
1) Activities for vocabulary development through matching words with pictures and sentence completion.
2) Activities for vocabulary development through synonyms, antonyms, homonyms, word meanings and classes, definitions, multiple meaning words, word usage and context clues.

Treasure Mountain
Author: none listed (1997)
Publishing Co.: The Learning Company
Contents: Educational computer game involving reading and vocabulary.

Words Their Way
Author: Bear, D.R, Invernizzi, M., Templeton, S., and Johnston, F. (1996)
Publishing Co.: Prentice Hall, Inc. 2000 edition published by Merrill.
Contents:
Activities for matching words to pictures.
Activities for sorting semantic concepts.

APPENDIX 6.3. SUGGESTED MATERIALS TO STRENGTHEN THE CONTEXT PROCESSOR

Any book the student is reading
Any of the student's written language

100% Punctuation
Authors: LoGiudice, C., & LoGiudice, M. (1998)
Publishing Co.: LinguiSystems
Contents: Activities for increasing punctuation skills in the following: capitalization, end marks, apostrophes, commas, hyphens, quotation marks, colons and semicolons, and italics and underlining.

100% Punctuation Lite
Authors: LinguiSystems staff (2000)
Publishing Co.: LinguiSystems
Contents: Activities for increasing punctuation skills in the following: capitalization, end marks, apostrophes, commas, quotation marks, letters, abbreviations, colons and semicolons.

Bring the Classics to Life
Authors: various (Various dates)
Publishing Co.: Edcon
Contents: Classics written in lower readibility. Teaches students to learn vocabulary and use context clues.

Capitalization
Authors: Remedia staff (no date)
Publishing Co.: Remedia Publications
Contents: Activities to reinforce and enrich language skills in capitalization.

Cloze Reading
Authors: Remedia staff (no date)
Publishing Co.: Remedia Publications
Contents: Activities to reinforce and enrich language skills in capitalization.

Next Stop: Reading in Different Genres
Author: Auger, T. (2001)
Publishing Co.: Educators Publishing Service
Contents: Teaches young readers how to recognize different literary genres and story conventions.

Punctuation
Authors: Remedia staff (no date)
Publishing Co.: Remedia Publications
Contents: Activities to reinforce and enrich language skills in punctuation.

Reading Milestones
Author: Quigley, S.P, McAnally, P.L., Rose, S. & King, C.M. (2001)
Publishing Co.: Pro-Ed
Contents: Activities for increasing the ability to inferring word meaning through context.

Read, Write and Type: a Program on CD
Authors: The Learning Company (1997)
Publishing Co.: The Learning Company staff
Contents:
1) Activities linking speech sounds to typing to let students write anything they can say.
2) 6 engaging activities at each of 40 levels that build reading and phonics skills as students write on the computer.
3) Lifelike talking hands that provide spoken help, demonstrate each keystroke, and guide students through the learning process.

Skill Booster Series

Authors: Remedia staff (no date)

Publishing Co.: Remedia Publications

Contents: Activities for increasing knowledge of prefixes and suffixes.

Wordly Wise 3000, A,B,C

Authors: Hodkinson, K., & Adams, S. (2001)

Publishing Co.: Educators Publishing Service

Contents: Teaches vocabulary by giving students the opportunity to read words in meaningful context, to write them in sentences, and to recognize their meaning in a series of interesting exercises.

Writing Blaster: a program on CD

Authors: Davidson & Associates staff (1998)

Publishing Co.: Davidson & Associates

Contents:

1) Activities for writing complete sentences and paragraphs.

2) Activities for writing to communicate an idea.

3) Activities for using descriptive words.

4) Activities for using capital letters and punctuation.

CHAPTER

7

Some Final Considerations

OUTLINE

I.   WHAT IS GOOD INSTRUCTION?

ASHA Guidelines (2001) proposed that in keeping with IDEA97, speech–language specialists need to offer curriculum-relevant therapy. They need to modify the general curriculum and instruction and provide "direct, explicit instruction targeting reading and writing for students with language disorders to help them gain access to the general curriculum" (p. 15). According to the guidelines, for students with language based reading problems, good literacy instruction is:

> *Outcome oriented:* literacy curriculum is usually based on state-developed content standards and benchmarks (see section II in this chapter).

> *Comprehensive:* to include those aspects research has deemed necessary for literacy achievement at various levels including phonological awareness, print awareness, word recognition, comprehension, and authentic use.

> *Balanced:* having a blend of all the components needed for literacy such as reading decoding, fluency, reading comprehension, spelling, and written composition. It is essential that one area does not become the entire focus of the literacy program.

> *Contextualized:* problems students have in written language must be addressed specifically but "the overall context of authentic use of literacy skills in real reading and real writing tasks must be maintained in a complete program" (p. 21).

> *Age-appropriate:* educational activities need to be developmentally and age appropriate.

> *Recursive:* because literacy acquisition involves learning about different components of the process spanning over many years, certain elements must be addressed repeatedly with varying levels of complexity.

> *Direct:* needing explicit face-to-face instruction.

> *Explicit:* clear and detailed with step-by-step instruction.

> *Intense:* instruction that is frequent and engaging with follow-up guided-practice and independent practice activities. The student must be actively involved in the instructional sessions.

Scaffolded: instruction that facilitates students as they transition from what they know to what they must learn. Questioning and modeling are used to help students focus on cues they have previously missed.

Informative: apprising students of what they already know and what they need to learn in the process of literacy acquisition.

Corrective: informing students as to what they need to do to correct their errors and improve performance (pp. 21-22).

II. CURRICULUM-BASED IEP GOALS TO SUPPORT LITERACY

To facilitate the use of suggestions offered in this book, the focus of this chapter section is on using curriculum standards to write curriculum relevant IEP goals. Literacy goals can come from any state's Reading/Language Arts Framework, available through each state's board of education and online. See, for instance: *http://www.teacher.com/sdoe.htm   http://K-6educators.about.com/msubusa.htm* or *http://www.indiana.edu/~eric_rec/gninf/standards.html*

I found wide variation in the listings. Some states posted general standards while others posted very specific standards.

When viewing the standards, the subject area for literacy is *Language Arts*, which is typically divided into a number of strands such as: reading, literature, writing, listening, speaking, and viewing. Content standards are broad statements of what students are expected to know and be able to do (Kendall & Marzano, 1994), for example: "The student demonstrates emergent literacy through developing concepts about print." Standards are divided into benchmarks that are more specific statements of expected or anticipated performance at various developmental levels or grades (Ehern, 1999). For example: "The student demonstrates various strategies to comprehend printed material." The following examples from various states demonstrate some differences in how the standards are presented.

Included in **Arkansas'** listing:

Subject Area: Language Arts

Strand 2: Reading

Content Standard 1: Students will comprehend, evaluate, and respond to the world of literature and other kinds of writing which reflect their own cultures and developing viewpoints as well as those of others.

Grades K–4 student learning expectations:

R.1.1. Demonstrate understanding of the relationship between written and oral language.

R.1.2. Demonstrate and use concepts of print such as directionality, spacing, punctuation, and configuration in developmentally appropriate ways.

R.1.3. Recognize and associate letters and sounds.

R.1.4. Use phonetic skills to decode words.

R.1.5. Use major cueing systems such as phonetic, syntactic, and semantic to decode and construct meaning.

R.1.6. Expand vocabulary through reading.

R.1.7. Understand the goal of reading is to construct meaning.

R.1.8. Understand that reading is communication between the author and the reader.

R.1.9. Establish purposes for reading such as enjoying, learning, modeling, sharing, performing, investigating, and solving problems.

R.1.10. Use relationships between words and sentences, sentences and paragraphs, and paragraphs and whole pieces to understand text.

R.1.11. Use prior knowledge to extend reading ability and comprehension.

R.1.12. Use specific strategies such as making comparisons, predicting outcomes, drawing conclusions, identifying the main ideas, and understanding cause and effect to comprehend a variety of literary genres from diverse cultures and time periods.

R.1.13. Understand that texts have different purposes, such as: persuading, informing, entertaining, and instructing.

Assessment can be accomplished: S: statewide; T: teacher made tests; PO: portfolio; PR: project; C: checklist; O: observation; PE: performance; E: exhibition; D: demonstration; LJ: log/journal; W: writing.

Florida's listing provided succinct grade level expectations. For instance:

Subject Area: Language Arts

Strand A: Reading

Standard 1: The student uses the reading process effectively.

Benchmark LA.A.1.1.1: The student predicts what a passage is about based on its title and illustrations.

Grade Level Expectations. The student in:

Kindergarten: uses titles and illustrations to make oral predictions.

First: uses prior knowledge, illustrations, and text to make predictions.

Second: uses prior knowledge, illustrations, and text to make and confirm predictions.

Benchmark LA.A.1.1.2: The student identifies words and constructs meaning from text, illustrations, graphics, and charts using the strategies of phonics, word structure, and context clues.

Grade Level Expectations: The student in:

Kindergarten:

1. Understands how print is organized and read (for example, locating print on a page, matching print to speech, knowing parts of a book, reading top-to-bottom and left-to-right, sweeping back to left for the next line).
2. Knows the names of the letters of the alphabet, both upper and lower case.
3. Knows the sounds of the letters of the alphabet.
4. Understands the concept of words and constructs meaning from shared text, illustrations, graphics, and charts.
5. Understands basic phonetic principles (for example, knows rhyming words; knows words that have the same initial and final sounds; knows which sound is in the beginning, middle, end of a word; blends individual sounds into words).
6. Understands that print conveys meaning.

First Grade:

1. Uses basic elements of phonetic analysis (for example, hears, segments, substitutes, and blends sounds in words).
2. Uses sound/symbol relationships as visual cues for decoding.
3. Uses beginning letters (onsets) and patterns (rhymes) as visual cues for decoding.
4. Uses structural cues to decode words (for example, word order, sentence boundaries).
5. Uses context clues to construct meaning (meaning cues) for example, illustrations, knowledge of the story and topic.

6. Cross checks visual, structural, and meaning cues to figure out unknown words.

Second Grade:

1. Blends sound components into words.
2. Applies knowledge of beginning letters (onsets) and spelling patterns (rhymes) in single and multisyllable words as visual cues for decoding.
3. Uses a variety of structural cues (for example, word order, prefixes, suffixes, verb endings) to decode unfamiliar words.
4. Uses a variety of context cues (for example illustrations, diagrams, information in the story, titles and headings, sequence) to construct meaning (meaning cues).
5. Cross-checks visual, structural, and meaning cues to figure out unknown words.
6. Uses context cues to define multiple meaning words.

Idaho includes the following under language/communication standards for Kindergarten:

Subject Area: Language Arts/Communication

Strand: Reading

Standard 01: The student will read a variety of traditional electronic materials for information and understanding.

Content Knowledge and Skills: Using decoding and word-recognition strategies to fluently read kindergarten materials.

Phonics/Phonemic Awareness

1. Using various techniques, identify and/or name two or more words that rhyme:
   Complete phrases and sentences with rhyming words
   Produce a word that rhymes with a given word
   Recognize if two or more one-syllable words rhyme

2. Using varied techniques, orally segment:
   Sentences into words
   Syllables into sounds
   Words into syllables and sounds

3. Orally blend phonemes into words

Phonics

1. Recognize names of upper and lower case letters
2. Associate letters to letter sounds
3. Identify beginning, middle, and ending letters in a word

Concepts About Print

identify front of book
attend to print
use picture clues to support text
use story language
know where to start reading
move left to right across print
make return sweep to next line of text
match word by word
understand first and last of text, top and bottom of page, and order of pages for turning
read left page before right page
identify one or two letters; first and last letter, and capital letters; point to specific letter when requested

With these examples of the variation that exists in literacy standards, how might we incorporate a goal from this text into a curriculum-relevant IEP?

Ehern (1999) suggested that literacy intervention planning for speech–language specialists include the following concepts.

Curriculum: identify concepts, skills and strategies needed in literacy appropriate for student's grade level.

Underpinnings: analyze what the student will need to grasp to understand the curriculum.

Language disorder: describe the student's current needs and identify what cognitive–linguistic differences may interfere with his/her ability to learn the curriculum.

Describe student's literacy skills and predict what problems the student may have based on your knowledge of the student's language disorder.

Therapy targets: to include long-term goal; how the speech–language specialist will collaborate on the development of IEP goals and objectives; and a plan for curriculum-relevant therapy objectives.

Assistance to teachers: offer curriculum modifications and assist teachers in their planning to include modifications and to foster generalization of remedial goals.

By way of illustration, I selected a standard from the California curriculum for kindergarten reading and used parts of Ehern's format:

Subject Area: Language Art

Strand: Reading

Grade: Kindergarten

Standard 1.0: Word analysis, fluency and systematic vocabulary development

Benchmark: Student knows about letters, words, and sounds. They apply this knowledge to read simple sentences. Grade level expectations are listed under Concepts About Print and Phonemic Awareness. Because I selected a phonemic awareness goal to illustrate, I will list the expectations as they appear in the California Reading/Language Arts Framework (1999).

Phonemic Awareness:

1.7 Track (move sequentially from sound to sound) and represent the number, sameness/difference, and order of two and three isolated phonemes (e.g., /f, s, th/, /j, dz/).

1.8 Track (move sequentially from sound to sound) and represent changes in simple syllables and words with two and three sounds as one sound is added, substituted, omitted, shifted, or repeated (e.g., vowel–consonant, consonant–vowel, or consonant–vowel–consonant).

1.9 Blend vowel–consonant sounds orally to make words or syllables.

1.10 Identify and produce rhyming words in response to an oral prompt.

1.11 Distinguish orally stated one-syllable words and separate into beginning or ending sounds.

1.12 Track auditorily each word in a sentence and each syllable in a word.

1.13 Count the number of sounds in syllables and syllables in words.

I would suggest that the following topics and information be included in this kindergarten student's IEP considering Ehern's suggestions:

What the student must already be/know:

> Phonologically aware at the word and syllable level.
> Has concepts about print.
> Tracks and represents the number, sameness/difference and order of 2 and 3 isolated phonemes.
> Tracks and represents changes in simple syllables and words with 2 and 3 sounds as one sound is added, substituted, omitted, shifted or repeated.
> Blends vowel–consonant sounds orally to make words or syllables.

What the student cannot do yet:

> Distinguish orally stated one-syllable words and separate into beginning or ending sounds.
> Track auditorily each word in a sentence and each syllable in a word.
> Count the number of sounds in syllables and syllables in words.

The underlying language problem: Phonological processing problem affecting one or all of the following areas:

> Phonological coding in memory holding onto sounds
> Expressive phonological coding including oral–motor sequencing skills
> Phonological coding for word retrieval
> Phonological awareness

Long-term therapy goal: The student will be able to correctly identify and produce rhyming words in response to an oral prompt. This can be found in this book in Chapter 5 under Intentional Acts Inherent in Phonological Awareness Training: Section IIB. Goal 6.

> Rationale: This target is the 10th of 18 needed by kindergarten students to become successful readers as identified by California Language Arts Content Standards for Kindergarten Reading (Standard 1).
> To be accomplished by: 11/15____
> To be observed by: SLS, RSP, and classroom teacher.

Short-term therapy objectives:

> The student will listen to speech–language specialist read nursery rhymes and other books containing rhyme.
>
> The student will respond to specific teaching techniques and correction procedures regarding identifying and producing rhyme.
>
> The student will correctly identify 8 of 10 rhyming words when given an oral prompt, for example, "Do these 2 words rhyme?"
>
> The student will correctly produce 8 of 10 rhyming words when given an oral prompt: for example, "What word rhymes with 'cat.'?"

III. POSSIBLE COLLABORATION

As interest about the role of the speech–language specialist in literacy has increased over the past ten years, I have had the good fortune of presenting workshops throughout the United States. The issue that always arises, and leads to interesting discussions, is simply: **so who does what?** I have learned much by listening to suggestions by our colleagues working in school settings, and I have attempted to incorporate these in the following discussion.

Adams' model of reading acquisition was introduced in Chapter 2 of this book and referred to in the subsequent assessment and intervention chapters. Because it is built around four processors, this model seems helpful when considering issues surrounding how educators can work together most efficiently and effectively in their support of literacy. There, of course, can be no **one** answer to the division of labor in teaching literacy because of the diversity of our work settings and the diversity of our learners.

A. Phonological processor.

> The goals suggested in Chapter 5 can be implemented by a number of individuals such as parents, teachers, speech–language specialists, and resource specialists. The speech–language specialist works most directly with young children who have developmental language impairments. Because of their backgrounds in linguistics, phonetics, language acquisition, and childhood language disorders, speech–language specialists represent a critical and natural bridge to training of other educators and others as well as implementing phonological awareness training to students on their caseloads and/or in classroom environments. The speech–language specialist is strategically positioned to screen, assess, and teach/remediate phonological awareness skills. The addition of phonological awareness testing to this special-

ist's assessment battery is entirely appropriate because of the oral–written language continuum and because early oral language problems so frequently evolve into later reading, writing, spelling problems. It would seem the natural linkage for the speech–language specialist to implement phonological awareness training, and for the resource specialist to follow up with explicit phonics instruction.

In his position as director of the National Institute of Child Health and Human Development (NICHD), Lyon (1997) considered speech–language specialists as "gems" in the shift toward integrating phonological awareness training into reading. Lyon noted that the nature of speech–language specialists' curriculum and clinical training prepares them to integrate practice with theory. They "know how to interpret the data, know the importance of phonological awareness, . . . (and) need to explicitly and daily translate what they know about language and reading to teachers" (p. 5). The training can be done on an individual basis or in a group setting. Ball (1997) suggested that when teachers incorporate sound-based activities through books providing play with rhyme, alliteration, and invented spellings, "they seize (the) opportunity to heighten for some children the connections between sound and print" (p. 23). Ideally, phonological awareness and naming speed will be included among the language domains assessed by the speech–language specialist. Goals that target these two areas are therefore within the speech–language specialist's scope of practice.

B. Orthographic processor.

As we transition from strengthening the phonological processor into strengthening the orthographic processor, we necessarily move into print. Again, depending on the work setting, goals in Chapter 6 can be variously shared. Beyond enhancing phonological processing and awareness skills, speech–language specialists can continue to support literacy by connecting phonemes and graphemes (see Chapter 6, Goal 1). Because automaticity is critical in literacy acquisition, the speech–language specialist can target increasing rapid naming of sublexical units through timed exercises with word families (See Chapter 6, section II.A. Goal 1).

C. Meaning and context processors.

Because students with language and reading problems also present with a myriad of reading comprehension problems, increasing the efficiency of the meaning and context processors is a concern to the classroom teacher, the speech–language specialist, reading specialist, and the resource specialist. Reading specialists and resource specialists have the necessary background training to target the orthographic, meaning and context processors. Goals targeting word attack and recognition skills, structured analysis, phonics, use of context clues, dictionary skills, outlining, and note-taking are among those the RSP might include to support literacy. According to ASHA Guidelines (2001) it is the responsibility of speech–language specialists:

> to identify inadequate language skills in authentic activities that they can become the targets of focused instruction. Although intervention aimed at developing word- and sentence-level skills may be isolated at times for purposes of developing explicit awareness and/or practicing to a particular standard, for the most part such skills should be taught, to the degree possible, in the contexts of authentic literate language uses. Students also need experiences with different genres and text structures. Activities should be designed specifically to teach students with special needs to apply new knowledge and skills in functional contexts for authentic reading, writing, listening, speaking, and thinking purposes. Contextualized activities should not be saved for the last "carry over" stages of intervention. They play an important role in the development of new skills and their becoming automatized from the earliest sessions of treatment (p. 17).

Catts et al. (2001) suggested that students with speech and language problems who are "high" risk for reading problems may benefit from the following service delivery model:

The speech–language specialist works with students on a pull-out (away from the class) basis in addition to literacy targets taught within the classroom.
Phonological awareness training is included among literacy standards.
Vocabulary, grammar, pragmatics also need to be targeted.
Classroom content materials should be used in the teaching of other language areas.

Catts et al. (2001) recommended students with speech and language problems who are "low" risk for reading problems may benefit from the following delivery model:

The speech–language specialist works with the classroom teacher on literacy goals and then the speech–language specialist is faded from the classroom.
Phonological awareness training is included among literacy standards.

Sound letter correspondences are introduced.
Classroom reading activities are intensified through teacher time and
encouragement for these students.

Many educational team members I have interacted with explain that
they have divided the assessment of literacy-related skills in the following way.

> The speech–language specialist assesses oral language including
> listening comprehension,   phonological awareness, and rapid
> automatized naming.
> The resource-specialist assesses word attack, word identification,
> reading comprehension, and aspects of written language formula-
> tion.

They integrate their assessment results to identify:

> *Students with oral language problems* in areas such as semantics,
> syntax, and phonology. These are students traditionally found to
> qualify for speech–language services.
> *Students with significant oral language problems* and/or phonologi-
> cal awareness and/or rapid automatized naming problems. These
> students will develop later reading/writing problems.
> *Students with minimal oral language problems*, and/or phonological
> awareness and/or rapid automatized naming problems. These stu-
> dents are likely to develop later reading/writing problems.
> *Students with grade level or above listening comprehension* and below
> grade level reading comprehension need to be assessed further.
> Listening and reading comprehension should be equivalent to each
> other. If listening comprehension is higher than reading compre-
> hension, we need to look further at how various oral language
> influences are operating to contribute to lowered reading compre-
> hension.

IV. A PERSONAL STORY

I hope the numerous suggestions for assessment and teaching that I've
included in this book help in the technical side of your work with developmental reading disabilities. None of those suggested tests, goals, activities, or materials will do justice if we focus solely on them and minimally
on our students' understanding and acceptance of their language-learning
challenges. Through the years I have observed what happens to students as
they get trapped in the cascading downward spiral of failure. If, in our zeal

to accomplish our oral–written language goals, we stop listening to our students, then we have not finished our jobs. In the first chapter of this book I recalled the stories of two students I know and I now want to include a story about Brandon, who, as a seventh grader, wanted to tell me about how angry his parents became as his learning problems escalated over the course of three years (from fourth to seventh grade).

My interpretation of the intent in Brandon's written story is indicated by brackets.

Brandon's Story

4th grade

"4th grade is when I could remember [first recall I had problems]. At the beginning of 4th grade it was fine. It couldn't be better, until the end of the year. My parents got short with me because I fell behind in math, and it progressed until the year ended, and then cooled down.

5th grade

started out bad because I didn't like anybody so I pretended I was sick all the time when I really wasn't. And [my] parents got very mad at me for that. But when I did go to school the kids picked on me because I didn't go to school alot. So I think that's when I started to get shy and passive. My parents did not like that so they yelled at me but it did not work because I knew inside that all they want[ed] me [to do is try] trying my best and that's what I was doing. [The yelling part also made me get passive so that didn't help any.] I would of told them what was going on at school but they wouldn't believe me because I hated school there [the school he was attending]. By now I was almost afraid to tell the truth and talk to anybody [friends, family, parents] about anything cause I was afraid they would yell at me.

6th grade

Every test you got lower [than] 70% [on] you have to get the test signed. So by the time I got comfortable [I was] already too far [behind and] the class was ahead of me. So I tried my best. [I got a] 50% of [on the] test [and so that meant I] was failing so I had to get it signed and I wouldn't give it to my dad, cause he would get upset so I gave [the] tests to my mom through 6–7 [grades] to sign. One day it was a conversation that practically turned into a disaster. It was about truth [even though I was telling the truth], honesty, and why I didn't give him the tests to sign. So I told him. By now it was the end of 6th and I was exhaust[ed] and I was in a [hole] for about 3 years, afraid to talk but even worse. . .

7th grade

[I did] a couple [of] big reports and I didn't do [so] well on them. It was like that the whole year. At the middle of the year I was so overwhelmed and behind [and] I started to give up slowly, but surely. I was over-whelmed. By now my mom didn't care how I did. My dad still didn't understand why I was doing so bad. So I gave up. The only reason I passed 7th grade is I was going to another school that is special."

When Brandon told me this story during one of my last sessions with him, I asked him why he felt comfortable telling me his story. He said it was because I kept "piecing things together," and because "you stood up to my dad one time when he started to get mad at me." This is a lesson I'll never forget. Remember to keep talking to your students about how they are doing. Talk with students about what their perceptions are of their work, including what's getting stronger and what still needs work. I use graphs to help visually explain to students what areas are strong and those that we need to work on. Together we place dots on each subtest grade-level equivalence achieved by the student during assessment. As we work together, I ask students to put new dots on graphs to indicate growth in various areas, and in this way, I find that, to a far greater extent, they become partners with me.

V. FUTURE DIRECTIONS

The purposes of this book were threefold. First, a rationale for the speech–language specialist's role in treating developmental reading disabilities was discussed. Second, assessment measures for identifying reading problems and differentiating among developmental reading disabilities and underlying factors were presented. Third, specific teaching goals, activities, and materials were outlined. In the final chapter of the first edition of this book I presented a number of unresolved issues. Interestingly, although great progress has been made in our understanding of developmental reading disabilities, many of the same issues I mentioned in the first edition remain unresolved. I will summarize and update those issues here.

A. Need for Appropriate Tests and Training Materials.

Results of follow-up studies repeatedly indicate that many young children with oral language problems are dismissed from speech–language-specialists' caseloads and are re-identified in the second to fourth grades, because they are experiencing increasingly complex problems across the school curriculum. What is missing from the screening and/or assessment battery used by speech–language specialists? Are measures available to assess skills needed in the classroom to identify students at risk for later academically based learning problems? If measures used by specialists do not identify these students, what combination of existing standardized and nonstandardized subtests might be used in conjunction with a student's portfolio with samples of classroom work? If tests and subtests are not available, what measures can be used to define the nature and extent of early problems in phonological awareness, auditory memory, word finding, speech perception and production, syntactic/morphologic processing and production, and early decoding? When will our educational system realize that strictly adhering to the IQ-discrepancy model for identifying at-risk students is tantamount to putting on blindfolds? Would it not make far greater sense to identify needs and support literacy in preschool and the early elementary years rather than continue the usual practice of waiting until the gap between students' IQ and academic abilities widens and they fall hopelessly behind their classmates across the curriculum? What *possible* sense does this make?

The good news is, since the first edition of this book, the combination of tests to use for identifying students at risk for oral–written literacy problems is in place (see Chapter 4 and the earlier section in this chapter on "possible collaboration.") The frustration lies in carving out the time for sharing the assessment load and interpreting the results. I frequently begin my workshops with overheads, slides, or powerpoint stating: In the beginning there was voice, fluency, articulation and language. And now there's AAC ADD CP ADHD CAPD DAS FAE/FAS HOH LLD ESL MR PDD-NOS SLI SPD TBI (to mention a few entries in our alphabet soup). And we have to think about: IDEA IEPs IFSPS ITPs and whether we are going to work in PULL-OUT SIT-IN MAINSTREAM COLLABORATE CONSULT LEARNING SKILL CENTERS HOME BASED OR FULL INCLUSION... and now you're asking us to teach reading!!! The answer to this question is a resounding NO! But I am convinced that as we continue to educate each other as to our roles and responsibilities in literacy, we will arrive at the solution.

B. Therapy and Teaching Materials That Support Literacy and the Curriculum.

In Chapters 5 and 6, teaching goals, suggested activities, and materials were outlined. These should be incorporated into language therapy with at-risk and identified preschool, elementary-aged, and older students, to facilitate literacy skills. Rather than worksheets and time-consuming, unnecessary, games and gameboards, materials should include books, crayons, pencils, paper, markers, white boards, literacy-based computer programs, and curriculum relevant goals. The ASHA (2001) Guidelines included the following suggested materials to use with younger students. When working on concepts of phonology and skill in phonological processing include nursery rhymes, alliteration, poems, fingerplays, chants, television jingles, and rhymes for children's names (p.5). When the focus is on alphabetic/letter knowledge include the following: "naming letters, numbers and frequent words; using letter blocks, finger painting, or sponge letters to make words; sorting pictures that begin with the same letter; and making lists of words that begin with the same letter" (p. 5). When working to increase a student's sense of story, use wordless books; predictable stories with repetitive themes and rhyme sequences; books with familiar daily sequences of events; and familiar stories and tales.

C. Increasing Public Awareness.

The public needs to be educated about emergent literacy, the oral and written language continuum, and the importance of early identification of language problems. And while progress has been made since the first edition of this book, there still remains much confusion as to when a problem is significant enough and which professional works with what. Articles need to appear in magazines for parents and in professional journals for nurses, pediatricians, otolaryngologists, family practitioners, psychologists, regular and special educators, speech–language specialists, and audiologists. State, federal, and professional agencies and organizations should develop brochures; promote informational workshops; and run advertisements on television, radio, and other telecommunication informational systems to publicize the overt and subtle symptoms in children at risk for oral and written language problems. The importance of middle ear problems, late onset or slow development of speech, difficulty following directions, and so on, must be emphasized as possible indicators of oral and, subsequently, written language problems. Language disabilities will not disappear. Thus parents concerned about their children's slow speech and language-learning development should *never* hear "he'll outgrow it," "boys will be boys," "come back and see me in 6 months," "she knows about second-grade information but just doesn't have the nuts and bolts yet," or "reading problems can't be diagnosed until third or fourth grades."

D. Transdisciplinary Training Across Professional Fields.

Casby's (1988) survey (reviewed in Chapter 1) indicated that, although many speech–language specialists recognize they need to be involved in treating developmental reading disabilities, 52% of the respondents reported that their knowledge about the oral-to-written language connection came from independent study and experience and not their university training programs. Eighty-nine percent of those interviewed expressed a need for in-service training on this important topic. Has much changed since Casby's survey? The speech–language specialists in Conner/Coover's (2001) survey were least comfortable with the following competencies:

Supervising and planning for speech assistants

Teaching the writing process

Determining augmentative communication options

Teaching alternative reading programs and strategies

Understanding and integrating the general education language arts curriculum into therapy

Acting as a resource to other school staff

Participating as a member of school-based committees (p. 19).

I believe much *has* changed since the first edition of this book, and I think it is vitally important that we do not misinterpret our charge. "Support literacy" is far different than knowing how to teach writing or teaching alternative reading programs. The term "literacy" needs to be regarded in its broader sense to include oral and written language, and this definition needs to be infused across curriculum provided through our university training programs. Existing language or curriculum courses should be modified to include acquisition of reading, information on specific and nonspecific reading disabilities, and how to assess and remediate these problems. Existing graduate language practicum and methods courses should be modified to include phonological awareness and other emergent literacy activities as part of the long range plan for at-risk children demonstrating subtle or overt oral language problems. Courses on assessment should emphasize the use of static and dynamic measures.

Opportunities should be provided for dialogue among future professionals, including students in nursing, medicine, regular and special education, psychology, speech–language pathology, and audiology. Rather than randomly coming together after graduation as practitioners serving children with language-learning problems, training should occur during graduate school to provide interaction among students and faculty from various disciplines to promote a transdisciplinary approach. The curriculum should include concepts common to all disciplines involved and incorporate the specialized approaches of each. Observation of master teachers and clinicians serving students with language-based reading problems should be available during student teaching, and opportunities to practice their skills within teams should be available during student teaching placements. Sharing coursework and practical experiences will foster closer working relationships among these professionals following graduation. Finally, according to the ASHA (2001) Guidelines, speech–language specialists have responsibilities to:

> help university program faculty provide effective instructional methods and examples for preparing professionals to work in school-based and other pediatric-practice settings. Ongoing professional development programs is also necessary to assist practitioners already working in the field to assure the necessary knowledge and skills to implement ... literacy roles and responsibilities ... (p. 23).

VI. SUMMARY

My focus has been to view developmental oral and written language problems on a continuum and to regard assessment and treatment as an ongoing process. Using a model of reading acquisition that encompasses phonology, orthography, meaning and context sets the stage for looking at the varied components that must be considered in the support of literacy.

There is *no silver bullet* in remediation of developmental reading disabilities. To focus solely on the phonological aspects of reading would result in students with good decoding skills but mediocre reading comprehension. To target only the visual aspects of reading would result in increased letter–word identification, but students would still need to learn how to decode print. And to overemphasize reading comprehension and use of contextual cues would result in students knowing about words and context cues in those books. What about the vast numbers of books they will encounter in their educational careers? We must adopt a model of reading acquisition and continue to revisit that model so as to not get stuck emphasizing one aspect of reading to the exclusion of the other important aspects.

Finally, we must continue to teach each other. The best use of our professional energies will be in training each other in techniques that work. Practitioners must continue to share their expertise and report their results. The more transdisciplinary the approach to assessment and treatment, the more students with oral–written language problems will benefit. When old views are replaced by new ones, and when territorial issues are put aside, professionals involved with students who demonstrate oral–written language problems agree that our mission is a common one—to help our students learn, grow, and take their places in society as literate adults.

VII. CLINICAL COMPETENCIES.

To provide appropriate instruction to support literacy the teacher/clinician/student will demonstrate the following competencies:

A. Understand what good literacy instruction is.

B. Collaborate with other professionals in teaching/remediating the phonological, orthographic, meaning and context processors.

C. Explain what needs to be considered in the future for speech/language specialists in the support of literacy.

APPENDIX A

Informal Measures to Use in Assessment

I. BALL, E.W. (1993).

Table A-1. Developmental Scoring For Invented Spellings.

Points	Level	Characteristics	Example
0	Prephonemic (random string)	Know how letters are formed and that letters represent language. However, they string letters together in an unsystematic fashion because they have not realized yet the alphabetic principle.	BMKGTO (candy) FMTXBR (train)

Table A–1. Developmental Scoring For Invented Spellings (continued).

Points	Level	Characteristics	Example
1	Early phonemic spelling (sparse single, phoneme representations)	Have an early understanding of the alphabetic principle and attempt to represent phonemes in words with letters. May follow their representations with a random string of letters.	
		Phonemic representations may be correct or made with a phonetically related letter (letters that are related to the articulatory features of the conventional phoneme or that contain the phoneme in the letter's name; e.g., H representing ch). Representations are sparse.	P (piano) J (train)
2	Early phonemic spelling++ or letter-name spelling	Typically, more than one phoneme is represented, but there is not the one-to-one correspondence seen in letter-name spelling.	TA (train) PTE (pretty)
3	Letter-name	More than one phoneme is represented with phonetically related or conventional letters, and there is a one-to-one correspondence.	TAN (train) LAP (lamp)
		However, consonant digraphs (e.g., ch, sh, th, ph) are represented by one letter, nasals are dropped near medial vowels and unstressed vowels (schwa) are not represented.	HARE (cherry) YET (went) LETL (little)
		Letter-name spellers frequently use the sounds of the names of letters to represent particular phonemes, and lax (or short) vowels often are represented by long vowels with the same tongue positions (e.g., short e as in edge is represented by the letter a, short i with the letter e, short u with the letter o and short o with the letter i.	HEM (him)

Table A–1. Developmental Scoring For Invented Spellings (continued).

Points	Level	Characteristics	Example
4	Transitional (easy to read)	This level goes beyond the one-to-one correspondence between sounds and letters and includes many of the features of conventional spelling. However, these conventional spellings may be applied uncertainly or overextended.	TRANE (train)
		The influence of print is evident at this stage because the transitional speller is a reader. We may see all the correct letters of a word but not in the correct order.	NIHGT (night)
		Derivational spelling might be included at this level—that is, spellings that indicate an awareness that the spelling of a particular word reflects, or is derived from, the morpheme.	EXPLANATION (explanation)
5	Conventional	Correct spelling	

Note: ++ = advanced stage of early phonetic spelling.

Source: From "Assessing Phoneme Awareness" by E. W. Ball, 1993, p. 133. *Language, Speech, and Hearing Services in Schools, 24.* Reprinted with permission.

II. PARIS, S. (1991). AN EXAMPLE OF A THINK-ALONG PASSAGE (TAP, PP. 49–50).

A. Devising a Passage.

Paris adapted a Heath Reading Strategies Assessment (1991) passage, "The Peabody Ducks," but explained that any regular curriculum material from basal readers or content area texts may be used to devise a think-along passage (TAP). Comprehension questions are devised to assess a student's ability to identify topics or themes in a passage, make predictions, monitor meaning of novel words, make inferences and summarize key ideas. Metacognitive questions are designed to examine strategies the student did or might use. The examiner should present the student with the passage and picture and then ask questions 1a, 1b, and 2a (see below). The student should then finish reading the passage and answer questions 3 to 5 (see below) asked by the examiner.

B. Scoring.

The questions are judged "Right" or "Wrong," and the examiner must use his or her judgment in assessing the correctness of the student's response.

After the student is presented with the printed material and corresponding picture, the examiner asks/scores the following questions.

Monitoring meaning	Strategies:	Observed	Notes
3a. What do you think "trat" (a word in Peabody Ducks) means in the sentence you read?	Uses context cues	_____	_____
	Substitution looks or sounds similar	_____	_____
	Mentions others as resources	_____	_____
	Mentions dictionary as resource	_____	_____
	Other	_____	_____

3b. How could you tell?

If you don't know, how could you find out?

Making inferences	Strategies:	Observed	Notes
4a. Why do you think Edward Pembroke uses a cane?	Infers based on text cues	_____	_____
	Infers based on prior knowledge	_____	_____
	Scans forward	_____	_____
4b. How did you decide this?	Rereads	_____	_____
	Other	_____	_____

Summarizing	Strategies:	Observed	Notes
5a. If you wanted to tell your friends about this story, what would you tell them?	Retells mostly main ideas	_____	_____
	Retells mostly details	_____	_____
	Organizes ideas in recall	_____	_____

Summarizing	Strategies:	Observed	Notes
5b. How did you decide what things to tell them?	Expresses opinions or reactions	_____	_____
	Connects to personal experiences	_____	_____
	Uses genre/structures to help recall	_____	_____
5c. If you don't know, how do you think you could decide?	Displays appropriate affect	_____	_____
	Other	_____	_____

III.   ROSNER, J. (1979). TEST OF AUDITORY ANALYSIS SKILLS

The test starts off with two demonstration items that are intended to show the child what he is expected to do. The first (item A) goes like this: "Say cowboy." Now pause and allow him to respond . . . Then say: "Now say it again but don't say boy." Give him time to respond. (The correct answer, of course, is cow.)

If he gets this one correct, move on to the second demonstration item. If he does not get item A correct, see if you can explain it to him. However, if it requires more than a simple explanation, stop testing.

The second demonstration item (item B) is "Say steamboat." (Pause—wait for his response.) "Now say it again, but don't say steam."

If he answers both demonstration items correctly, start the test with item 1. If he does not answer both demonstration items correctly, do not administer any more items.

NOTE: Do not give him hints with your lips. Speak distinctly, but do not stress any particular sounds. In other words, do not give him any additional information that might make the task easier. Certainly, you want the child to do well, but not at the expense of looking better on the test than he really is. The results would be misleading and deprive him of the chance to learn the skills needed for reading and spelling . . . Remember, when you get to the items that ask the child to "Say the word, but don't say /.../ [a single sound]" you are to say the sound of the letter, not the letter name.

Item	Question	Correct Response
A Say cowboy	Now say it again but don't say boy	cow
B Say steamboat	Now say it again but don't say steam	boat
1 Say sunshine	Now say it again but don't say shine	sun
2 Say picnic	Now say it again but don't say pic	nic
3 Say cucumber	Now say it again but don't say cu (q)	cumber
4 Say coat	Now say it again but don't say /k/	oat (the k sound)
5 Say meat	Now say it again but don't say /m/	eat (the m sound)
6 Say take	Now say it again but don't say /t/	ache (the t sound)
7 Say game	Now say it again but don't say /m/	gay
8 Say wrote	Now say it again but don't say /t/	row
9 Say please	Now say it again but don't say /z/	plea
10 Say clap	Now say it again but don't say /k/	lap
11 Say play	Now say it again but don't say /p/	lay
12 Say stale	Now say it again but don't say /t/	sale
13 Say smack	Now say it again but don't say /m/	sack

Stop testing after two successive errors—two incorrects in a row—and record the number of the last correct item before those two errors. That is his TAAS score. For example, if he was correct with items 1, 2, 3, 4, and 5, then incorrect on items 6 and 7, his TAAS score would be 5. If he was correct on 1, 2, and 3, incorrect on 4, correct on 5 and 6, then incorrect on 7 and 8, his TAAS score would be 6.

Interpreting the test results

Now you have to determine whether the child's performance was adequate for his grade level. Make note of his score—the last item he answered correctly before he produced two wrong answers in succession—and relate it to the following chart.

To read the chart, locate the child's score in the left-hand column. Opposite that number is the grade level of children who customarily earn this score. For example, if the child's score is 3, we would expect him to be in kindergarten. If he is in kindergarten, you can assume that his auditory perceptual skills are normal. If he is in preschool, he is probably precocious. If, on the other hand, he is in first grade or beyond, you can assume that his auditory perceptual skills are inadequate and, as such, are contributing to his school learning problem.

What if his score is 9? Then his auditory perceptual skills can be considered satisfactory if he is in the first grade or below. If he is in a higher grade, his performance on the TAAS is to be considered substandard.

As you can see from the chart, no item in the TAAS—not even the final ones—should be too difficult for a child in the third grade or above. If it is, it again indicates inadequate auditory perceptual skills.

TAAS Score	Expected for Children in:
1	Kindergarten
2	Kindergarten
3	Kindergarten
4	Grade 1
5	Grade 1
6	Grade 1
7	Grade 1
8	Grade 1
9	Grade 1
10	Grade 2
11	Grade 2
12	Grade 3
13	Grade 3

Source: Reprinted with permission from Rosner, 1979, pp. 47–49.

APPENDIX B

Summary of Goals Suggested in This Book

Goals That Target the Phonological Processor

I. IF THE STUDENT'S ABILITY TO USE THE PHONETIC/PHONO-LOGICAL CODE TO HOLD SOUNDS AND WORDS IN MEMORY IS WEAK, TEACHING GOALS MAY INCLUDE ANY OF THE FOLLOWING, THE FIRST SIX OF WHICH ARE FREQUENTLY REFERRED TO AS AUDITORY PROCESSING/PERCEPTUAL SKILLS.

- Goal 1: To increase auditory decoding through decreasing phonemic discrimination problems.

- Goal 2: To increase auditory decoding through decreasing temporal pattern recognition/use problems.

- Goal 3: To decrease auditory processing problems secondary to auditory figure/ground problems.

- Goal 4: To decrease auditory processing problems secondary to auditory selective attention problems.

- Goal 5: To decrease auditory processing problems secondary to poor auditory memory.

- Goal 6: To decrease auditory processing problems through increasing binaural integration (a.k.a. auditory closure/synthesis).

- Goal 7: To increase simple receptive language.

- Goal 8: To increase listening comprehension.

- Goal 9: To increase verbal repetition.

II. IF THE STUDENT'S ABILITY TO USE THE PHONOLOGICAL CODE IN PHONOLOGICAL AWARENESS IS IMPAIRED, TEACHING GOALS MAY INCLUDE ANY OF THE FOLLOWING:

- Goal 1: To increase phonological awareness at the word level: implicit teaching.

- Goal 2: To increase phonological awareness at the word level: explicit teaching.

- Goal 3: To increase phonological awareness at the syllable level: implicit teaching.

- Goal 4: To increase phonological awareness at the syllable level: explicit teaching.

- Goal 5: To increase phonological awareness at the phoneme level: implicit teaching.

- Goal 6: To increase phonological awareness at the phoneme level: explicit teaching.

III. IF THE STUDENT'S ABILITY TO USE THE PHONOLOGICAL CODE IN VERBAL OUTPUT IS WEAK, TEACHING GOALS MAY INCLUDE ANY OF THE FOLLOWING:

- Goal 1: To increase oral vocabulary.

- Goal 2: To increase syntax/morphology.

- Goal 3: To increase oral narrative skills.

- Goal 4: To increase ability to say complex words.

- Goal 5: To decrease use of phonological processes/deviations.

IV. IF THE STUDENT'S ABILITY TO USE THE PHONOLOGICAL CODE IN WORD RETRIEVAL IS WEAK, TEACHING GOALS MAY INCLUDE ANY OF THE FOLLOWING:

- Goal 1: To increase isolated word finding abilities.

- Goal 2: To increase word finding abilities in discourse.

V. IF THE STUDENT'S ABILITY TO USE THE PHONOLOGICAL CODE IN READING IS WEAK, TEACHING GOALS MAY INCLUDE:

- Goal 1: To increase auditory processing and phonological awareness abilities.

- Goal 2: To increase word attack skills.

Methods That Target the Orthographic Processor

I. IF THE STUDENT'S ABILITY TO USE THE ORTHOGRAPHIC PROCESSOR IS WEAK, TEACHING GOALS MAY INCLUDE ANY OF THE FOLLOWING:

- Goal 1: To increase phonological awareness skills at the phoneme level using print.

- Goal 2: To increase visual discrimination abilities to facilitate use of the orthographic processor.

- Goal 3: To increase rapid naming of sublexical units, that is, word families/word parts/ phonograms/ or onset–rimes, to increase word identification and fluency in reading, and to increase spelling of words.

- Goal 4: To increase word attack, word identification, and spelling abilities through exposure to increasingly complex print.

Methods That Target the Meaning Processor

I. **IF THE STUDENT'S ABILITY TO USE THE MEANING PROCESSOR IS WEAK, TEACHING GOALS MAY INCLUDE ANY OF THE FOLLOWING:**

- Goal 1: To increase reading comprehension: teaching active strategies before reading.

- Goal 2: To increase reading comprehension: teaching active strategies during reading.

- Goal 3: To increase reading comprehension: teaching active strategies after reading.

Methods That Target the Context Processor

I. **IF THE STUDENT'S ABILITY TO USE THE CONTEXT PROCESSOR IN READING IS WEAK, TEACHING GOALS MAY INCLUDE ANY OF THE FOLLOWING:**

- Goal 1: To increase strategic use of context cues in reading.

- Goal 2: To increase understanding and recognition of morphological aspects of words: roots, prefixes, and suffixes, i.e., to increase structural analysis.

II. IF THE STUDENT'S ABILITY TO USE THE CONTEXT PROCESSOR IN WRITING IS WEAK, TEACHING GOALS MAY INCLUDE ANY OF THE FOLLOWING:

- Goal 1: To increase written language formulation.

- Goal 2: To increase syllabication and spelling abilities.

- Goal 3: To increase capitalization and punctuation.

- Goal 4: To increase proofreading.

APPENDIX C

Phonological Awareness Training Program

This appendix provides a synopsis of the activities included in the explicit teaching of phonological awareness activities described in Chapter 5. Three levels were developed.

Level I.   Increasing word awareness: dividing sentences into words.

Level II.   Increasing syllable awareness: dividing words into syllables

Level III.   Increasing sound awareness: dividing syllables onset and rime; and dividing syllables into phonemes.

Each level of the training program included two sections.

1. **Listening activities** to increase a student's attention to the sound structure of the language. These activities were meant to enhance a student's phonological awareness abilities at the implicit level.

2. Activities for deliberate manipulation of words, syllables, and phonemes to increase the student's ability to play with, that is, to analyze the sounds of language, thereby providing explicit phonological awareness training. Because there is a developmental progression of phonological awareness activities progressing from the word to the syllable to the phoneme level, the user is encouraged to begin with the word level, if the student needs to begin here, and progress to the syllable and finally to the phoneme level. Activities included in each of the three sections have been arranged according to level of difficulty. For instance, some of the activities included under the *phoneme* section include lower level implicit activities such as rhyming in patterns and alliteration, to higher, more explicit level activities including providing initial and final sounds in words, segmenting sounds, replacing sounds within words, pig Latin, and finally phoneme switching (switching the first two phonemes in words, for example, "bad wolf" becomes "wad bolf").   It is suggested that the user begin with the first activity level under each category and move through the activities in the suggested sequence.   However, as with all other developmental milestones, children will vary in their acquisition of phonological awareness and consequently respond to activities listed later in a section before the more basic activities. Activities included in this book include the following.

I. PHONOLOGICAL AWARENESS ACTIVITIES AT THE WORD LEVEL: EXPLICIT TEACHING

Identifying Words and Sentences. As you read to the student ask him or her to point to words and sentences. Explain that the first word in a sentence begins with a capital letter and that sentences end with punctuation marks, "period/the dot." Show the student how words are separated on the page by the spaces between them.

Explaining Words and Sentences. The student explains how we can tell when there is a word or sentence on the page and gives some information about what a word and/or a sentence is.

Filling in Words as Adult Reads. Omit words as you read and allow time for the student to "read" the omitted words.

Counting Words Heard or Seen. Ask the student to count the number of words he or she hears/sees as you read from a book. Provide blocks for the student to tap/count and then ask the student to tell you the number of words/blocks counted.

Rearranging Words to Make Sentences. To increase the student's semantic–syntactic and memory abilities, provide increasingly longer sentences with the words out of order. Ask the student to rearrange the words so they make sense.

II. PHONOLOGICAL AWARENESS ACTIVITIES AT THE SYLLABLE LEVEL: EXPLICIT TEACHING

Syllable Tapping in Poems and Rhymes. Nursery rhymes are used and the student is asked to tap each syllable on his or her knees or on the table.

Differentiating Real Compound Words from Nonreal, Compound Words. The student is asked to indicate when a word is "real," for example, "Is baseball a word?" Is "ballbase a word?"

Differentiating Real, Noncompound Words from Nonreal, Noncompound Words. As in the activity previously described using non-compound words, the student is asked to identify real and nonreal words, for example, "Is quickly a word?" "Is ly-quick a word?" Nonsense words are used here and in later activities in this program to promote generalization of phonological awareness ability, not just word knowledge.

Identifying the Missing Syllable. Ask the student to name each of two pictures shown, for example, "cow" and "boy." Then, ask the student to identify which part of the word is missing when you cover one picture, for example, the cow. Fade the use of pictures when the child understands the task.

Syllable Counting. Ask the student to count the number of syllables in words as you read words. Use blocks if the student needs tangible manipulatives to help count.

Deleting a Syllable. The student is asked to say a word, for example, "butterfly," then is asked to say it again but to leave out a specified part of the word, for example, "don't say butter," or "don't say fly."

Defining Syllables. The student is taught that a syllable is a part of a word and is asked to provide the same definition. It may help the student's understanding to show the pieces of a 3- to 4-piece puzzle. Like a part of a puzzle, a syllable is a part of a word.

Identifying the Common (Hidden) Syllable in Words. The student is asked to tell if a particular syllable is heard in words, for example, "Is the word 'dog' in the word 'doghouse'?" "Is it in hotdog?" "Is it in housepet?"

Adding a Syllable. Ask the student to add another part (prefix or suffix) to the word you say, for example, "add '-ing' to the end of 'begin.'" Increasingly complex words—"photo, photograph, photographer, photography, photographic" can facilitate phonological maturity (see Chapter 2).

Substituting a Syllable. Ask the student to substitute (replace) a part of a word, for example, ask the student to say "baseball." Then, instead of "base" say "basket."

Reversing Syllables in Compound Words. Ask the student to reverse or switch the parts in a compound word, for example, "Switch the two parts of 'horsefly'" (flyhorse).

Reversing Syllables in Noncompound, Bisyllabic Words. As in the previous task, using noncompound, two-syllable words, ask the student to reverse or switch the parts, for example, "Switch the two parts of 'flower'" (erflow).

III. PHONOLOGICAL AWARENESS ACTIVITIES AT THE PHONEME LEVEL: EXPLICIT TEACHING

Blending sounds in monosyllabic words divided into onset–rime beginning with two consonant cluster. Ask the student to put sounds together to make a word, for example, "Say /sp/ /ot/ to make a word."

Blending Sounds in Monosyllabic Words Divided Into Onset–Rime Beginning with a Single Consonant. Ask the student to put sounds together to make a word, for example, "h + ot."

Sound Play–Initial Sound. Tell the student you are going to play a game making up new words for pictures or objects. For example, label things in the room by making them all begin with the /b/ sound. "Chair" becomes "bair," "desk" becomes "besk."

Sound Play–Final Sound. Tell the student you are going to play a game making up a new language by adding a sound to the end of words that name things in the room, for example, "desky" or "lampy" (Catts, 1991b).

Supplying the Rhyming Word in Known Nursery Rhymes. Read a nursery rhyme known by the student, for example, "Humpty Dumpty." Read it again leaving out certain rhyming words and ask the student to fill in the missing word, for example, "Humpty Dumpty sat on a wall" "Humpty Dumpty had a great _____" (student supplies "fall").

Producing Rhyme Using Content Words. Ball (1993) found that "the ability to provide rhymes on demand is relatively low in terms of explicitness and is easy to assess" (p. 133). Ask the student to generate a word that rhymes with a word you say, for example, "Tell me a word that rhymes with 'cat'."

Producing Rhyme Using Noncontent Words. As in the previous task, use noncontent words, for example, "Tell me a word that rhymes with 'of.'"

Recognizing Rhyme. Ask the student if two words rhyme, for example, "Does 'cat' rhyme with 'hat'?" "Does 'cat' rhyme with 'coat'?"

Sound Categorization or Identifying Rhyme Oddity. Ball (1993) explained that "categorizing words by rhyme requires the child to group words together that contain the same rhyme" (p. 24). Bradley and Bryant (1983, 1985) referred to this as an "oddity task." Ball (1993) provided the following example:

Children are presented with four pictures of objects, three of which rhyme and one that is the "odd one out." (With younger children, it is suggested that two rhyming pictures and one nonrhyming picture be used.) After naming each of the pictures, children must select the card that does not belong with the others because it does not rhyme (p. 24).

Matching Rhyme. Ask the student to choose one of three words that rhyme with a stimulus word (e.g., "Which word rhymes with coat? 'boat,' 'cat,' 'dog'?")

Sound Matching. Ask the student to identify which of two to four words begin with a particular sound, for example, "Which words begin with the /s/ sound: sink, soup, soap, cat." Do this with pictures, if needed, and then repeat the activity without pictures.

Generating Words Beginning with a Particular Sound. Ask the student to tell you one to four word(s) that start(s) with a certain phoneme, for example, "the /k/ sound."

Blending Three Continuous Sounds to Form a Monosyllabic Word. Ask the student to put three sounds together to make a word, and then to tell you what the word is. For example, ask the student to "say sssss-aaaa—mmmmm. What's the word?" Choose words beginning with continuant sounds, for example, /m/, /n/, /s/, /f/, /sh/, /th/, /r/, /h/, /l/, and /w/.

Blending Three Noncontinuous Sounds to Form a Monosyllabic Word. Ask the student to put sounds together to make a word, and then to tell you what the word is. For example, ask the student to "Say c-a-t. What's the word?" Choose words beginning with noncontinuant sounds, for example, /p/, /b/, /t/, /d/, k/, and /g/.

Supplying the Initial Sound. Ask the student to tell you what sound is missing in the beginning of one of the words you say, for example, "Can, -an. What sound do you hear in 'can' that is missing in '-an'?"

Supplying the Final Sound. Ask the student to tell you what sound is missing at the end of one of the words you say, for example, "Can, Ca- What sound do you hear at the end of 'can' that is missing in 'ca-'?"

Judging the Initial Consonant Same. Ask the student to identify which of three to four words begins with the same sound heard in the beginning of a stimulus word. For example, "Which word begins with the same first sound you hear in 'cat?': 'boat,' 'hat,' 'cow.'"

Judging the Final Consonant Same. Ask the student to identify which of three to four words ends with the same sound heard in the end of a stimulus word. For example, "Which word ends with the same sound you hear at the end of cat? 'cow,' 'hat,' 'dog.'"

Identifying Initial (Continuant) Sound. Ask the student to identify what sound is heard at the beginning of one to four stimulus word(s). For example, "What is the first sound you hear in 'mom,' 'me,' 'moo,' 'mine'?" (Choose words beginning with continuant sounds—/m/, /n/, /s/, /r/, /f/, /h/, /l/, /v/, /w/, and /z/.)

Identifying the Initial (Stop) Sound. Ask the student to identify what sound is heard at the beginning of one to four stimulus word(s). For example, "What is the first sound you hear in these words, 'put,' 'pet,' 'pat,' 'pot'?" (Choose words beginning with stop sounds—/p/, /b/, /t/, /d/, /k/, and /g/.)

Identifying the Initial Consonant Different (also referred to as a phonological oddity task). Ask the student to identify which one of three to four words begins with a different sound. For example, "Which word has a different beginning sound? 'bat,' 'horse,' 'ball,' 'banana.'"

Identifying the Final Consonant Different. Ask the student to identify which one of three to four words ends with a different sound. For example, "Which word has a different ending sound? 'cat,' 'coat,' 'dog,' 'sit.'"

Substituting the Initial Sound. Ask the student to change the first sound in a word. For example, "Say cat. Now say it with a /s/ instead of /k/ in the beginning."

Substituting the Final Sound. Ask the student to change the last sound in a word, for example, "Say cat. Now say it with an /n/ instead of /t/ at the end."

Matching the Initial Sound-to-Word Using Real, Content Words. Ask the student to tell you if a word begins with a particular sound. Suggest either the correct or incorrect answer. For example, "Does cat begin with /k/?" or "Does cat begin with /t/?"

Matching the Initial Sound-to-Word Using Nonreal or Noncontent Words. Ask the student to tell you if a word begins with a particular sound. Suggest either the correct or incorrect answer. For example, "Does gat begin with /g/?" or " Does gat begin with /m/?"

Matching the Final Sound-to-Word Using Real, Content Words. Ask the student to tell you if a word ends with a particular sound suggesting either the correct or incorrect answer, for example, "Does cat end with /t/?" or "Does cat end with /g/?"

Matching the Final Sound-to-Word Using Nonreal or Noncontent Words. Ask the student to tell you if a word ends with a particular sound. Suggest either the correct or incorrect answer. For example, "Does gat end with /t/?" or "Does gat end with /b/?"

Segmenting the Initial Sound in Real, Content Words. Ask the student to identify the first sound in a word. For example, "What's the first sound in cat?" Segmenting the first or last sound (C:VC or CV:C) is easier for students than segmenting the word into three separate sounds C:V:C

Segmenting the Initial Sound in Nonreal or Noncontent Words. Ask the student to identify the first sound in a word, for example, "What's the first sound in gat?"

Segmenting the Final Sound in Real Content Words. Ask the student to identify the last sound in a word, for example, "What's the last sound in cat?"

Segmenting the Final Sound in Nonreal or Noncontent Words. Ask the student to identify the last sound in a word. For example, "What's the last sound in gat?"

Segmenting the Middle Sound in Real, Content Words. Ask the student to identify the middle sound in a word. For example, "What's the middle sound in cat?"

Segmenting the Middle Sound in Nonreal or Noncontent Words. Ask the student to identify the middle sound in a word. For example, "What's the middle sound in gat?"

Counting and Segmenting All Sounds in Real, Content Words. Ask the student to identify all sounds in a word. Begin with three-sound monosyllabic words. For example, "How many sounds do you hear in the word 'cat'?" or "What three sounds do you hear in the word cat?"

Counting and Segmenting All Sounds in Nonreal or Noncontent Words. Ask the student to identify all sounds in a word. Begin with three-sound monosyllabic words. For example, "What three sounds do you hear in the word zog?"

Deleting the Initial Sound. Ask the student to omit the first sound of a word. For example, "Say cat. Say it again but don't say /k/."

Deleting the Final Sound. Ask the student to omit the last sound of a word. For example, "Say cat. Say it again but don't say /t/."

Deleting Sounds Within Words. Ask the student to omit a sound in a word. For example, "Say slip. Say it again but don't say /l/."

Substituting Sounds in Words. Ask the student to substitute a sound in a word. For example, "Say slip. Say it again but instead of /l/ say /k/."

Saying Words Backward or Sound Reversing. Ask the student to say words backwards. For example: "If we say 'tall' backward, the word is 'lot.'"

Switching First Sounds in Words. Ask the student to switch the first sounds in two words. For example: "If we switch the first sounds in 'feet sank' the new words are 'seet fank.'"

Learning a "Secret Language," for Example, "Pig Latin." Ask the student to put the first consonant of a word at the end and add a long /a/ sound, for example, "lamp" becomes "amplay."

APPENDIX D

Books to Use in Phonological Awareness Training

Some of the books I use in work with students having developmental reading disabilities are listed here under 9 headings.

Books with alliteration
Books with assonance
Books with figurative language or riddles
Books with manipulation or fingerplays
Books with no words
Books with patterning/repetitive/predictable text
Books with poems or rhymes
Books with sound
Miscellaneous children's books mentioned in this text

BOOKS WITH ALLITERATION (SAME CONSONANT AT BEGINNING OF STRESSED SYLLABLES)

Adshead, P. S. (1993). *One odd old owl.* New York: Discovery Toys, Inc. by Child's Play (International) Ltd.

Base, G. (1986). *Animalia.* New York: Harry N. Abrams, Inc., Publishers.

Base, G. (1987). *Jabberwocky.* New York: Harry N. Abrams, Inc., Publishers.

Base, G. (1992). *The sign of the seahorse: A tale of greed and high adventure in two acts.* New York: Harry N. Abrams, Inc., Publishers.

Bayer, J. (1984). *A my name is alice.* New York: Dial Books.

Berenstain, S., & Berenstain, J. (1971). *The Berenstain's B Book.* New York: Random House.

Brown, M.W. (1993). *Four fur feet.* New York: Doubleday.

Carle, E. (1974). *All about arthur (an absolutely absurd ape).* New York: Franklin Watts.

Carter. D. (1990). *More bugs in boxes.* New York: Simon and Schuster.

Cole, J., & Calmenson, S. (1993). *Six sick sheep: 101 Tongue twisters.* New York: Beech Tree.

Collins, B., & Calmenson, S. (1993). *Six sick sheep: 101 tongue twisters.* New York: Morrow, Williams & Co.

De Regniers, B., Moore, E., White, M., & Carr, J. (1988). *Sing a song of popcorn.* New York: Scholastic.

Edwards, P. D. (1996). *Some smug slug.* New York: HarperTrophy.

Edwards, P. D. (1999). *The wacky wedding: A book of alphabet antics.* New York: HarperTrophy.

Geisel, T. S., & Geisel, A. S. (l963). *Dr. Seuss's ABC.* New York: Beginner Books, A division of Random House.

Gordon, J. (1991). *Six sleepy sheep.* New York: Puffin Books.

Hague, K. (1984). *Alphabears.* New York: Henry Holt.

Jonas, A. (1997). *Watch William walk.* New York: Greenwillow.

Lester, A. (1998). *Alice and Aldo.* Boston: Houghton Mifflin.

London, J. (1992). *Froggy gets dressed.* New York: Viking.

Mosel, A. (1968). *Tikki tikki tembo.* New York: Scholastic.

Most, B. (1998). *A trio of triceratops.* San Diego: Harcourt.

Obligado, L. (1983). *Faint frogs feeling feverish and other terrifically tantalizing tongue twisters.* New York: Viking.

Pelham, D., & Formena, M. (1988). *Worms wiggle.* New York: Simon & Schuster.

Wiesner, D. (1992). *June 29, 1999.* New York: Clarion Books: A Division of Houghton Mifflin Company.

BOOKS WITH ASSONANCE (REPETITION OF SIMILAR VOWEL SOUNDS IN STRESSED SYLLABLES)

Clements, A. (1997). *Double trouble in walla walla.* New York: Wm. Morrow & Co. Inc.

Geisel, T. S., & Geisel, A. S. (1960). *Green eggs and ham by Dr. Seuss.* New York: Beginner Books, A division of Random House.

Geisel, T. S., & Geisel, A. S. (1963). *Hop on pop by Dr. Seuss.* New York: Beginner Books, A division of Random House.

Geisel, T. S., & Geisel, A. S. (1965). *Fox in socks by Dr. Seuss.* New York: Beginner Books, A division of Random House.

Geisel, T. S., & Geisel, A. S. (1974). *There's a wocket in my pocket by Dr. Seuss.* New York: Beginner Books, A division of Random House.

Gerstein, M. (1999). *The absolutely awful alphabet.* San Diego: Harcourt.

Most, B. (1996). *Cock-a-doodle-moo!* San Diego: Harcourt Brace.

Serfozo, M. K. (1988). *Who said red?* New York: Macmillan.

Shaw, N. (1986). *Sheep in a jeep.* Boston, MA: Houghton, Mifflin.

Shaw, N. (1989). *Sheep on a ship.* Boston, MA: Houghton, Mifflin.

Strauss, B. & Friedlana, H. (1987). *See you later alligator: A first book of rhyming word-play.* Los Angeles, CA: Price Stern Sloan.

BOOKS WITH FIGURATIVE LANGUAGE AND RIDDLES

Doolittle, J. H. (1991). *Dr. DooRiddles: Associate reasoning activities.* Pacific Grove, CA: Midwest Publications.

Gwynne, F. (1970). *The king who rained.* New York: Scholastic Inc.

Gwynne, F. (1976). *A chocolate moose for dinner.* New York: Scholastic Inc.

Gwynne, F. (1988). *A little pigeontoed.* New York: Scholastic Inc.

Maestro, G. (1989). *Riddle roundup.* New York: Clarion Books.

Most, B. (1991). *Pets in trumpets and other word-play riddles.* San Diego, CA: Harcourt Brace Jovanovich, Publishers.

Weinberg, L. (1993). *Guess a rhyme.* New York: Random House.

BOOKS WITH MANIPULATION AND FINGERPLAYS

Ahlberg, J. & Ahlberg, A. (1986). *The jolly postman or other people's letters.* Boston, Little, Brown.

Ahlberg, J. & Ahlberg, A. (1991). *The jolly Christmas postman.* Boston, MA: Little, Brown.

Ball, S. (1981). *Crocguphant: A flip-flap-book.* Bridgeport, CT: W J Fantasy, Inc.

Ball, S. (1985). *Porguacan: A flip-flap-book.* Bridgeport, CT: W J Fantasy, Inc.

Christelow, E. (1989). *Five little monkeys jumping on the bed.* New York: Scholastic, Inc.

Cole, J. & Calmeson, S. (1991). *The eentsy, weentsy spider: Fingerplays and action rhymes.* New York: William Morrow.

Hart, M. (1987). *Fold-and-cut stories and fingerplays.* Belmont, CA: David S. Lake Publishers.

Hill, E. (1980). *Where's spot?* New York: G. P. Putnam's Sons.

LeSieg, T. (1989). *The pop-up mice of Mr. Brice.* New York: Random House.

Moerbeek, K. (1988). *Who's peeking at me: A pop up book.* Santa Monica, CA: Price Stern Sloan.

Myers, B. (1988). *Mixed up rhymes: A mix-and-match book.* New York: Scholastic.

Pienkowski, J. (1989). *Oh my a fly: Pop and rhyme.* Los Angeles, CA: Price Stern Sloan.

Sanders, G. (1992). *The mix and match book of dinosaurs.* New York: Simon & Schuster.

Scott, L. B. & Thompson, J. J. (1960). *Rhymes for fingers and flannelboards.* St. Louis, MO: Webster Publishing Company.

Van Scoy K., & Whithead, R. (1971). *Literature games.* Belmont, CA: Fearon Publishers.

Wirth, M., Stassevitch, V., Shotwell, R., & Stemmler, P. (1983). *Musical games, fingerplays, and rhythmic activities for early childhood.* West Nyack, NY: Parter Publishing.

BOOKS WITH NO WORDS

Day, A. (1985). *Good dog, Carl.* New York: Green Tiger Press.

Day, A. (1989). *Carl goes shopping.* New York: Green Tiger Press.

Mayer, M. (1967). *A boy, a dog, and a frog.* New York: Dial Books for Young Readers.

Mayer, M. (1969). *Frog, where are you?* New York: Dial Books for Young Readers.

Mayer, M. (1971). *A boy, a dog, a frog, and a friend.* New York: Dial Books for Young Readers.

Mayer, M. (1973). *Frog on his own.* New York: Dial Books for Young Readers.

Mayer, M. (1974). *Frog goes to dinner.* New York: Dial Books for Young Readers.

Mayer, M. (1976). *Hiccup.* New York: Dial Books for Young Readers.

Mayer, M. (1977). *Oops.* New York: Dial Books for Young Readers.

Mayer, M. (1977). *One frog too many.* Penguin Putnam Books for Young Readers.

Turk, H. (1983). *Max the art lover.* Boston, MA: Neugebauer Press.

Turk, H. (1983). *Raking leaves with Max.* Boston, MA: Neugebauer Press.

Turk, H. (1984). *Happy birthday Max.* Boston, MA: Neugebauer Press.

Turk, H. (1984). *Max packs.* Boston, MA: Neugebauer Press.

Turk, H. (1985). *Friendship Max*. Boston, MA: Neugebauer Press.

Turk, H. (1986). *A fright for Max*. Boston, MA: Neugebauer Press.

Wiesner, D. (1991). *Tuesday*. New York: Clarion Books.

BOOKS WITH PATTERNING/REPETITIVE/PREDICTABLE TEXT

Ahlberg, J., & Ahlberg, A. (1980). *Funnybones*. New York: Greenwillow Books.

Banks, K. (1988). *Alphabet soup*. New York: Alfred A. Knopf.

Beaton, C. (1999). *One moose, twenty mice*. New York: Barefoot.

Brett, J. (1985). *Annie and the wild animals*. Boston, MA: Houghton Mifflin.

Brett, J. (1989). *The mitten*. New York: G. P. Putnam's Sons.

Brett, J. (1991). *Berlioz the bear*. New York: G. P. Putnam's Sons.

Carle, E. (1969). *The very hungry caterpillar*. New York: Philomel Books.

Carle, E. (1984). *The very busy spider*. New York: Philomel Books.

Carle, E. (1987). *Have you seen my cat?* New York: Scholastic, Inc.

Carle, E. (1990). *The very quiet cricket*. New York: Philomel Books.

Carle, E. (1994). *Today is monday*. New York: Philomel Books.

Carle, E. (1997). *From head to toe*. New York: Scholastic, Inc.

Carle, E. (1998). *Hello, fox*. New York: Simon & Schuster.

Dragonwagon, C. (1999). *This is the bread i baked for ned*. New York: Aladdin.

Eastman, P. D. (1960). *Are you my mother?* New York: Beginner Books, A division of Random House.

Geisel, T. S., & Geisel, A. S. (1960). *One fish, two fish, red fish, blue fish by Dr. Seuss*. New York: Beginner Books, A division of Random House.

Larranaga, A. M. (1999). *The big wide-mouthed frog*. Cambridge, MA: Candlewick.

Lawson, J. (1997). *Kate's castle*. Toronto, Canada: Stoddart.

Lewison, W. C. (1992). *Buzz said the bee*. New York: Scholastic.

London, J. (1992). *Froggy gets dressed*. New York: Viking.

London, J. (1996). *I see the moon and the moon sees me*. New York: Viking.

Lopshire, R. (1960). *Put me in the zoo*. New York: Beginner Books, A Division of Random House, Inc.

Martin, B. (1967). *Brown bear, brown bear, what do you see?* New York: Henry Holt.

Martin, B. (1991). *Polar bear, polar bear, what do you hear?* New York: Henry Holt.

Martin, J., & Archambault, J. (1988). *Listen to the rain*. New York: Henry Holt.

McClintock, M. (1958). *A fly went by*. New York: Random House.

Mosel. A. (1968). *Tiki tiki tembo*. New York: Scholastic Inc.

Reiser, L. (1998). *Cherry pies and lullabies*. New York: Greenwillow.

Wood, A. (1984). *The napping house*. New York: Harcourt Brace Jovanovich.

Wood, A. (1985). *King bidgood's in the bathtub*. New York: Harcourt Brace Jovanovich.

Wood, A. (1991). *Piggies*. Orlando, FL: Harcourt Brace Jovanovich.

Wood, J. (1992). *Moo moo, brown cow*. San Diego: Gulliver/Harcourt.

Yang, B. (1999). *Chili-chili-chin-chin*. San Diego: Silver Whistle/Harcourt.

Young, J. (1990). *A million chameleons*. Boston, MA: Little, Brown.

BOOKS WITH POEMS AND RHYMES

Adshead, P. S. (1993). *One odd old owl*. New York: Discovery Toys, Inc.

Ahlberg, J., & Ahlberg, A. (1986). *Each peach, pear, and plum*. New York: Puffin Books by Penguin Group.

Beil, K.M. (1998). *A cake all for me!* New York: Holiday House

Berenstain, S., & Berenstain, J. (1968). *The bears' vacation*. New York: Beginner Books, A division of Random House, Inc.

Berenstain, S., & Berenstain, J. (1978). *The spooky old tree*. New York: Beginner Books, A division of Random House, Inc.

Blackstone, S. (1999.) *Bear's busy family*. New York: Barefoot.

Blackstone, S. (1999.) *Bear in a square*. New York: Barefoot.

Brown, M. (1980). *Finger plays*. New York: E. P. Dutton.

Brown, M. (1985). *Hand rhymes*. New York: E. P. Dutton.

Buller, J., & Schade. S. (1988). *I love you, good night*. New York: Simon and Schuster.

Bunting, E. (1999). *Butterfly house*. New York: Scholastic.

Butler, D. (1991). *Higgledy piggledy hobbledy hoy*. New York: Greenwillow Books.

Cameron, P. (1968). *I can't said the ant*. New York: Scholastic.

Carlstrom, N. W. (1998). *It's about time, jesse bear, and other rhymes*. New York: Aladdin.

Cole, J. (1989). *Anna Banana: 101 jump-rope rhymes*. New York: Beech Tree.

Colgin, M. L. (1982). *One potato, two potato, three potato, four: 165 chants for children*. Mt. Ranier, MD: Gryphon House.

Degan, B. (1983). *Jamberry*. New York: Harper & Row.

Deming, A. G. (1994). *Who is tapping at my window?* New York: Penguin.

Emberley, B. (1987). *Drummer hoff*. New York: Simon & Schuster.

Emberley, B. (1992). *One wide river to cross*. Boston: Little, Brown.

Farber, N. (1997). *The boy who longed for a lift*. New York: HarperCollins.

Fox, M. (1998). *Boo to a goose*. New York: Dial.

Galdone, P. (1968). *Henny penny*. New York: Scholastic.

Geisel, T. S., & Geisel, A. S. (1957). *Cat in the hat by Dr. Seuss*. New York: Beginner Books, A division of Random House.

Geisel, T. S., & Geisel, A. S. (1958). *Cat in the hat comes back by Dr. Seuss*. New York: Beginner Books, A division of Random House.

Geisel, T. S., & Geisel, A. S. (1970). *Mr. Brown can moo! can you? by Dr. Seuss*. New York: Beginner Books, A division of Random House.

Geisel, T. S., & Geisel, A.S. (1978). *I can read with my eyes shut! by Dr. Seuss*. New York: Beginner Books, A division of Random House.

Geisel, T. S., & Geisel, A. S. (1989). *The sneetches and other stories by Dr. Seuss.* New York: Beginner Books, A division of Random House.

Goldstone, B. (1998). *The beastly feast.* New York: Holt.

Grossman, B. (1997). *The bear whose bones were jezebel jones.* New York: Dial.

Hawkins, C., & Hawkins, J. (1986). *Tog the dog.* New York: G.P. Putnam's Sons.

Hayles, M. (1998) *Beach play.* New York: Holt.

Hood, T. (1999). *Before I go to sleep.* New York: Morrow.

Hymes, L., & Hymes, J. (1964). *Oodles of noodles.* New York: Young Scott Books.

Jabar, C. (1991). *Bored blue? Think what you can do.* Boston, MA: Little, Brown.

Knowles, S. (1997). *Edwina the emu.* New York: HarperTrophy.

Knowles, S. (1998). *Edward the emu.* New York: HarperTrophy.

Krauss, R. (1985). *I can fly.* New York: Goldon Press.

Lear, E. (1997). *A was once an apple pie.* Cambridge, MA: Candlewick.

Lewison, W. (1992). *Buzz said the bee.* New York: Scholastic.

Marshak, S. (1999). *The absentminded fellow.* New York: Farrer, Straus & Giroux.

Martin, B. (1996). *"Fire! fire!" said mrs. mcguire.* San Diego: Harcourt.

Martin, M. J. (1996). *From anne to zach.* Honesdale, PA: Boyds Mills.

Martin, B., & Archambault, J. (1989). *Chicka chicka boom boom.* New York: Simon & Schuster Books for Young Readers.

Martin, B., & Kellogg, S. (1999). *A beast story.* San Diego: Harcourt.

Marzollo, J. (1989). *The teddy bear book.* New York: Dial.

Mcgrath, B. (1999). *The baseball counting book.* Watertown, MA: Charlesbridge.

Milgrim, D. (1998). *Cows can't fly.* New York: Viking.

Moss, J. (1992). *The Sesame Street book of poetry.* New York: Random House.

Mother Goose nursery rhymes illustrated by Eric Kincaid. (1986). Newmarket, England: Brimax Books.

Murphy, M. (1999). *My puffer train.* Boston: Houghton Miffliln.

Ochs, C. P. (1991). *Moose on the loose.* Minneapolis, MN: Carolrhoda books.

Otto, C. (1991). *Dinosaur chase*. New York: HarperTrophy.

Parry, C. (1991). *Zoomerang-a-boomerang: Poems to make your belly laugh*. New York: Puffin Books.

Pomerantz, C. (1993). *If I had a paka*. New York: Mulberry.

Rosen, M. (1989). *We're going on a bearhunt*. New York: Margaret K. McEderry Books.

Schwart, A. (1992). *And the green grass grew all around: Folk poetry from everyone*. New York: HarperCollins.

Shaw, N. (1989). *Sheep on a ship*. Boston, MA: Houghton Mifflin.

Silverstein, S. (1964). *A giraffe and a half*. New York: HarperCollins.

Slepian, J. & Seidler, A. (1967). *The hungry thing*. New York: Scholastic.

Slepian, J. & Seidler, A. (1990). *The hungry thing returns*. New York: Scholastic.

Smath, J.(1998). *Yum, yum, all done*. New York: Grosset and Dunlap.

Sorting. (1993). Lincolnwood, IL: Publications International.

Teague, M. (1997). *Baby tamer*. New York: Scholastic.

Tell me more Mother Goose nursery rhymes illustrated by Eric Kincaid. (1986). Newmarket, England: Brimax Books.

Vozar, D. (1993). *Hungry wolf! A nursery rap*. New York: Bantam Doubleday Dell Publishing Group.

Weissman, J. (1991). *Rhymes, higglety pigglety pop!* Overland Peak, KS: Miss Jackie Music Co.

Wellington, M. (1997). *Night house bright house*. New York: Dutton.

Westcott, N. B. (1988). *The lady with the alligator purse*. Boston: Little, Brown.

What's different? (1993). Lincolnwood, IL: Publications International, Ltd.

Winthrop, E. (1986). *Shoes*. New York: HarperTrophy.

Young, J. (1990). *A million chameleons*. Boston: Little, Brown.

BOOKS WITH SOUND

Cherdiet, J. (1993). *The magic fish rap.* New York: Scholastic.

Follow that squeak with Mickey Mouse. (1983). New York: Penguin Books.

Korman, J. (1991). *The circus comes to town.* Golden Sound Story: TinyToon Adventures. Racine, WI: Western Publishing Co. (or any other Sight 'N' Sound Books).

Old MacDonald had a farm. (1992). Lincolnwood, IL: Publications International.

MISCELLANEOUS CHILDREN'S BOOKS MENTIONED IN THIS TEXT

Brown, M. (1986). *Arthur's nose.* Boston: Little, Brown.

Gackenbach, D. (1977). *Harry the terrible whatzit.* New York: Clarion Books.

Heilbroner, J. (1962). *This is the house where Jack lives.* New York: Harper & Row.

Keats, E. J. (1986). *The snowy day.* New York: Puffin Books.

McQueen, L. (1987). *Little red hen.* New York: Scholastic, Inc.

Morrissey, D. (1994). *Ship of dreams.* New York: Abrams.

Numeroff, L. J. (1985). *If you give a mouse a cookie.* New York: HarperCollins Books.

Waber, B. (1972). *Ira sleeps over.* Boston: Houghton Mifflin.

APPENDIX E

Sources For
Teaching Materials

Academic Press
Address: 525 B Street, Suite 1900, San Diego, CA 92101-4495
Telephone (619) 699-6403
E-mail: ap@acad.com
Website: *www.academicpress.com/textbooks*

American Guidance Service, Inc.
Address: 4201 Woodland Road, Circle Pines, MN 55104-1796
Telephone: 1-800-328-2560
E-mail: customerserve@agsnet.com
Website: American Guidance Service Inc

Brookes Publishing Co.
Address: P.O. Box 10624, Baltimore, MD 21285-0624
Telephone: 1-800-638-3775
E-mail: custserv@brookespublishing.com
Website: *www.pbrookes.com*

Cognitive Concepts
Address: 990 Grove Street, Evanston, IL 60201
Telephone: 1-888-328-8199
Email: support@earobics.com
Website: *www.cogcon.com*

Davidson & Associates
Address: 4100 W. 190th St., Torrance, CA 90504
Telephone: 1-800-545-7677
E-mail: sales@education.com
Website: *http://www.education.com*

Discovery Toys, Inc.
Address: 6400 Bresa Street, Livermore, CA 94550
P.O. Box 5023 Livermore, CA 94551
Telephone: 1-800-426-4777
E-mail: dt@discoverytoys.net
Website: Discovery Toys

Educators Publishing Service, Inc.
Address: 31 Smith Place Dept. T3., Cambridge, MA 02138-1089
Telephone: 1-800-225-5750
E-mail: epsbooks@epsbooks.com
Website: *www.epsbooks.com*

Janelle Publications, Inc.
Address: P.O. Box 811, 1189 Twombley Rd., DeKalb, IL 60115
Telephone: 1-800-888-8834. FAX: 1-815-756-4799
E-mail: info@janellepublications.com
Website: *www.janellepublications.com/order*

Imaginart
Address: 307 Arizona Street, Bisbee, AZ 85603
Telephone: 1-800-828-1376
E-mail: imaginart@compuserv.com
Website: *www.imaginartonline.com*

Kendall/Hunt Publishing Company
Address: 2460 Kerper Boulevard, P.O. Box 539 Dubuque, IA 52004-0539
Telephone: (563) 589-1000
E-mail: webmaster@kendallhunt.com
Website: *www.kendallhunt.com*

LinguiSystems
Address: 3700 4th Avenue, East Moline, IL 61244
Telephone: 1-800-PRO-IDEA
E-mail: linguisys@aol.com
Website: *http://linguisystems.com*

Prentice-Hall, Inc.
Address: One Lake Street, Upper Saddle River, NJ 07458
Telephone: 1-800-282-0693
Website: *www.prenhall.com*

PRO-ED, Inc.
Address: 8700 Shoal Creek Boulevard, Austin, TX 78757-6897
Telephone: 1-800-897-3202
E-mail: info@proedinc.com
Website: *www.proedinc.com*

Psychological and Educational Publications, Inc.
Address: P.O. Box 520, Hydesville, CA 95547-0520
Telephone: 1-800-523-5775
E-mail: none
Website: none

Remedia Publications
Address: 15887 N. 76th Street #120, Scottsdale, AZ 85258
Telephone: 1-800-826-4740
E-mail: customerservice@rempub.com
Website: *www.rempub.com*

Riverside Publishing
Address: 425 Spring Lake Drive, Itasca, IL 60143-2079
Telephone: 1-800-323-9540
E-mail: rpwebmaster@hmco.com
Website: *www.riversidepublishing.com*

Scholastic Books
Address: P.O. Box 7502, Jefferson City, MO 65102
Telephone: 1-800-325-6149
Website: *www.scholastic.com*

Slosson Education Publications, Inc.
Address: P.O. Box 280, East Aurora, NY 14052-0280
Telephone: 1-888-756-7766
E-mail: slosson.com
Website: *www.slosson.com*

Spencer Learning
Address: 7770 Regents Road, Suite 113 PMB 622, San Diego, CA 92122
Telephone: 1-858-455-9818
E-mail: mail@spencerlearning.com
Website: *www.spencerlearning.com*

Sopris West
Address: 1140 Boston Avenue, Longmont, CO 80501
Telephone: (303) 651-2829
E-mail: webmaster@sopriswest.com
Website: *www.sopriswest.com*

Stoelting Co.
Address: 620 Wheat Lane, Woodlake, IL 60191
Telephone: (630) 860-9700
E-mail: info@stoeltingco.com
Website: *www.stoeltingco.com*

Super Duper Publications
Address: P.O. Box 24997, Greenville, SC 29616
Telephone: 1-800-277-8737
E-mail: custserv@superduperinc.com
Website: *www.superduperinc.com*

Teacher Created Materials, Inc.
Address: 6421 Industry Way, Westminster, CA 92683
Telephone: 1-800-662-4321
E-mail: custserv@teachercreated.com
Website: *www.teachercreated.com*

The Guilford Press
Address: 72 Spring Street, New York, NY 10012
Telephone: 1-800-365-7006
E-mail: webmaster@guilford.com
Website: *info@guilford.com*

The Learning Company, Inc.
Address: One Athenaem Street, Cambridge, MA 02142
Telephone: (617) 761-3000
E-mail: webmaster@learningco.com
Website: *www.learningco.com*

The Psychological Corporation
Address: P.O. Box 708906, San Antonio, TX 78270
Telephone: 800-872-1726
E-mail: customer_care@harcourt.com
Website: *www.PsychCorp.com*

The Speech Bin
Address: 1965 Twenty-Fifth Avenue, Vero Beach, FL 32960
Telephone: 1-800-4-SPEECH
E-mail: info@speechbin.com
Website: *www.speechbin.com*

Thinking Publications
Address: 425 Galloway Street, P.O. Box 163, Eau Claire, WI 54702-0163
Telephone: 1-800-225-4769
E-mail: custserv@ThinkingPublicatins.com
Website: *wwwThinkingPublications.com*

Thomson Delmar Learning
Address: 5 Maxwell Dr., Clifton Park, NY 12065-2919
Telephone: 1-800-355-9983
E-mail: custom@swpco.com
Website: *http://www.delmarhealthcare.com*

Western Psychological Services
Address: 12031 Wilshire Blvd., Los Angeles, CA 90025-1251
Telephone: 1-800-648-8857
E-mail: custsvc@wpspublish.com
Website: *www.wpspublish.com*

References

Aaron, P. G. (1989). *Dyslexia and hyperlexia: Diagnosis and management of developmental reading disabilities.* Norwell, MA: Kluwer Academic Publishers.

Aaron, P. G., & Joshi, R. M. (1992). *Reading problems: Consultation and remediation.* New York: The Guilford Press.

Adams, M. J. (1990). *Beginning to read: Thinking and learning about print.* Cambridge, MA: The MIT Press.

Adams, M. J., Foorman, B. R., Lundberg, I., & Beeler, T. (1998). The elusive phoneme: Why phonemic awareness is so important and how to help children develop it. *American Educator, 22,* 18-22.

Alegria, J., Pignot, E., & Morais, J. (1982). Phonetic analysis of speech and memory codes in beginning readers. *Memory and Cognition, 10,* 451-456.

American Hyperlexia Association. *http://www.hyperlexia.org/aha*

Aram, D. (1997), Hyerlexia: Reading without meaning in young children. *Topics in Language Disorders, 17,* 1-13.

ASHA Guidelines (2001): *Roles and responsibilities of speech-language pathologists with respect to reading and writing in children and adolescents.* Washington, DC: American Speech-Language-Hearing Association.

Ball, E.W. (1993). Assessing phoneme awareness. *Language, Speech, and Hearing Services in the Schools, 24,* 130-139.

Ball E. (1997). Phonological awareness: Implications for whole langage and emergent literacy programs. *Topics in Language Disorders 17,* 14-26.

Ball, E. W., & Blachman, B.A. (1988). Phoneme segmentation training: Effect on reading readiness. *Annals of Dyslexia, 38,* 208-225.

Ball, E. W., & Blachman, B. A. (1991). Does phoneme awareness training in kindergarten make a difference in early word recognition and developmental spelling? *Reading Research Quarterly, 26,* 49-66.

Barrett, M., Huisingh, R., Zachman, L., Blagden, C., & Orman, J. (1992). *The Listening Test.* East Moline, IL: LinguiSystems.

Bashir, A. S., & Scavuzzo, A. (1992). Children with language disorders: Natural history and academic success. *Journal of Learning Disabilities, 25,* 53-65.

Baumann, J. F., Jones, L. A., & Seifert-Kessell, N. (1993). Using think alouds to enhance children's comprehension monitoring abilities. *The Reading Teacher, 47,* 184-193.

Bear, D. R. Invernizzi, M., Templeton, S. & Johnston, F. (1996). *Words their way: Word study for phonics, vocabulary, and spelling.* Columbus, OH: Prentice Hall.

Bebko, R. R., Alexander, J., & Doucet, R. (2001). *Language! roots* (2nd ed.). Longmont, CO: Sopris West.

Bedi, G. C. (1994). *Low–level visual and auditory processing in dyslexic readers.* Unpublished doctoral dissertation, City University of New York.

Begley, S. (1994). Why Johnny and Joanie can't read. *Newsweek.* New York: Newsweek Inc.

Bellis, T. J. (2001). *Assessment and management of auditory processing disorders.* Presented at California Speech-Language-Hearing Association Annual State Conference. Monterey, CA.

Benson, D. F. (1994). *The neurology of thinking.* New York: Oxford University Press, Inc.

Benton, A. L. (1973). The measurement of aphasic disorders. In A. C. Velasquez (Ed.), *Aspectos pathalogicos del language.* Lima, Peru: CentroNeuropsychologico.

Berthoud-Papandropoulou, I. (1978). An experimental study of children's ideas about language. In A. Sinclair, R. J. Jarvella, & W. J. M. Levelt (Eds.), *The child's conception of language* (pp. 55-64). Berlin: Springer Verlag.

Bird, J., Bishop, D. V. M., & Freeman, N. H. (1995). Phonological awareness and literacy development in children with expressive phonological impairments. *Journal of Speech and Hearing Research, 38* , 446-462.

Bishop, D. V. M. (1983). *Test for the Reception of Grammar.* Manchester, England: University of Manchester.

Bishop, D. V. M. (1997). *Uncommon understanding: Development and disorders of language comprehension in children.* Psychology Press Limited: United Kingdom.

Bishop, D. V. M., & Edmundson, A. (1987). Language–impaired 4-year olds: Distinguishing transient from persistent impairment. *Journal of Speech and Hearing Disorders, 52,* 156-173.

Blachman, B. A. (1991). Early intervention for children's reading problems: Clinical applications of the research in phonological awareness. *Topics in Language Disorders, 12,* 51-65.

Blachman, B. A. (1994a). Early literacy acquisition: The role of phonological awareness. In G. P. Wallach & K. G. Butler (Eds.), *Language learning disabilities in school-age children and adolescents: Some principles and applications* (pp. 253-274). New York: Macmillan.

Blachman, B. A. (1994b). What have we learned from longitudinal studies of phonological processing and reading and some unanswered questions: A response to Torgesen, Wagner, and Rashotte. *Journal of Learning Disabilities 27,* 287-291.

Blake-Davies, K. (1994). *Training of phonological awareness skills by a speech-language specialist to improve the emergent reader's decoding skills.* Unpublished master's thesis, California State University, Sacramento.

Blockcolsky, V. D., Frazer, J. M., & Frazer, D. H. (1987). *40,000 selected words: Organized by letter sound and syllable*. Tucson, AZ: Communication Skill Builders.

Bos, C. S., & Vaughn, S. (1988) *Strategies for teaching students with learning and behavior problems*. Boston, MA: Allyn & Bacon.

Boudera, D. M., & Hedberg, N. L. (1999). A comparison of early literacy skills in children with specific language impairment and their typically developing peers. *American Journal of Speech-Language Pathology, 8*, 249-260.

Bowers, P. G., & Wolf, M. (1993). Theoretical links between naming speed, precise timing mechanisms and orthographic skill in dyslexia. *Reading and Writing: An Interdisciplinary Journal, 5*, 69-85.

Bowey, J. A., & Tunmer, W. E. (1984). Word awareness in children. In W. E. Tunmer, C. Pratt, & M. L. Herriman (Eds.), *Metalinguistic awareness in children: Theory, research, and implications* (pp. 73-91). New York: Springer-Verlag.

Bradley, L., & Bryant, P. (1983). Categorizing sounds and learning to read: A causal connection. *Nature, 30*, 419-421.

Bradley, L., & Bryant, P. (1985). *Rhyme and reason in reading and spelling*. Ann Arbor: University of Michigan Press.

Brady, S. A. (1991). The role of working memory in reading disability. In S. A. Brady, & D. P. Shankweiler (Eds.), *Phonological processes in literacy: A tribute to Isabelle Y. Liberman* (pp. 129-152). Hillsdale, NJ: Lawrence Erlbaum.

Brady, S. A. (1997). Ability to encode phonological representations. In B. Blachman (Ed.), *Foundations of reading acquisition and dyslexia: Implications for early intervention* (pp. 21-47). Hillsdale, NJ: Lawrence Erlbaum.

Bransford, J. D., Delclos, V., Bristow, P. S. (1985). Are poor readers passive readers? Some evidence, possible explanations, and potential solutions. *The Reading Teacher, 39*, 318-325.

Brody, S. (1991). *Brody reading materials*. Milford, NH: Brody Books.

Brown, L., Sherbenou, R. J., & Johnsen, S. K. (1992). *Test of Nonverbal Intelligence—2*. Austin, TX: Pro-Ed.

Brown, V. L., Hammill, D. D., & Wiederholt, J. L. (1994). *Test of Reading Comprehension—3*. San Antonio, TX: The Psychological Corporation.

Butler, K. G. (1999). Foreword. *Topics in Language Disorders, 20*, iv-v.

Butler, K. G. (1999). From oracy to literacy: Changing clinical perceptions. *Topics in Language Disorder, 20*, 14-32.

Butler, K. G. (2000). From the editor. *Topics in Language Disorders, 21*, iv-v.

California Department of Education. (1994). *I can learn: A handbook for parents, teachers, and students*. Sacramento: CA: California Department of Education.

Casby, M. (1988). Speech-language pathologists' attitudes and involvement regarding language and reading. *Language, Speech, and Hearing Services in Schools, 19*, 352-361.

Catts, H. W. (1989). Speech production deficits in developmental dyslexia. *Journal of Speech and Hearing Disorders, 54*, 422-428.

Catts, H. W. (1991a). *Early identification and remediation of reading disabilities.* Short course presented at the annual convention of the American Speech-Language-Hearing Association, Atlanta, GA.

Catts, H. W. (1991b). Facilitating phonological awareness: Role of speech-language pathologists. *Language, Speech, and Hearing Services in Schools, 22,* 196-203.

Catts, H. W. (1993). The relationship between speech-language impairments and reading disabilities. *Journal of Speech and Hearing Research, 36,* 948-958.

Catts, H. W., Fey, M. C., Zhang, X., & Tomblin, J. B. (2001). Estimating the risk of future reading difficulties in kindergarten children: A research–based model and its clinical implementation. *Language, Speech, and Hearing Services in Schools, 32,* 38-50.

Catts, H. W. & Kamhi, A. G. (1999). Causes of reading disabilities. In H. W. Catts & A. G. Kamhi (Eds.), *Language and reading disabilities* (pp. 95-127). Needham Heights, MA: Allyn & Bacon.

Catts, H. W. & Kamhi, A. G. (2000). *Language and reading.* Needham Heights, MA: Allyn & Bacon.

Cecil, N. L. (1990). Child's play: An important precursor to literacy. In N. L. Cecil (Ed.), *Literacy in the '90s* (pp. 23-27). Dubuque, IA: Kendall/Hunt Publishing Company.

Chall, J. S. (1983). *Stages of reading development.* New York: McGraw-Hill.

Cheek, E. H., Flippo, R. F., & Lindsey, J. D. (1997). *Reading for success in elementary schools.* Chicago: Brown & Benchmark.

Cherdiet, J. (1993). *The magic fish rap.* New York: Scholastic Inc.

Clark–Klein, S. M. (1994). Expressive phonological deficiencies: Impact on spelling development. *Topics in Language Disorders, 14,* 40-55.

Clay, M. M. (1984). *Reading: The patterning of complex behavior* (2nd ed). Auckland, New Zealand: Heinemann Educational Books.

Clay, M. M. (1991). Introducing a new storybook to young readers. *The Reading Teacher, 45,* 264-273.

Coles, G. (1987). *The learning mystique.* New York: Pantheon Books.

Coltheart, M. (1986). Graphemics and visual word recognition. In G. Augst (Ed.), *New trends in graphemics and orthography.* Berlin: deGruyter.

Conner, T. N. & Coover, A (2001). Self–reported competencies: Survey of speech-language pathologists in a public school setting. *Advance for Speech-Language Pathologists & Audiologists.* Merion Publications, Inc.: King of Prussia, PA.

Cruickshank, W. M. (1986). Foreword. In G. T. Pavlidis & D. F. Fisher (Eds.), *Dyslexia: Its neuropsychology and treatment* (pp. xiii-xvi). New York: John Wiley.

Culatta, B., Page, J., & Ellis, J. (1983). Story retelling as a communicative performance screening tool. *Language, Speech, and Hearing Services in Schools, 14,* 66-74

Cunningham, P. M. & Cunningham, J. W. (1992). Making words: Enhancing the invented spelling-decoding connection. *The Reading Teacher, 46,* 106-115.

Cunningham, A. E., & Stanovich, K. E. (1997). Early reading acquisition and its relation to reading experience and ability ten years later. *Developmental Psychology, 33,* 934-945.

Cushen–White, N. (2000). The slingerland multisensory structured language approach. *The International Dyslexia Association Northern California Branch Winter Newsletter, 4-6.*

Damico, J. S. (1988). The lack of efficacy in language therapy: A case study. *Language, Speech, and Hearing Services in Schools, 19,* 51-66.

DeFries, J. C., Olson, R. K., Pennington, B. F., & Smith, S. D. (1991). Colorado reading project: An update. In D. D. Duane & D. B. Gray (Eds.), *The reading brain: The biological basis of dyslexia* (pp. 53-88). Parkton, MD: York Press.

DeGoes, C., & Martiew, M. (1983). Young children's approach to literacy. In M. Martlew (Ed.), *The psychology of written language-developmental and educational perspectives.* Chichester: John Wiley.

DeKerckhove, D. & Lumsden, C. (1987) (Eds.). *The alphabet and the brain.* New York: Springer-Verlag.

Denckla, M. B. (1987). Quoted in *Update,* Preview Issue. Chevy Chase, MD: National Institute of Dyslexia.

Denckla, M. B. (1993). A neurologist's overview of developmental dyslexia. In P. Tallal, A. M. Galaburda, R. R. Llinas, & C von Euler (Eds.), *Annals of the New York Academy of Sciences, Vol. 682. Temporal information processing in the nervous system: Special reference to dyslexia and dysphasia* (pp. 23-26). New York: The New York Academy of Sciences.

Denckla, M. B. & Rudel, R. G. (1976). Rapid automatised naming: Dyslexia differentiated from other learning disabilities. *Neuropsychologia, 14,* 471-479.

Dickinson, D. & McCabe, A. (1991). The acquisition and development of language: A social interactionist account of language and literacy development. In J. F. Kavanagh (Ed.), *The language continuum: From infancy to literacy* (pp. 1-40). Parkton, MD: York Press.

Donahue, M. (1986). Linguistic and communicative development in learning disabled children. In S. Ceci (Ed.), *Handbook of cognitive, social, and neuropsychological aspects of learning disabilities* (pp. 263-289). Hillsdale, NJ: Lawrence Erlbaum Associates.

Donnelly, K., Thomsen, S., Huber, L., & Shoemer, D. (1992). *More than words: Activities for phonological awareness and comprehension.* Tucson, AZ: Communication Skill Builders.

Dunn, L. M. & Markwardt, F. C. (1970). *Peabody Individual Achievement Test.* Circle Pines, MN: American Guidance Service, Inc.

Ehern, B. J. (1994). New directions for meeting the academic needs of adolescents with language learning disabilities. In G. P. Wallach & K. G. Butler (Eds.), *Language learning disabilities in school-age children and adolescents: Some principles and applications* (pp. 393-417). New York: Macmillan.

Ehern, B. J. (1999). *Using curriculum standards to define language therapy and SLP roles in literacy.* ASHA Convention, San Francisco, CA.

Ehri, L. C. (1992). Review and commentary: Stages of spelling development. In S. Templeton & D. R. Bear (Eds.), *Development of orthographic knowledge and the foundations of literacy: A memorial festschrift for Edmund H. Henderson* (pp. 307-332). Hillsdale, NJ: Lawrence Erlbaum.

Elkonin, D.B. (1973). U.S.S.R. In J. Downing (Ed.), *Comparative reading* (pp. 551-579). New York: Macmillan.

Ellis, W. (1997). Phonological awareness. *NICHCY News Digest, 25,* 13-15.

Evans, J. E. (1983). *An uncommon gift.* Philadelphia, PA: The Westminster Press.

Evers, A., Gilligan, S., & Wernig, M. (1994). *Demystifying personal mysteries: Helping children understand their learning disabilities.* Presented at the annual conference of the National Orton Dyslexia Society. Los Angeles, CA.

Farnham-Diggory, S. (1990). Foreword. In R. B. Spalding & W. T. Spalding (Eds.), *The writing road to reading* (pp. 1-12). New York: Quill William Morrow.

Fischer, K. M., & Hansen, M. P. (1989). *Plays for reading aloud: The Book of Three.* New York: Walker & Company.

Fletcher, S. G. (1972). Time-by-count test of diadochokinetic syllable rate. *Journal of Speech and Hearing Research, 15,* 763-770.

Fletcher, J. M., Morris, R., Lyon, G. R., Stuebing, K. K., Shaywitz, S. E., Shankweiler, D. P., Katz, L., & Shaywitz, B. A. (1997). Subtypes of dyslexia: An old problem revisited. In B. A. Blachman (Ed.), *Foundations of reading acquisition and dyslexia: Implications for early intervention* (pp. 95-114). Hillsdale, NJ: Lawrence Erlbaum Associates.

Foorman, B. R., Francis, D. J., & Fletcher, J. M. (1997). NICHD early interventions project. *Perspectives, 23,* 2-5.

Fowler, A. (1991). How early phonological development might set the stage for phoneme awareness. In S. Brady & D. Shankweiler (Eds.), *Phonological processes in literacy: A tribute to Isabelle Y. Liberman* (pp. 97-117). Hillsdale, NJ: Lawrence Erlbaum Associates.

Fox, B. & Routh, D. K. (1984). Phonemic analysis and synthesis as word attack skills: Revisited. *Journal of Educational Psychology, 76,* 1059-1061.

Freil-Patti, S. (1994). Auditory linguistic processing and language learning. In G. P. Wallach & K. G. Butler (Eds.), *Language learning disabilities in school-age children and adolescents: Some principles and applications* (pp. 373-392). New York: Macmillan.

Frith, U. (1985). Beneath the surface of developmental dyslexia. In K. Patterson, J. Marshall, & M. Coltheart (Eds.), *Surface dyslexia* (pp. 301-330). London: Lawrence Erlbaum.

Frith, U. (1986). A developmental framework for developmental dyslexia. *Annals of Dyslexia, 36,* 69-81.

Galaburda, A. M. (1991). Anatomy of dyslexia: Argument against phrenology. In D. D. Duane, & D. B. Gray, (Eds.), *The reading brain: The biological basis of dyslexia* (pp. 119-131). Parkton, MD: York Press.

Galaburda, A. M. & Livingstone, M. (1993). Evidence for a magnocellular defect in developmental dyslexia. In P. Tallal, A. M. Galaburda, R. R. Llinas, & C. von Euler (Eds.), *Annals of the New York Academy of Sciences, Vol. 682. Temporal information processing in the nervous system: Special reference to dyslexia and dysphasia* (pp. 70-82). New York: The New York Academy of Sciences.

Galaburda, A. M., Menard, M. T., & Rosen, G. D. (1994). Evidence for aberrant auditory anatomy in developmental dyslexia. *Proceedings of the National Academy of Sciences, 91*, 8010-8013.

Gardner, M. F. (1990). *Expressive One-Word Picture Vocabulary Test—Revised.* Austin, TX: Pro-Ed.

Gardner, M .F. (1991). *Receptive One-Word Picture Vocabulary Test—Revised.* Austin, TX: Pro-Ed.

Gardner, M. F., & Brownell, R. (1983). *Expressive One-Word Picture Vocabulary Test: Upper Extension.* Austin, TX: Pro-Ed.

Gardner, M. F., & Brownell, R. (1987). *Receptive One-Word Picture Vocabulary Test: Upper Extension.* Austin, TX: Pro-Ed.

Gebers, J. (1995). *Books are for talking too: A sourcebook for using children's literature in speech-language remediation.* Tucson, AZ: Communication Skill Builders.

Geisel, T. S. *Green eggs and ham by Dr. Seuss* (1960). New York: Random House

Gerber, A. (1993). Cognition and information processing. In A. Gerber (Ed.), *Language-related learning disabilities: Their nature and treatment* (pp. 63-104). Baltimore, MD: Paul H. Brookes.

German, D. J. (1990). *Test of adolescent/adult word finding.* Chicago, IL: Riverside Publishing Company.

German, D. J. (1991). *Test of Word Finding in Discourse.* Allen, TX: DLM Teaching Resources.

German, D. J. (2000). *Test of Word Finding—2.* Austin, TX: Pro-Ed.

German, D. J. (2001a). *Child word finding: Bridging assessment and intervention.* Paper presented at the California Speech-Language-Hearing Annual State Conference, Monterey, CA.

German, D. J. (2001b). *It's on the tip of my tongue: Word–finding strategies to remember names and words you often forget.* Chicago: Word Finding Materials, Inc.

Gillon, G. T. (2000). The efficacy of phonological awareness intervention for children with spoken language impairment. *Language, Speech, and Hearing Services in Schools, 31*, 126-141.

Goldman, R., & Fristoe, M. (1986). *Goldman-Fristoe Test of Articulation.* Circle Pines, MN: American Guidance Service.

Goldman, R., Fristoe, M., & Woodcock, R. W. (1974). *Goldman-Fristoe-Woodcock Auditory Skills Test Battery.* Circle Pines, MN: American Guidance Service.

Goldman, R., Fristoe, M., & Woodcock, R. W. (1990). *Goldman-Fristoe-Woodcock Test of Auditory Discrimination.* Austin, TX: Pro-Ed.

Goldsworthy, C. (1996). *Developmental reading disabilities: A language based treatment approach.* San Diego: Singular Publishing, Inc.

Goldsworthy, C. (1998). *Sourcebook of phonological awareness training: Children's classic literature.* San Diego: Singular Publishing, Inc.

Goldsworthy, C. (2001). *Sourcebook of phonological awareness training: Children's core literature.* San Diego: Singular Publishing, Inc.

Goldsworthy, C., & Pieretti, R. (2003). *Sourcebook of phonological awareness training: Children's core literature: Grades 3–5.* Clifton Park: Delmar Thomson Learning.

Gombert, J. E. (1992). *Metalinguistic development.* London: Harvester-Wheatsheaf.

Goswami, U. & Mead, F. (1992). Onset and rime awareness and analogies in reading. *Reading Research Quarterly, 27,* 153-162.

Gough, P. B., & Juel, C. (1991). The first stages of word recognition. In L. Rieben & C. A. Perfetti (Eds), *Learning to read: Basic research and its implications* (pp. 47-56). Hillsdale, NJ: Lawrence Erlbaum.

Gough, P. P. & Tunmer, W. (1986). Decoding, reading, and reading disability. *Remedial and Special Education, 7,* 6-10.

Greene, J. (1993). Systematic phonology: The critical element in teaching reading and language to dyslexics. In S. F. Wright, & R. Groner (Eds.), *Facets of dyslexia and its remediation, Vol. 3* (pp. 541-549). Amsterdam: North-Holland Elsevier.

Greene, J. F. & Woods, J. F. (2000). *J & J language readers.* Longmont, Co: Sopris West.

Greene, V. E., & Enfield, M. L. (1991). *Project read.* Bloomington, MN: Language Circle Enterprise.

Griffith, P. L. & Olson, M. W. (1992). Phonemic awareness helps beginning readers break the code. *The Reading Teacher, 45,* 516-523.

Grossen, B. (1997). *A synthesis of research on reading from the National Institute of Child Health and Human Development.* http://www.nrrf.org/synthesis_research.htm

Haasbrouck, J., and Tindal, G. (1992). Curriculum-based oral reading fluency norms for students in grades 2 through 5. *Teaching Exceptional Children:* 41-44.

Harbers, H.M., Paden, E.P., & Halle, J.W. (1999). Phonological awareness and production: Changes during intervention. *Language, Speech, and Hearing Services in Schools, 30,* 50-60.

Hatcher, P. J. (1994). *Sound linkage: An integrated programme for overcoming reading difficulties.* London, England: Whurr.

Healy, J. M. (1990). *Endangered minds: Why children don't think and what we can do about it.* New York: Simon & Schuster.

Healy, J. M. (1998). *Failure to connect: How computers affect our children's minds—for better and worse.* New York: Simon & Schuster.

Healy, J. M. & Aram, D. (1986). Hyperlexia and dyslexia: A family study. *Annals of Dyslexia, 36,* 237-252.

Helm-Estabrooks, N., Nicholas, M., & Morgan, A. (1989). *Melodic Intonation Therapy program.* San Antonio, TX: Special Press.

Helm-Estabrooks, N., & Albert, M. L. (1991). *Manual of aphasia therapy.* Austin, TX: Pro-Ed.

Henderson, E. H. (1992). The interface of lexical competence and knowledge of written words. In S. Templeton & D. R. Bear (Eds.), *Development of orthographic knowledge and the foundations of literacy: A memorial festschrift for Edmund H. Henderson* (pp. 1-30). Hillsdale, NJ: Lawrence Erlbaum Associates.

Henk, W. A., Helfeldt, J. P. & Platt, J. M. (1986). Developing reading fluency in learning disabled students. *Teaching Exceptional Children, 18,* 202-206.

Henry, M. K. & Redding, N. C. (1990). *Tutor.* Los Gatos, CA: LexPess.

Hinshelwood, J. (1917). *Congenital word-blindness.* London: Lewis.

Hodson, B. W. (1986). *The Assessment of Phonological Processes—Revised.* Austin, TX: Pro-Ed.

Hodson, B., & Edwards, M. (1997). Appendix A: Glossary in *Educational perspectives in applied phonology* (pp. 225-232). Gaithersburg, MD: Aspen Publishers, Inc.

Hodson, B. W., & Paden, E. (1991). *Targeting intelligible speech: A phonological approach to remediation,* (2nd ed.). Austin, TX: Pro-ED.

Hoffman, P. R. (1990). Spelling, phonology, and the speech-language pathologist: A whole language perspective. *Language, Speech, and Hearing Services in Schools, 21,* 238-243.

Hook, P. E. & Jones, S. D. (2002). The importance of automaticity and fluency for efficient reading comprehension. *http://www.resourceroom.net/Sharestrats/2002automaticity.asp* Also Appeared in *Perspectives, (2002), 28,* (1), 9–14.

Hooper, S. R. & Willis, W. G. (1989). *Learning disability subtyping: Neuropsychological foundations, conceptual models and issues in clinical differentiation.* New York: Springer-Verlag.

Hulquist, A. M. (1997). Orthographic processing abilities of adolescents with dyslexia. *Annals of Dyslexia, 47,* 89-116.

Hutson-Nechkash, P. (2001) *Narrative toolbox: Blueprints for storybuilding.* EauClaire, WI: Thinking Publications.

International Dyslexia Association: General information about dyslexia (2000).
http://www.ldonline.org/ld_indepth/reading-4.html
http://www.ldonline.com/ld_indepth/process_deficit/capd_paton.html

Javins, J. (1993). Personal communication.

Jenkins, R., & Bowen, L. (1994). Facilitating development of preliterate children's phonological abilities. *Topics in Language Disorders, 14,* 26-39.

Jenkins, R., Heliotis, J. D., Stein, M. L., & Haynes, M. C. (1987). Improving reading comprehension by using paragraph restatements. *Exceptional Children, 54,* 54-59.

Kameenui, E. J., & Simmons, D. C. (1990). *Designing instructional strategies: The prevention of academic learning problems.* Columbus, OH: Merrill.

Kamhi, A. G. & Catts, H. W. (1989). Language and reading: Convergences, divergences, and development. In A. G. Kamhi & H. W. Catts (Eds.), *Reading disabilities: A developmental language perspective* (pp. 1-34). Needham Heights, MA: Little, Brown.

Kamhi, A. G., & Catts, H. W. (1999). Language and reading: Convergences and divergences. In H. W. Catts & A. G. Kamhi (Eds.), *Language and reading disabilities* (pp. 1-24). Needham Heights, MA: Allyn & Bacon.

Kamhi, A. G., Catts, H. W., & Mauer, D. (1990). Explaining speech production deficits in poor readers. *Journal of Learning Disabilities, 23*, 632-636.

Kamhi, A. G., & Hinton, L. N. (2000). Learning to read and learning to spell: Two sides of a coin. *Topics in Language Disorders, 20*, 37-49

Kaplan, E., Goodglass, H., & Weintraub, S. (1983). *The Boston Naming Test.* Philadelphia: Lea & Febiger.

Katz, J., Stecker, N. and Henderson, D. (1992). *Central auditory processing: A transdisciplinary view.* St. Louis, MO: Mosby.

Kavanagh, J. F. (1991). Preface. In J. F. Kavanagh (Ed.), *The language continuum: From infancy to literacy* (pp. vii-ix). Parkton, MD: York Press.

Kavanagh, J. F., & Truss, T. (1988). *Learning disabilities: Proceedings of the National Conference.* Parkton, MD: York Press

Keller, W. D. (1992). Auditory processing disorder or attention-deficit disorder? In J. Katz, N. A. Stecker, & D. Henderson (Eds.), *Central auditory processing: A transdisciplinary view* (pp. 107-114). St. Louis, MO: Mosby–Year Book.

Kendall, J. S., & Marzano, R. J. (1994). *The systematic identification and articulation of content standards and benchmarks.* Aurora, CO: McREL.

Kent, R. D. (1990). The fragmentation of clinical service and clinical science in communicative disorders. *National Student Speech Language Hearing Association Journal, 17*, 4-16.

Kent, R. D. (1992). Phonological development as biology and behavior. In R. S. Chapman (Ed.), *Processes in language acquisition and disorders* (pp. 67-85). St. Louis, MO: Mosby-Year Book.

Klein, J. O. (1986). Risk factors for otitis media in children. In J. F. Kavanagh (Ed.), *Otitis media and child development* (pp. 45-51). Parkton, MD: York Press.

Koppenhaver, D. A., Coleman, P. P., Kalman, S. L., & Yoder, D. E. (1991). The implications of emergent literacy research for children with developmental disabilities. *American Journal of Speech-Language Pathology, 1*, 38-44.

Kuhl, P. K. (1988). Auditory perception and the evaluation of speech. *Human Evolution, 3*, 19-43.

Lance, D. M., Swanson, L. A., & Peterson, H. A. (1997). A validity study of an implicit phonological awareness paradigm. *Journal of Speech, Language, and Hearing Research, 40*, 1002-1010.

Larsen, S. C. & Hammill, D. D. (1994). *Test of Written Spelling—3.* Austin, TX: Pro-Ed.

Lavoi, R. (2001). *Batteries not included.* Presentation for Northern California Dyslexia Association. San Francisco, CA.

Lee, C. M. & Jackson, R. F. (1992). *Faking it: A look into the mind of a creative learner.* Portsmouth, NH: Boynton/Cook.

Levelt, W. J. M. (1989). *Speaking, from intention to articulation.* Cambridge, MA: MIT Press.

Leverett, R. G. & Diefendorf, A. O. (1992). Students with language deficiencies: Suggestions for frustrated teachers. *Teaching Exceptional Children,* 24, 30-35.

Levine, M. D. (1993). *All kinds of minds: A young student's book about learning abilities and learning disorders.* Cambridge, MA: Educators Publishing Service.

Lewis, B. A., Freebairn, L. A., & Taylor, H. G. (2000). Follow-up of children with early expressive phonology disorders. *Journal of Learning Disabilities, 33,* 433-444.

Liberman A. M. (1997). How theories of speech affect research in reading and writing. In B. A. Blachman (Ed.) *Foundations of reading acquisition and dyslexia: Implications for early intervention* (pp. 320). Hillsdale, NJ: Lawrence Erlbaum Associates.

Liberman, I. Y. (1983). A language-oriented view of reading and its disabilities. In H. R. Myklebust (Ed.), *Progress in learning disabilities* (5, 81-101). New York: Grune & Stratton.

Liberman, I. Y., Liberman, A. M., Mattingly, I. G., & Shankweiler, D. (1980). Orthography and the beginning reader. In J. F. Kavanagh & R. Venezky (Eds.), *Orthography, reading, and dyslexia* (pp. 137-153). Baltimore, MD: University Park Press.

Liberman, I. Y., Rubin, H., Duques, S. & Carlisle, J. (1985). Linguistic abilities and spelling proficiency in kindergartners and adult poor readers. In D. B. Gray & J. F. Kavanagh (Eds.), *Biobehavioral measures of dyslexia* (pp. 163-176). Parkton, MD: York Press.

Liberman, I. Y., & Shankweiler, D. (1991). Phonology and beginning reading: A tutorial. In L. Rieben & C. A. Perfetti (Eds.), *Learning to read: Basic research and its implications* (pp. 3-17). Hillsdale, NJ: Lawrence Erlbaum Associates.

Liberman, I. Y., Shankweiler, D., Fischer, F. W., & Carter, B. (1974). Explicit syllable and phoneme segmentation in the young child. *Journal of Experimental Child Psychology, 18,* 201-212.

Llinas, R. R. (1993). Is dyslexia a dyschronia? In P. Tallal, A. M. Galaburda, R. R. Lllinas, & C. von Euler (Eds.), *Annals of the New York Academy of Sciences Vol. 682 Temporal information processing in the nervous system: Special reference to dyslexia and dysphasia* (pp. 48-56). New York: The New York Academy of Sciences.

Locke, J. L. (1993). *The child's path to spoken language.* Cambridge, MA: Harvard University Press.

Locke, J. L. (1997). A theory of neurolinguistic development. *Brain and Language, 58,* 265-326.

Logan, R. K. (1986). *The alphabet effect.* New York: St. Martin's Press.

Lombardino, L., Bedford, T., Fortier, C., Carter, J., & Brandi, J. (1997). Invented spelling: Developmental patterns in kindergarten children and guidelines for early literacy intervention. *Language, Speech, and Hearing Services in Schools, 28,* 333-343.

Lubs, H., Duara, R., Levin, B., Jallad, B., Lubs, M. L., Rabin, M., Kushch, A, & Gross-Glenn, K. (1991). Dyslexia subtypes: Genetics, behavior, and brain imaging. In D. D. Duane & D. B. Gray, (Eds.), *The reading brain: The biological basis of dyslexia* (pp. 89-118). Parkton, MD: York Press.

Lucker, J. R., and Wood, D. (2000). Auditory processing disorders. *http://www.ncapd.org/APD%20.../decoding_problems.htm*

Lundberg, I. (1988). Preschool prevention of reading failure: Does training in phonological awareness work? In R. L. Masland & M. W. Masland (Eds.), *Preschool prevention of reading failure* (pp. 163-176). Parkton, MD: York Press.

Lyon, G. R. (1995a). *Dyslexia and its relation to disorders of attention: Recent NIH/NICHD findings.* Paper presented at the annual convention of the California Speech-Language-Hearing Association. San Diego, CA.

Lyon, G. R. (1995b). Toward a definition of dyslexia. *Annals of Dyslexia, 4,* 3-27. National Center for Learning Disabilities.

Lyon, G. R. (1997). "SLPS play key role," Seymour tells NIH conference on ld. *ASHA Leader, 2,* 1-5.

Magnusson, E., & Naucler, K. (1990). Reading and spelling in language-disordered children—linguistic and metalinguistic prerequisites: Report on a longitudinal study. *Clinical Linguistics and Phonetics, 4,* 49-61.

Manis, F. R., Szeszulski, P. A., Holt, L. K., & Graves, K. (1990). Variation in component word recognition and spelling skills among dyslexic children and normal readers. In T. H. Carr & B. A. Levy (Eds.), *Reading and its development: Component skills approaches* (pp. 207-259). New York: Academic Press.

Maria, K. (1990). *Reading comprehension instruction: Issues & strategies.* Parkton, MD: York Press.

Mather, N. (2001). *The rol of orthografe in dislexea.* Presented at the International Dyslexia Association 52nd Annual Conference, Albuquerque, New Mexico.

Mather, N. & Lachowicz, B. L. (1992). Shared writing: An instructional approach for reluctant writers. *Teaching Exceptional Children, 27,* 26-30.

Maxwell, S. E. & Wallach, G. P. (1984). The language-learning disabilities connection: Symptoms of early language disability change over time. In G. P. Wallach & K. G. Butler (Eds.), *Language learning disabilities in school-age children* (pp. 15-34). Baltimore, MD: Williams & Wilkins.

Mayer, C. (2001). *Assessing central auditory processing and interpreting the results.* A workshop presented by Department of Speech Pathology & Audiology, California State University, Sacramento.

McCabe, A., & Rollins, P. R. (1994). Assessment of preschool narrative skills. *American Journal of Speech-Language Pathology, 3,* 45-56.

Mc Cardle, P., Cooper, J. A., Houle, G. R., Karp, N., & Paul–Brown, D. (2001). Emergent and early literacy: Current status and research directions—introduction. *Learning Disabilities Research & Practice, 16*(4), 183-185.

McGregor, K. K. (1994). Use of phonological information in a word-finding treatment for children. *Journal of Speech and Hearing Research, 37,* 1381-1393.

McGuiness, C., & McGuinnes, G. (1998). *Reading reflex: The foolproof phonographix method for teaching your child to read.* New York: Simon & Schuster.

Menyuk, P. (1991). Metalinguistic abilities and language disorder. In J. Miller (Ed.), *Research on child language disorders: A decade of progress* (pp. 387-397). Austin, TX: Pro-Ed.

Menyuk, P. (1992). Relationship of otitis media to speech processing and language development. In J. Katz, N. A. Stecker, & D. Henderson (Eds.), *Central auditory processing: A transdisciplinary view* (pp. 187-198). St. Louis, MO: Mosby Year Book.

Merzinich, M. (1996). *Neurological bases of fastforword training for language learning impaired children* (pp. 8/1-8/5). San Francisco: Scientific Learning Corporation.

Meyer, M. S., & Felton, R. H. (1999). Repeated reading to enhance fluency: Old approaches and new directions. *Annals of Dyslexia, 49*, 283-306.

Meyer, M. S., Wood, F. B., Hart, L. A., & Felton, R. H. (1998). Selective predictive value of rapid automatized naming in poor readers. *Journal of Learning Disabilities, 31*, 106-118.

Moats, L. (1997). With use by permission of author.

Mody, M., Studdert–Kennedy, M., & Brady, S. (1997). Speech perception deficits in poor readers: Auditory processing or phonological coding? *Journal of Experimental Child Psychology, 64*, 199-231.

Morgan, W. P. (1896). A case of congenital word-blindness. *British Medical Journal, 2*, 1368.

Nelson, N. W. (1993). *Childhood language disorders in context: Infancy through adolescence.* New York: Macmillan.

Nelson, N. W. (1994). Curriculum-based language assessment and intervention across the grades. In G. P. Wallach & K. G. Butler (Eds.), *Language learning disabilities in school-age children and adolescents: Some principles and applications* (pp. 104-131). New York: Macmillan.

Never ending stories (1993). Martinez, CA: Discovery Toys.

Newcomer, P. L. (1990). *Diagnostic Achievement Battery—2.* Austin, TX: Pro-Ed.

Newcomer, P. L., & Hammill, D. D. (1988). *Test of Language Development: Primary—2.* Austin, TX: Pro-Ed.

New Standards Primary Literacy Committee (1999). *Reading & writing grade by grade: Primary literacy standards for kindergarten through third grade.* Pittsburgh: National Center on Education and the Economy and the University of Pittsburgh.

NICHD (2000). *Why children succeed or fail at reading: Research from NICHD's program in learning disabilities.* http://www.nichd.nih.gov/publications/pubs/readbro.htm

Nicholson, T. (1997). Closing the gap on reading failure: Socal background, phonemic awareness, and learning to read. In B. A. Blachman (Ed.) *Foundations of reading acquisition and dyslexia: Implications for early intervention* (pp. 381-408). New Jersey: Lawrence Erlbaum Associates.

Nicolson, R. I. & Fawcett, A. J. (1995). Reaction times and dyslexia. *Quarterly Journal of Experimental Psychology, 47*, 29-48.

Norris, J. A. (1991). From frog to prince: Using written language as a context for language learning. *Topics in Language Disorders, 12*, 66-81.

Obregon, M., & Wolf, M. (1995). *A fine-grained analysis of serial naming duration patterns in developmental dyslexia.* Poster presented at the Society for Research in Child Development Indianapolis, IN.

O'Connor, R. E., Jenkins, J. R., Leicester, N., & Slocum, T. A. (1993). Teaching phonological awareness to young children with learning disabilities. *Exceptional Children, 59,* 532-546.

Ojemann, G. A. (1990). Organization of language derived from investigations during neurosurgery. *Neuroscience, 2,* 297-305.

Orton, J. (1968). Treatment needs of the child with developmental dyslexia. In A. H. Keeney & V. T. Keeney (Eds.), *Dyslexia, diagnosis and treatment of reading disorders* (pp. 131-136). St. Louis, MO: C.V. Mosby..

Papandropoulou, I., & Sinclair, H. (1974). What is a word? Experimental study of children's ideas on grammar. *Human Development, 17,* 241-258.

Paris, S. G. (1991). Assessment and remediation of metacognitive aspects of children's reading comprehension. *Topics in Language Disorders, 12,* 32-50.

Paul, R. (2001). *Language disorders from infancy through adolescence* (2nd ed.). St. Louis, MO: Mosby.

Pennington, B. F. (1991). (Ed.) *Reading disabilities: Genetic and neurological influences.* Dordrecht, The Netherlands: Kluwer.

Perfetti, C. A. (1991a). On the value of simple ideas in reading instruction. In S. A. Brady & D. P. Shankweiler (Eds.), *Phonological processes in literacy: A tribute to Isabelle Y. Liberman* (pp. 211-218). Hillsdale, NJ: Lawrence Erlbaum Associates.

Perfetti, C. A. (1991b). Representations and awareness in the acquisition of reading competence. In L. Rieben & C. A. Perfetti (Eds.), *Learning to read: Basic research and its implications* (pp. 33-46). Hillsdale, NJ: Lawrence Erlbaum Associates.

Pickering, J. S. (1993a). *Auditory Discrimination and Memory, Intermediate/Advanced.* Dallas, TX: The June Shelton School and Evaluation Center.

Pickering, J. S. (1993b). *Auditory Discrimination and Memory for Pre-School Children and First Grades.* Dallas, TX: The June Shelton School and Evaluation Center.

Pickering, J. S. (1994, November). *Phonological awareness: Academic application of sound segmentation and synthesis.* Presented at the annual conference of The National Orton Dyslexia Society, Los Angeles, CA.

Pieretti, R. A. (2001). *Double–deficit reading disorders: A bottom–up perspective.* Unpublished master's thesis. California State University, Sacramento.

Pritchard, R. (2001). *Strategic teaching and learning.* Workshop presented to Kern County Consortium SELPA. Bakersfield, CA

Quigley, S. P., McAnally, P. L., Rose, S. & King, C. M. (2001). *Reading Milestones.* Austin, TX: Pro-Ed.

Rae, C., Martin, A. L., Dixon, R. M., Blamire, A. M., Thompson, C. H., Styles, P., Talcott, J., Richardson, A. J., and Stein, J. F. (1998). Metabolic abnormalities in developmental dyslexia detected by 1H magnetic resonance spectroscopy. *Lancet, 351,* 1849-52.

Reed, M. A. (1989). Speech perception and the discrimination of brief auditory cues in phonological processing. *Reading & Writing: An Interdisciplinary Journal, 2,* 1-25.

Rees, N. (1974). The speech pathologist and the reading process. *ASHA, 16,* 255-258.

Reid, D. K., Hresko, W. P., & Hammill, D. D. (1991). *Test of Early Reading Ability—2.* Austin TX: Pro-Ed.

Reitsma, P. (1984). Sound priming in beginning readers. *Child Development, 55,* 406-423.

Richards, K. B., & Fallon, M. O. (1988). *Audio workbook for the verbally apraxic adult.* Tucson, AZ: Communication Skill Builders.

Richardson, E., & DiBenedetto, B. (1991). Acquiring the linguistic code for reading: A model for teaching and learning. In J. K. Kavanagh (Ed.), *The language continuum: From infancy to literacy* (pp. 63-114). Parkton, MD: York Press.

Richman, L. (1995). *Peaceful coexistence.* American Hyperlexia Association. *http://www.hyperlexia.org/aha_winter9697.html*

Roberts, B. (1992). The evolution of the young child's concept of a word as a unit of spoken and written language. *Reading Research Quarterly, 2,* 125-138.

Roberts, J. E. & Medley, L. P. (1995). Otitis media and speech-language sequelae in young children: Current issues in management. *American Journal of Speech-Language Pathology, 4,* 15-24.

Rosen, G. D., Fitch, R. H., Clark, M. G., Lo Turco, J. J., Sherman G. F., & Galaburda, A. M. (2001). Animal models of developmental dyslexia: Is there a link between neocortical malformations and deficits in fast auditory processing? In M. Wolf (Ed.), *Dyslexia, fluency and the brain,* (pp. 129-157) Timonium, MD: York Press, Inc.

Rosner, J. (1979). The Test of Auditory Analysis Skills. In J. Rosner: *Helping children overcome learning difficulties,* (2nd ed., pp. 46-49). New York: Walker Publishing.

Rumsey, J. M. & Eden, G. (1998). Functional neuroimaging of developmental dyslexia: Regional cerebral blood flow in dyslexic men. In B. K. Shapiro, P. J. Accardo, & A. J. Capute (Eds.), *Specific reading disability: A view of the spectrum,* (pp. 935-962). Timonium MD: York Press, Inc.

Sawyer D. J. (1992). Language abilities, reading acquisition, and developmental dyslexia: A discussion of hypothetical and observed relationships. *Journal of Learning Disabilities, 25,* 82-95.

Sawyer, D. J. (1994, November). *Phonological awareness training in intervention programs for adolescents and adults.* Presented at the annual conference of the National Orton Dyslexia Society, Los Angeles, CA.

Scanlon, D. M., & Vellutino, F. R. (1997). Instructional influences on early reading success. *Perspectives, 23,* Baltimore, MD: The International Dyslexia Association.

Scarborough, H. S. (1990). Very early language deficits in dyslexic children. *Child Development, 61,* 1728-1743.

Scarborough, H. S. & Dobrich, W. (1990). Development of children with early language delay. *Journal of Speech and Hearing Research, 33,* 70-83.

Schwartz, R. & Leonard, L. (1982). Do children pick and choose? An examination of phonological selection and avoidance in early lexical acquisition. *Journal of Child Language, 9*, 319-336.

Semel, E., Wiig, E. H., & Secord, W. (1987). *Clinical Evaluation of Language Fundamentals—Revised*. San Antonio, TX: The Psychological Corporation.

Semel, E., Wiig, E. H., & Secord, W. (1995). *Clinical Evaluation of Language Fundamentals—3*. San Antonio, TX: The Psychological Corporation.

Shankweiler, D. P. (1991). The contribution of Isabelle Y. Liberman. In S. A. Brady & D. P. Shankweiler (Eds.), *Phonological processes in literacy: A tribute to Isabelle Y. Liberman* (pp. xiii-xvii). Hillsdale, NJ: Lawrence Erlbaum Associates.

Shankweiler, D. P., Crain, S., Brady, S., & Macaruso, P. (1992). Identifying the causes of reading disability. In P. B. Gough, L. C. Ehri, & R. Treiman (Eds.), *Reading acquisition* (pp. 275-305). Hillsdale, NJ: Lawrence Erlbaum Associates.

Shaywitz, S. E. (1998). Dyslexia. *The New England Journal of Medicine, 338*, 307-312.

Shaywitz, S. E., Shaywitz, B. Z., Pugh, K. R., Fulbright, R. K., Constable, R. T., Mencl, W. B., Shankweiler, D. P., Liberman, A. M., Skudlarski, P., Fletcher, J. M., Katz, L., Marchione, K. E., Lacadie, C., Gatenby, C., and Gore, J. C. (1998). Functional disruption in the organization of the brain for reading in dyslexia. *Proceedings of the National Academy of Sciences of the United States of America, 95*, 2636-41.

Shriberg, L. D., & Austin, D. (1998). Comorbidity of speech-language disorder: Implications for a phenotype marker for speech delay. In R. Paul (Ed.), *Exploring the speech/language connection* (pp. 73-118). Baltimore: Brookes.

Silliman, E. R. & Wilkinson, L. C. (1994). Discourse scaffolds for classroom learning. In G. P. Wallach & K. G. Butler (Eds.), *Language learning disabilities in school-age children and adolescents: Some principles and applications* (pp. 27-52). New York: Macmillan.

Sipe, L. R. (1993). Using transformations of traditional stories: Making the reading-writing connection. *The Reading Teacher, 47*, 18-26.

Sloan, C. (1986). *Treating auditory processing difficulties in children*. San Diego, CA: College-Hill Press.

Smith, F. (1994). *Understanding reading: A psycholinguistic analysis of reading and learning to read*. Hillsdale, NJ: Lawrence Erlbaum Associates.

Smith, S. B., Simmons, D. C., & Kameenui, E. J. (1995). Synthesis of research on phonological awareness: Principles and implications for reading acquisition. Tech. Rep. No. 21. Eugene: University of Oregon, National Center to Improve the Tools of Education. *http://idea.uoregon.edu/~ncite/documents/techrep/tech21.html*

Snider, V. (1997). The relationship between phonemic awareness and later reading achievement. *The Journal of Educational Research, 90*, 203-211.

Snow, C. & Dickinson, D. (1991). Skills that aren't basic in a new conception of literacy. In A. Purves and E. Jennings (Eds.), *Literate systems and indi-*

vidual lives: Perspectives on literacy and schooling. Albany, NY: SUNY Press.

Snow C. E., Scarborough H. S., & Burns, M. S. (1999). What speech-language pathologists need to know about early reading. *Topics in Language Disorders, 20*, 48-58.

Snowling, M. J. (2000). *Dyslexia*. Malden, MA: Blackwell Publishers Inc.

Snyder, L. (1980). Have we prepared the language disordered child for school? *Topics in Language Disorders, 1*, 29-45.

Snyder. L. (1994, November). *Rapid naming abilities*. Presented at the annual conference of The National Orton Dyslexia Society, Los Angeles, CA.

Snyder, L. S. & Downey, D. M. (1995). Serial rapid naming skills in children with reading disabilities. *Annals of Dyslexia, 45*, 31-47.

Sparks, R. L. & Artzer, M. (2000). Foreign language learning, hyperlexia, and early word recognition. *Annals of Dyslexia, 50*, 189-212.

Stackhouse, J. (1997). Phonological awareness: Connecting speech and literacy problems. In B. W. Hodson & M. L. Edwards (Eds.), *Perspectives in applied phonology* (pp. 157-196). Gaithersburg, MD. Aspen.

Stackhouse, J., & Wells, B. (1991). Dyslexia: The obvious and hidden speech and language disorder. In M. Snowling & M. Thomson (Eds.), *Dyslexia: Integrating theory and practice* (pp. 185-194). London: Whurr.

Stahl, S. A., Osborn, J., & Lehr, F. (1990). *Beginning to read: Thinking and learning about print. A summary*. Full text by M. J. Adams. Cambridge, MA: The MIT Press.

Stanback, M. & Hansen, M. (1980). Integrative review of spelling. In *Integrative reviews of research Vol. l*, (pp. 135-200). New York: Teachers College, Institute for the Study of Learning Disabilities.

Stanovich, K. E. (1988). The right and wrong places to look for the cognitive locus of reading disability. *Annals of Dyslexia, 38*, 154-180.

Stanovich, K. E. (1991a). Changing models of reading and reading acquisition. In L. Rieben & C. A. Perfetti (Eds.), *Learning to read: Basic research and its implications* (pp. 19-32). Hillsdale, NJ: Lawrence Erlbaum Associates.

Stanovich, K. E. (1991b). Cognitive science meets beginning reading. *Psychological Science, 2*, 70-81.

Stanovich, K. E. (1994). Romance and reality. *The Reading Teacher, 47*, 280-290.

Stanovich, K. E. (2000). *Progress in understanding reading: Scientific foundations and new frontiers*. New York: The Guilford Press.

Stanovich, K. E., West, R. F., & Cunningham, A. E. (1991). Beyond phonological processes: Print exposure and orthographic processing. In S. A. Brady and D. P. Shankweiler (Eds.), *Phonological processes in literacy* (pp. 219-236). Hillsdale, NJ: Lawrence Erlbaum Associates.

Stein, J. (2001). The neurobiology of reading difficulties In M. Wolf (Ed.) *Dyslexia, fluency and the brain* (pp. 3-22). Timonium, MD: York Press, Inc.

Stoll, C. (1995). *Silicon snake oil*. New York: Anchor Books.

Stone, B., & Brady, S. (1995). Evidence for phonological processing deficits in less-skilled readers. *Annals of Dyslexia, 45*, 51-78

Stothard, S. E., Snowling, M. J., Bisop, D. V. M., Chipchase, B. B., & Kaplan, C. A. (1998). Language–impaired preschoolers: A follow–up into adolescence. *Journal of Speech-Language-Hearing Research, 41,* 407-418.

Strickland, D., & Cullinan, B. (1990). Afterword. In M. J. Adams, *Beginning to read: Thinking and learning about print* (pp. 425-434). Cambridge, MA: The MIT Press.

Sturomski, N. (1999). Teaching students with learning disabilities to use learning strategies. *http://www.ldonline.org/ld_indepth/teaching_techniques/nichcy_interventions.html.*

Swank, L. K. (1994). Phonological coding abilities: Identification of impairments related to phonologically based reading problems. *Topics in Language Disorders, 14,* 56-71.

Swinburne, L., & Bank, S. (1987). *Cloze stories for beginning readers: Book Two.* New York: Walker and Company.

Tallal, P. (1988). Developmental language disorders. In J. K. Kavanagh & T. J. Truss (Eds.), *Learning disabilities: Proceedings of the National Conference* (pp. 181-272). Parkton, MD: York Press.

Tallal, P. (1991). Back to the future: Research on developmental disorders of language. In J. Miller (Ed.), *Research on child language disorders: A decade of progress* (pp. 399-407). Austin, TX: Pro-Ed.

Tallal, P. (1993). Preface. In P. Tallal, A. M. Galaburda, R. R. Llinas, & C. von Euler (Eds.), *Annals of the New York Academy of Sciences, Vol. 682. Temporal information processing in the nervous system: Special reference to dyslexia and dysphasia* (p. ix). New York: The New York Academy of Sciences.

Tallal, P. (1996). *The role of temporal processing in developmental language-based learning disorders: Research and clinical implication* (pp. 7/1-7/15). San Francisco: Scientific Learning Corporation.

Tallal, P., Miller, S., & Fitch, H. (1993). Neurobiological basis of speech: A case for the preeminence of temporal processing. In P. Tallal, A. M. Galaburda, R. R. Llinas, & C von Euler (Eds.), *Annals of the New York Academy of Sciences Vol. 682. Temporal information processing in the nervous system: Special reference to dyslexia and dysphasia* (pp. 27-47). New York: The New York Academy of Sciences.

Tattershall, S. S. (1999). *Facilitating academic language comprehension: Why & how.* American Speech-Language-Hearing Association Annual Conference. San Francisco, CA.

Temple, C., Nathan, R., Temple, F., & Burris, N. A. (1993). *The beginnings of writing.* Boston, MA: Allyn & Bacon.

The Literacy Volunteer Connection (2001). *http://www.literacyvolunteer.com*

Toomey, M. M. (1989). *Morph-aid: A source of roots, prefixes and suffixes.* Cincinnati, OH: Circuit Publications.

Torgesen, J. K. (1998). Personal communication to Maryanne Wolf.

Torgesen, J. K. (1998). Catch them before they fall: Identification and assessment to prevent reading failure in young children. *American Educator. http://www.ldonline.ore/ld_indepth/reading/torgesen_catchthem.html*

Torgesen, J. K., & Mathes, P. G. (2000). *A basic guide to understanding, assessing, and teaching phonological awareness.* Austin, TX: Pro-Ed.

Torgesen, J. K., Rashotte, C. A., & Alexander, A. W. (2001) Principles of fluency instruction in reading: Relationships with established empirical outcomes. In M. Wolf (Ed.), *Dyslexia, fluency, and the brain*. (pp. 333-355). Timonium, MD: York Press, Inc.

Torgesen, J. K., & Wagner, R. K. (1994). *Comprehensive Tests of Phonological Processing—Experimental Version.* Unpublished manuscript, Florida State University, Tallahassee.

Torgesen, J. K., Wagner, R. K., & Rashotte, C. A. (1994). Longitudinal studies of phonological processing and reading. *Journal of Learning Disabilities, 27*, 276-286.

Torgesen, J. K., Wagner, R. K., & Rashotte, C. A. (1999). *Comprehensive Test of Phonological Awareness Abilities.* Austin, TX: ProEd.

Torgesen, J. K., Wagner, R. K., Rashotte, C. A., Burgess, S., & Hecht, S. (1997). Contributions of phonological awareness and rapid automatic naming ability to the growth of word-reading skills in second-to fifth-grade children. *Scientific Studies of Reading, 1*, 161-185.

Treiman, R. & Zukowski, A. (1991). Levels of phonological awareness. In S. A. Brady & D. Shankweiler (Eds.), *Phonological process in literacy: A tribute to Isabelle Y. Liberman* (pp. 67-83). Hillsdale, NJ: Lawrence Erlbaum Associates.

Trelease, J. (1984). *The read-aloud handbook*. New York: Penguin.

Trelease, J. (1995). *The new read-aloud handbook*. New York: Penguin.

Tuley, A. C. (1998). *Never too late to read: Language skills for the adolescent with dyslexia*. New York: York Press.

Ultimate Phonics (2000). San Diego, CA: Spencer Learning.

van Kleeck, A. (1990). Emergent literacy: Learning about print before learning to read. *Topics in Language Disorders, 10*, 25-45.

van Kleeck, A. (1994). Metalinguistic skills: Cutting across spoken and written language and problem-solving abilities. In G. P. Wallach & K. G. Butler (Eds.), *Language learning disabilities in school-age children* (pp. 128-153). Baltimore, MD: Williams & Wilkins.

Vellutino, F. R. (1993, November). *What speech and language therapists can do to facilitate assessment and remediation of reading difficulties*. Presented at the annual convention of the American Speech-Language-Hearing Association. Anaheim, CA.

Vellutino, F. R., & Scanlon, D. M. (1991). The preeminence of phonologically based skills in learning to read. In S. A. Brady and D. P. Shankweiler (Eds.), *Phonological processes in literacy* (pp. 237-252). Hillsdale, NJ: Lawrence Erlbaum Associates.

Vellutino, F. R., Scanlon, D., Sipay, E., Small, S., Pratt, A., Chen, R., & Denckla, M. (1996). Cognitive profiles of difficult-to-remediate and readily remediated poor readers. *Journal of Educational Psychology, 88*, 601-638.

Vellutino, F. R., Scanlon, D. M., Small, S. G., & Tanzman, M. S. (1991). The linguistic bases of reading ability: Converting written to oral language. *Text, 11*, 99-113.

Viall, J. T. (2000). "Shhh . . . don't talk about it" *Perspectives,* Winter, p. 3.

Vozar, D. (1993). *Hungry wolf! A nursery rap*. New York: Delacorte Press.

Wagner, R. K., and Torgesen, J. K. (1987). The nature of phonological processing and its causal role in the acquisition of reading skills. *Psychological
Bulletin, 101*, 192-212.

Watson, B. U. & Miller, T. K. (1993). Auditory perception, phonological processing and reading ability/disability. *Journal of Speech and Hearing
Research, 36*, 850-863.

Webster, P. E., Plante, A. S., & Couvillion, L. M. (1997). Phonological impairment and prereading: Update on a longitudinal study. *Journal of Learning
Disabilities, 30*, 365-375.

Wechsler, D. (1974). *Wechsler Intelligence Scale for Children—Revised*. NY:
Psychological Corporation.

Wechsler, D. (1989). *Wechsler Preschool and Primary Scale of Intelligence—
Revised*. NY: Psychological Corporation.

Wiederholt, J. L., & Bryant, B. R. (1992). *Gray Oral Reading Test—3*. Austin,
TX: Pro-Ed.

Wiig, E. H. & Semel, E. M. (1980). *Clinical Evaluation of Language Functions*.
Columbus, OH: Merrill.

Wilson, B. A. (1996). *The Wilson Reading System*. Millbury, MA: Wilson
Language Training.

Wing, C. S. (1990). A preliminary investigation of generalization to untrained
words following two treatments of children's word-finding problems.
Language, Speech, and Hearing Services in the Schools, 21, 151-156.

Wolf, M. (1991). Naming speed and reading: The contribution of the cognitive neurosciences.. *Reading Research Quarterly, 26*, 123-140.

Wolf, M. (1997). Phonological and naming-speed deficits. In B. A. Blachman
(Ed.) *Foundations of reading acquisition and dyslexia: Implications for early
intervention* (pp. 67-92). New Jersey: Lawrence Erlbaum Associates.

Wolf, M. (1998). *What time may tell: Towards a new conceptualization of developmental dyslexia*. Paper presented at the International Dyslexia
Association, San Francisco, CA.

Wolf, M. (1999). What time may tell: Towards a new conceptualization of
developmental dyslexia. *Annals of Dyslexia, 49*, 3-28.

Wolf, M. (2001). Preface: Seven dimensions of time. In M. Wolf (Ed.),
Dyslexia, fluency, and the brain (ix-xix). Timonium, MD: York Press, Inc.

Wolf, M & Bowers, P. (2000). The question of naming-speed deficits in developmental reading disabilities: An introduction to the double-deficit
hypothesis. *Journal of Learning Disabilities, 33*, 322-24.

Wolf, M., Miller, L., & Donnelly, K. (2000). Retrieval, automaticity, vocabulary
elaboration, orthography (RAVE–O). *Journal of Learning Disabilities, 33*,
375-386.

Wolf, M., & Obregon, M. (1989). *88 children in search of a name; A five-year
investigation of rate, word-retrieval, and vocabulary in reading development
and dyslexia*. Paper presented at Society for Research in Child
Development, Kansas City, MO.

Wolf, M., & Obregon, M. (1992). Early naming deficits, developmental
dyslexia, and a specific-deficit hypothesis. *Brain and Language, 42*, 219-
247.

Wolf, M., & Segal, D. (1992). Word finding and reading in the developmental dyslexias. *Topics in Language Disorders, 13*, 51-65.

Wolf, M., & Segal, D. (1999). Retrieval rate, accuracy and vocabulary elaboration (RAVE) in reading–impaired children: A pilot intervention programme. *Dyslexia, 5*, 1-27.

Wolff, P. (1993). Impaired temporal resolution in developmental dyslexia. In P. Tallal, A. Galaburda, R. Llinas, & C. von Euler (Eds.), Temporal information processing in the nervous system. *Annals of the New York Academy of Sciences, Vol. 682,* (pp. 87-103).

Woodcock, R. W. (1987). *Woodcock Reading Mastery Tests—Revised.* Circle Pines, MN: American Guidance Service.

Woodcock, R. W. (1991). *Woodcock Language Proficiency Battery—Revised.* Allen, TX: DLM Teaching Resources.

Yopp, H. (1992). Developing phonemic awareness. *The Reading Teacher, 45,* 696-703.

Yopp, H. & Troyer, S. (1992). *Training phonemic awareness in young children.* Unpublished manuscript.

Yopp, H. K., & Yopp, R. H. (1996). *Literature-based reading activities* (2nd ed.). Boston, MA: Allyn and Bacon.

Zeffiro, T. & Eden, G. (2000). The neural basis of developmental dyslexia. *Annals of Dyslexia, 50,* 3-30

Zentall, S. S. (1993). Research on the educational implications of attention deficit disorder. *Exceptional Children, 60,* 143-153.

Index

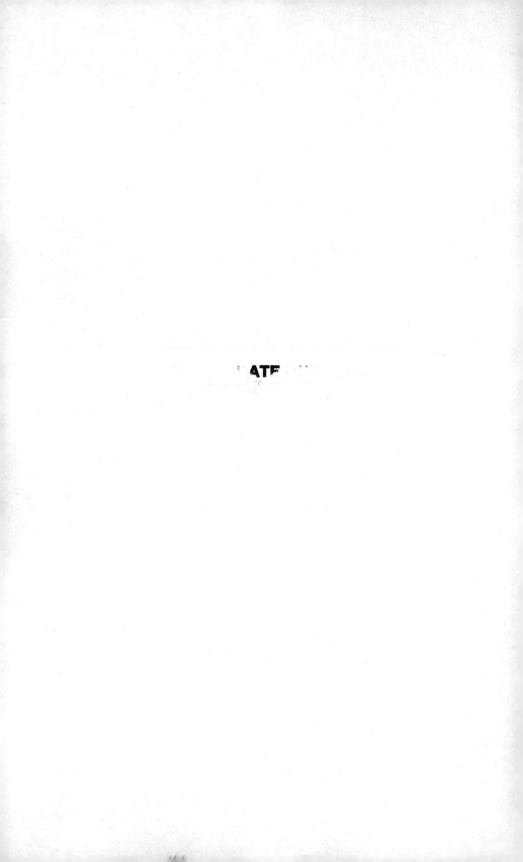
ATF